Hints and tips *from* times past

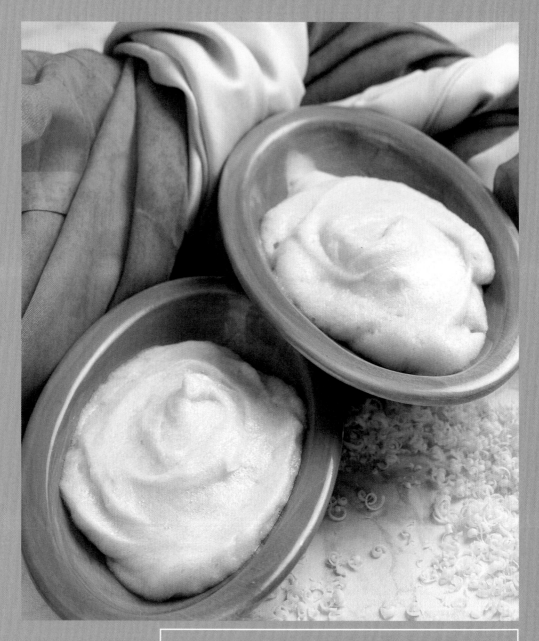

PUBLISHED BY
THE READER'S DIGEST ASSOCIATION LIMITED
LONDON • NEW YORK • SYDNEY • MONTREAL

Hints and tips *from* times past

HINTS AND TIPS FROM TIMES PAST

Adapted by Craft Plus Publishing Limited
from Grossmutters Hausmittel Neu Entdeckt
Published by Reader's Digest (Germany)
First edition copyright © 2000

Project Editor
Katharine Gurney

Designer
Tessa Dennison

Consultants
Dr Alan Lakin
Vincent Gradwell
Wendy Sweetser
Madeleine Barnard

Subeditor
Sue Churchill

Indexer
Laura Hicks

Translation
Book Creation Services Ltd

For The Reader's Digest, London

Project Editor
Rachel Warren Chadd

Art Editor
Jane McKenna

Proofreader
Barry Gage

Reader's Digest, General Books, London

Editorial Director
Cortina Butler

Art Director
Nick Clark

Executive Editor
Julian Browne

Publishing Projects Manager
Alastair Holmes

Development Editor
Ruth Binney

Picture Resource Manager
Martin Smith

Style Editor
Ron Pankhurst

visit our web site at
www.readersdigest.co.uk

Introduction

Drawing on past wisdom, but with the practicalities of today in mind, this book has advice on every area of home life. Its tips, natural remedies and recipes are the perfect antidote to our processed, pre-packaged age.

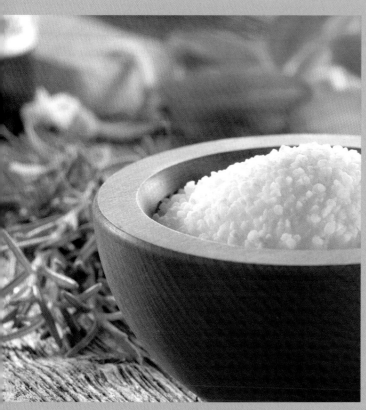

Everyday life has changed quite dramatically over the past 100 years – not least because chemical cleaners and convenience products have taken away much of the drudgery. But one price of progress has been the pollutants that damage the environment and our health.

Hints and tips from times past turns back the years to another age when only wholesome, natural ingredients were used.

Natural health arms you with herbal remedies to treat a variety of common ailments; **Beauty treatments** has lotions and potions to pamper you from top to toe. In **Around the house** you will discover how to create effective and environmentally friendly polishes and cleaning products, while **Kitchen secrets** is packed with delicious recipes from the past. **In the garden** outlines a wholly organic approach to growing home produce and traditional fragrant flowers. Finally, **Fact file** lists herbs and ingredients, explaining where to buy products that were once common but are less well known today.

With more than 1200 hints and tips, gleaned from generations of experience, this book is simply indispensable. And whether you prepare a tincture, face cream or polish, bottle fruit, or make a potpourri you can be sure that everything you use is part of a long household tradition – and naturally good.

Contents

4
Kitchen secrets

5
In the garden

6
Fact file

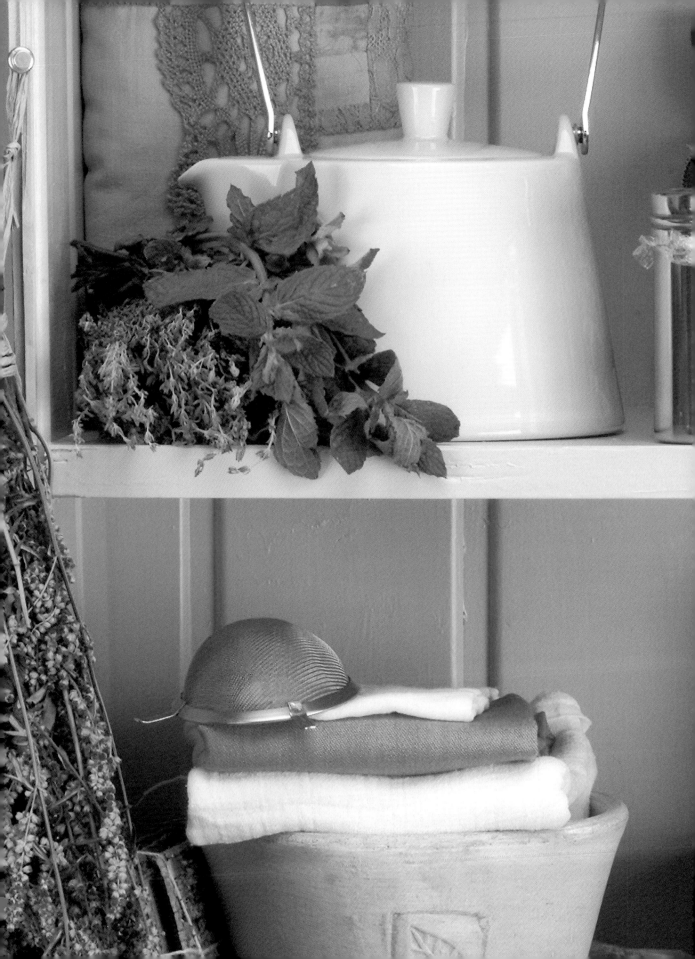

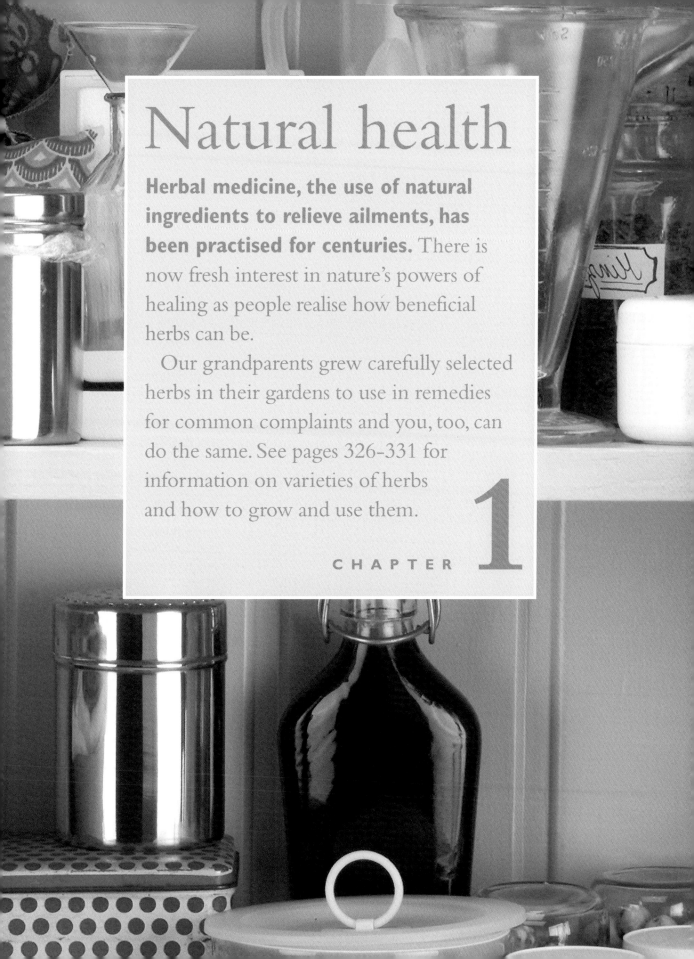

Natural health

Herbal medicine, the use of natural ingredients to relieve ailments, has been practised for centuries. There is now fresh interest in nature's powers of healing as people realise how beneficial herbs can be.

Our grandparents grew carefully selected herbs in their gardens to use in remedies for common complaints and you, too, can do the same. See pages 326–331 for information on varieties of herbs and how to grow and use them.

CHAPTER 1

Natural remedies for

Even minor ailments of the head make us feel wretched, whether it is a nagging headache or a sore throat. Use natural remedies to help to avoid or treat these health disorders.

Modern living with its stressful routines, polluted air and lack of time for relaxation makes us all vulnerable to irritating minor ailments, such as an aching head or a sore throat. Usually, there is nothing seriously wrong, and you won't need a doctor.

Instead, take a look at the way you live and make what changes you can. Also, think about using medicinal herbs to treat any problems and to help you to relax. Our grandparents knew all about soothing teas, inhalations, healing baths and compresses and have passed down recipes that can boost our well-being today.

Headaches

A headache is generally an indication that we are under par rather than a symptom of a serious illness. It may be a sign of stress, insufficient sleep or even just a change in the weather.

Tension headaches produce a dull, tight feeling in the head and are often due to eyestrain, bad posture or anxiety. Migraines cause severe pain, often coupled with nausea and vomiting.

Combat headaches by natural means, such as an arm bath or an onion compress (see Tried & Trusted, opposite). Try soothing herbal teas to help you to relax.

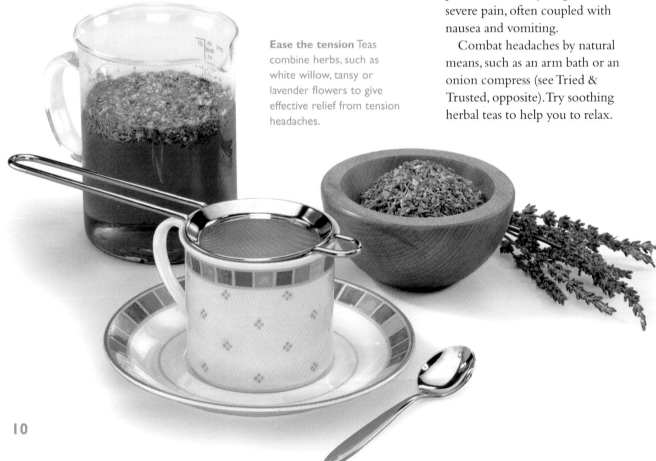

Ease the tension Teas combine herbs, such as white willow, tansy or lavender flowers to give effective relief from tension headaches.

a clear head

WHITE WILLOW AND SILVERWEED TEA

This tea gives effective pain relief. However, it can cause stomach irritation, so do not drink it if you suffer from stomach complaints.

25g (1oz) dried white
willow leaves
25g (1oz) dried silverweed
leaves
15g (½oz) dried marigold
flowers
500ml (18fl oz) water

Mix the herbs together and place 2 tablespoonfuls in a heatproof bowl. Boil the water and pour it over the herbs. Leave to infuse for 15 minutes, then strain the liquid.

If your headache is acute, drink one cup of tea immediately. If the pain is chronic, make up twice the amount of tea and drink throughout the day. If using this treatment for a long period of time, take a ten-day break every three weeks.

Take care

Always consult a doctor before trying natural remedies if you think the illness might be serious or if you are undergoing treatment for a medical or psychiatric condition.

LADY'S MANTLE AND MINT TEA

If you feel a migraine coming on, this tea can sometimes help to prevent it from getting a grip.

1 litre (1¾ pints) water
40g (1½oz) dried lady's
mantle leaves
15g (½oz) dried mint leaves

Pour the water into a saucepan. Bring to the boil, then add the herbs. Boil the mixture for 20 minutes.

Remove it from the heat and leave to infuse for 10 minutes. Strain the liquid through a fine sieve and drink one cup.

White willow

The main active ingredient in white willow is salicin, which has been used to relieve pain since the 17th century. Its synthetic derivative, aspirin, is used in many proprietary headache and fever remedies.

Tried & Trusted
Headache self-help

• Certain essential oils (aromatic plant extracts) have proved effective against headaches. Try rubbing just a few drops of peppermint oil onto your temples, forehead and the back of your neck – it can work wonders.

• Bathing one of your arms in cold water can prevent headaches from getting worse. Dip your arm in cold water for a few minutes and then dry it vigorously with a towel.

• A mustard footbath can ease your headache, too. Fill a bowl with hand-hot water and dissolve 2 tablespoons of dried mustard powder in it. Bathe your feet for 5 minutes, then rinse them using lukewarm water.

• If you are suffering pain at the back of your head, an onion compress may help. Slice a raw onion, put the slices on the back of your neck, cover them with a towel and fasten it around with a scarf to hold the compress in position. Leave it in place for 20 minutes, then rinse your skin with warm water.

St John's wort

This fragrant herb can be used to treat a whole range of disorders that cause headaches, such as stress or mild depression. Take it regularly as an infusion using 20g in 500ml water.

MEADOWSWEET TEA

This infusion helps to relieve the pain as well as the tension that is often the cause of a headache.

25g (1oz) dried meadowsweet flowers
25g (1oz) dried St John's wort flowers
25g (1oz) dried lady's bedstraw leaves
500ml (18fl oz) water

Mix the herbs together and place 2 tablespoonfuls in a heatproof bowl. Boil the water and pour it over the herbs. Leave to infuse for 15 minutes, then strain the liquid through a fine sieve.

If the pain is acute, drink one cup of tea immediately. If the pain is chronic, make up twice the amount of tea and drink throughout the day.

During a long-term treatment, take a ten-day break periodically. Caution: this tea may cause stomach irritation. Do not drink if pregnant.

Herbs, oils and spices for nasal complaints

The nose and sinuses are lined with a sensitive mucous membrane, whose job it is to filter, moisten and warm the air we breathe.

Since the blood vessels in the nasal mucous membrane are extremely fine, they can easily rupture, causing a nosebleed. Inflammation and swelling of the mucous membrane that result from infections can be very painful.

Nasal complaints are very common and usually linked to colds and hay fever. There are a variety of simple homemade remedies for treating them effectively.

Whether the problem is nosebleeds, sinusitis or just irritation, try some of these suggested medicinal herbs that can help without producing unpleasant side effects.

GINGER COMPRESS

Ginger is a versatile healing spice that stimulates circulation and helps to soothe sinus inflammations.

2-3 tablespoons freshly grated root ginger
250ml (9fl oz) water

Place the grated ginger in a muslin cloth and, using your hand, squeeze the juice into a saucepan. Add the water. Heat the liquid for a few minutes, then pour some of it onto a face flannel and place it over your forehead and nose.

Leave the flannel in place until it has cooled, then repeat the process until your skin reddens.

Pressure points Stop a nosebleed by using your fingers to apply pressure to the upper part of your nose.

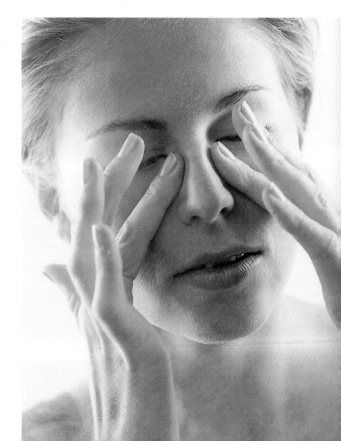

This nose rinse will help to reduce swelling and inflammation inside your nose.

750ml (1 pint 7fl oz) water
½ teaspoon dried horsetail 'needles' and stems

Pour the water into a saucepan and set it over the heat. Add the horsetail and boil briefly. Filter the liquid and leave to cool. Divide the solution into six to ten portions and sniff one portion through each nostril, three to five times a day.

OIL INHALATION TREATMENT

Essential oils can help to alleviate sinus problems.

1-2 drops eucalyptus oil
1-2 drops bergamot oil
  or
1-2 drops lavender oil

Drip the oils onto a cloth and inhale the scent. You can add these oils to your bath water, too.

Ginger

The ginger rhizome – an underground stem – stimulates blood circulation and thus promotes healing. It is native to Asia.

Tried & Trusted

Nosebleeds

- If your nose bleeds frequently, an onion treatment may help. Grate 1-2 raw onions, then press them through a sieve to extract the juice. Dilute the juice with a dash of vinegar. Use this solution every now and then as a preventive nose rinse.

- To stop a severe nosebleed, place an ice compress on the bridge of your nose, or a cold compress on the back of your neck for 5-10 minutes.

Sinus treatment

- Try this effective treatment for inflamed sinuses which will keep the mucous membranes moist and the blood circulating through your sinuses. Each morning sniff a mild saline solution (1 teaspoon of salt to 250ml (9fl oz) of water) through one nostril at a time.

- Camomile steam baths help to loosen phlegm and relieve inflammation of the sinuses. Add 2 tablespoons of dried camomile flowers to 500ml (18fl oz) of hot water in a heatproof bowl. Drape a towel over your head and bend over the bowl to inhale the steam.

- To relieve painful sinuses, you can also try bathing your feet in the evenings alternately in warm water at 38°C (100°F) for 5 minutes and then in cooler water at 18°C (64°F) for 10 seconds.

- At the first sign of a cold, relieve the symptoms by taking echinacea tablets and vitamin C. As products differ, refer to the manufacturer's instructions for the dosage.

Hay fever

- Honeycomb is a traditional remedy for hay fever. Chew a small piece for 20 minutes six times a day. Continue the treatment for at least three weeks.

- Cider vinegar is said to be a good remedy for hay fever. Try drinking 1 teaspoon of cider vinegar in a glass of water every morning.

- For long-term hay fever treatment, use fennel oil. The essential oil in the plant helps to balance the immune system. Refer to the manufacturer's instructions for the recommended dosage.

Help for sore eyes

The eyes are one of the body's most sensitive organs, yet they are regularly exposed to dust and pollution. Our grandparents' eyes had to cope with grime and smog but they didn't experience other modern-day problems that can make the eyes sore.

Dry air due to air-conditioning, working for a long time at a computer monitor or just being in a smoky environment can make the eyes sting and tire eye muscles.

For people prone to allergies, pollen can trigger conjunctivitis, and bacterial infections can result in an inflamed sebaceous palpebral gland, producing a sty on the edge of the eyelid.

Give stressed eyes a rest – get out in the fresh air and treat them to a natural rinse, compress or eye pack.

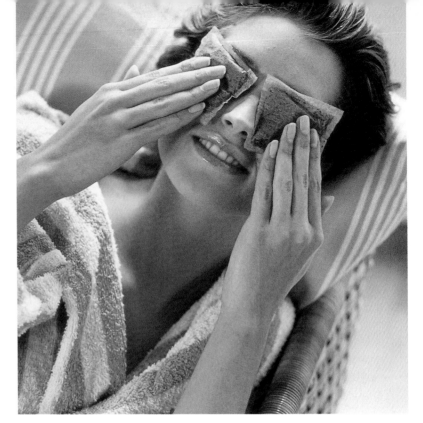

Simple soothers To make instant eye compresses, cool two used tea bags and place them over your closed eyelids.

SAGE COMPRESS

Commonly used in cooking, sage can also be used to reduce inflammation. Unlike camomile, which has similar properties, sage doesn't dry out the skin. Use this compress if you have conjunctivitis, or simply as a soothing eye pack.

1 tablespoon dried sage
250ml (9fl oz) water

Place the sage in a heatproof bowl. Boil the water and pour it over the herb. Leave to infuse for 10 minutes, then strain the liquid through a fine sieve. Dip a cotton-wool pad into the solution and place it on your closed eyelids. Regular sage compresses can reduce wrinkles.

PARSLEY EYE RINSE

This rinse is good for tired eyes. It also helps to clean the conjunctiva, the fine mucous membrane that lines the inner eyelid.

1 handful fresh parsley
750ml (1 pint 7fl oz) water

Rinse the parsley and place in a heatproof bowl. Boil the water and pour over the parsley. Leave to infuse for several hours, then strain the liquid through a sieve.

Fill an eye bath with the parsley rinse, bend your head forward, then press the eye bath firmly over the eye. Tip your head back, open your eye and, to rinse it thoroughly, look up and down and blink a few times. If necessary, use this rinse several times a day.

COOL QUARK EYE PACK

This eye pack alleviates pain and can help to reduce swelling if you have an inflamed eyelid.

3 tablespoons quark
juice of 1 lemon
1 tablespoon milk

Mix the ingredients together in a bowl, then spread half of the mixture onto a warm face flannel. Place the compress on your closed eyelid for 20 minutes. Repeat for the other eye.

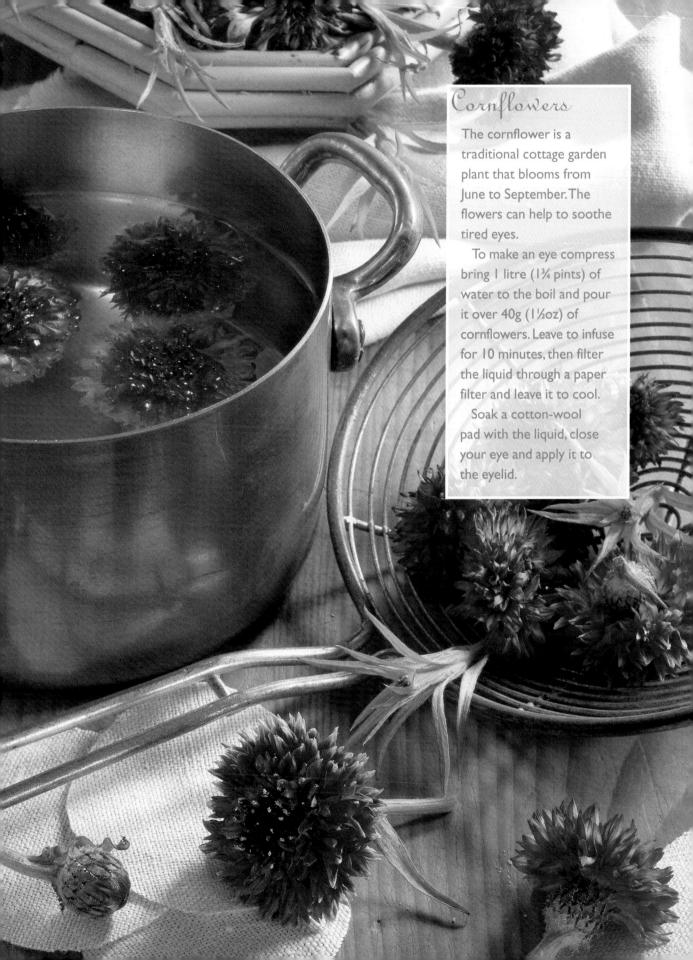

Cornflowers

The cornflower is a traditional cottage garden plant that blooms from June to September. The flowers can help to soothe tired eyes.

To make an eye compress bring 1 litre (1¾ pints) of water to the boil and pour it over 40g (1½oz) of cornflowers. Leave to infuse for 10 minutes, then filter the liquid through a paper filter and leave it to cool.

Soak a cotton-wool pad with the liquid, close your eye and apply it to the eyelid.

Coping with earache

Earache is generally caused by inflammation of the middle ear. In most cases a doctor should be consulted, not only because the pain can be excruciating, but also because the ear is so delicate and sensitive that expert advice is needed. But there are home remedies that can relieve the pain.

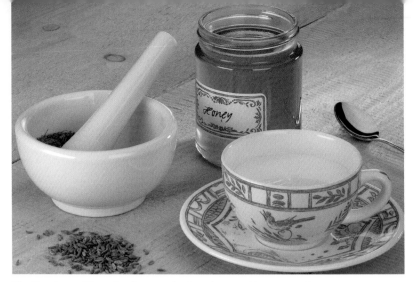

Healing brew Liquorice-flavoured aniseed tea and honey work well together to soothe a sore throat.

ONION WRAP

Onions have a range of healing properties and have long been used to treat earaches and other ailments.

I onion

Dice the onion and wrap a little in a gauze bandage. Place it on your aching ear and hold it in place with a crêpe bandage or a scarf.

MULLEIN OIL

Mullein oil can help to treat inflammations of the middle ear. It is also used to treat eczema.

I handful fresh mullein flowers
100ml (3½fl oz) olive oil

Slip the flowers into a bottle and pour the olive oil over them. Leave to infuse in a warm, sunny place for three to four weeks, shaking it thoroughly once a day.
    Strain the oil through a fine sieve and treat the affected ear with 3 drops each day.

ONION-MILK, THYME AND CLOVE TEA

The antiviral properties of onions can boost your immune system and help to fight an ear infection.

3 large onions
I clove
I teaspoon brown sugar
I sprig fresh thyme
water
½ cup milk

Chop the onions, including the skins. Place in a saucepan with the clove, sugar, thyme and sufficient water to cover the ingredients.
    Place the pan over the heat, cover and simmer for about 2 hours, occasionally topping up with a little more water.
    Press the mixture through a sieve. Heat the milk and mix with an equal quantity of the onion-juice liquid. This tea can be taken three times a day.

Throat complaints

A sore throat may be the start of a cold or throat infection, or just a result of straining your voice.
    Try a soothing tea first, but always call a doctor if a fever develops or severe red areas appear at the back of the throat.

ANISEED AND HONEY TEA

The seeds of the feathery anise plant have been used to make a comforting antiseptic tea since Egyptian times.

I teaspoon aniseed
600ml (I pint) water
honey to sweeten

Bruise the seeds using a pestle and mortar, then place them in a saucepan. Boil the water and pour it over the seeds. Simmer the mixture for 5-10 minutes. Strain the liquid through a fine sieve and sweeten it with the honey. Drink a cup of the tea immediately, while it is still hot.

Healthy teeth, strong gums and a fresh mouth

If you want healthy teeth and strong gums, good dental hygiene is essential. Regular care of your teeth will prevent tooth decay, inflammation of the gums and bad breath, which are all caused by the build-up of oral bacteria.

Make sure that you brush your teeth two or three times a day after meals and clean the gaps in between your teeth with dental floss. Frequent brushing and flossing will prevent tooth decay and receding gums.

Always replace your toothbrush every two months and make regular visits to your dentist.

Stress affects the mouth, too, and can lead to herpes and ulcers. A positive lifestyle and balanced diet will help to promote oral health.

SAVOY CABBAGE COMPRESS

You should get some relief from toothache within 30 minutes of using this treatment.

fresh savoy cabbage leaves

Cut out the thick stems in the cabbage leaves. Use a rolling pin to bruise and soften the leaves. Place the leaves on a linen cloth and hold it against your sore cheek.

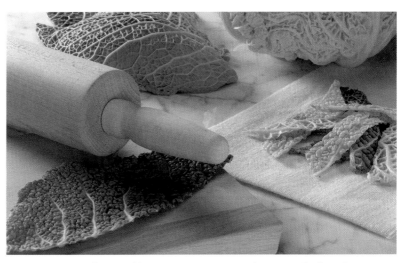

Toothache relief Savoy cabbage contains enzymes that can radically reduce swelling, which is why it has been used for centuries to combat toothache.

LEMON BALM TINCTURE

Cold sores are caused by a virus. Once you have caught it, you will repeatedly suffer from the infection, but lemon balm can help to stop the cold sore spreading.

15g (½oz) dried lemon
  balm leaves
100ml (3½fl oz) isopropyl
  alcohol

Place the ingredients in a bottle and seal. Leave them to infuse overnight. Dip a cotton bud into the mixture and dab a little of it on your affected lip. Repeat this several times a day. Never drink this tincture.

THREE-HERB TOOTH RINSE

If you often suffer from toothache, make up this rinse and keep it on hand for temporary relief.

25g (1oz) dried marjoram
  leaves
25g (1oz) dried rosemary
  leaves
25g (1oz) dried thyme leaves
1 litre (1¾ pints) vodka

Place the ingredients in a bottle and seal it with a cap or stopper. Leave to infuse for 15 days, then filter the liquid. Use the rinse twice a day or as needed.

Take care

It is dangerous to drink the three-herb tooth rinse because of its high alcohol content. Use it to rinse around your mouth and then spit it out. You must also make sure that isopropyl alcohol, as used in the lemon balm tincture, is never swallowed.

Breathing freely

The ability to breathe is something that most of us take for granted. But when breathing becomes difficult, due to a cold, a chest infection or asthma, there are traditional remedies that can help.

Our respiratory system is remarkably resistant to infections, resilient in extremes of weather and can even free itself from dust particles. But modern-day pollution and lifestyles put this natural resistance under pressure.

Several preventive measures can help to improve breathing and strengthen the respiratory organs. These include not smoking, eating a healthy diet and getting plenty of exercise.

Standing erect and using your full lung capacity can also help to contribute to a sense of well-being and increased vitality.

To help to treat or prevent respiratory diseases, try some of the tried-and-tested traditional remedies. Inhalations and teas can loosen stubborn phlegm and relieve inflammation. Such natural herb cures are often easier for our bodies to tolerate than modern pharmaceutical alternatives.

Restricted airways

There are many conditions that impede breathing. Most are caused by a viral or bacterial infection that affects the respiratory tract, resulting in anything from a heavy cold to a chest infection or bronchitis. The infection increases the amount of mucous material – catarrh or phlegm – produced by the cells lining the airways, and sometimes causes the lining to swell, restricting the airflow in and out of the lungs in a similar way to asthma.

Asthma can be brought on by allergies, infections, stress and anxiety; a natural predisposition to the disease also plays a role. People who suffer from asthma know just how dangerous attacks can be. Severe attacks can leave asthmatics feeling as if they are suffocating and are sometimes fatal.

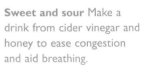

Sweet and sour Make a drink from cider vinegar and honey to ease congestion and aid breathing.

Asthma remedies

Asthmatics may find that breathing exercises and avoiding substances to which they are allergic brings some relief. There are also natural ingredients that help by relaxing bronchial muscles or by loosening phlegm if you have a cold.

CIDER VINEGAR AND HONEY

This drink may relax the bronchial muscles, help to loosen phlegm and relieve congestion.

2 teaspoons cider vinegar
1 teaspoon honey
250ml (9fl oz) water

Stir the vinegar and honey into the water and drink a glass of the mixture three times a day.

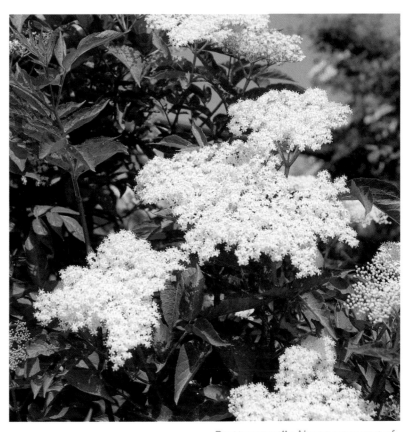

Pretty versatile Almost every part of the elder can be used medicinally.

ASTHMA TEA

The essential oil in thyme has antispasmodic and expectorant properties that can ease the symptoms of asthma.

55g (2oz) dried thyme leaves
15g (½oz) dried sundew leaves
25g (1oz) dried marjoram
  leaves
55g (2oz) dried masterwort
  leaves
250ml (9fl oz) water

Mix the herbs together and put 2 teaspoonfuls in a heatproof bowl. Boil the water and pour over the herbs. Leave to infuse for 5 minutes. Strain the liquid through a fine sieve. Drink 5-7 cups a day.

ELDERFLOWER AND COLTSFOOT TEA

Elderflowers reduce bronchial catarrh and help to ease breathing.

25g (1oz) dried elderflowers
25g (1oz) dried coltsfoot
  leaves
15g (½oz) dried mullein
  flowers
250ml (9fl oz) water

Mix the herbs together and put 1 teaspoonful in a saucepan. Boil the water and pour it over the herbs, then leave to infuse for 10 minutes. Strain the liquid through a fine sieve. Drink 5 cups of this tea a day; drink the last cup just before bedtime.

Preparing tea

Since the advent of the tea bag, strainers are much less widely used. However, they are perfect for straining infusions as they prevent pieces of leaves or flowers from floating in your herbal brew.

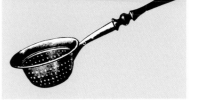

Bronchitis and stubborn coughs

Heavy, dry coughing can be a symptom of the common cold. Although irritating, it benefits the body by clearing the respiratory tracts. Natural remedies help this process by loosening the phlegm.

A dry cough accompanied by the need to gasp for air and chest pains may be a sign of bronchitis.

This is caused by a virus or by bacteria. If the symptoms do not improve in a day or so you should consult a doctor.

To combat a stubborn cough, turn to the traditional remedies: soak in a hot bath, mix and take natural cough remedies and drink plenty of fluids, ideally herbal teas.

CARROT SYRUP

Use organic carrots for this syrup to avoid any pesticides that may exacerbate your illness.

250ml (9fl oz) carrot juice
2 tablespoons honey
1 tablespoon water

Place the ingredients in a saucepan and boil the liquid until it forms a syrup. Take 3-4 teaspoons of the remedy each day.

LAVENDER AND MINT TEA

This tea soothes the respiratory tract and calms breathing.

15g (½oz) dried lavender
flowers
15g (½oz) dried black mint
1 litre (1¾ pints) water
honey to sweeten

Place the herbs in a heatproof bowl. Boil the water and pour over them. Leave to infuse for 5 minutes. Strain the liquid and sweeten as needed. Drink the tea three times a day.

CAMOMILE AND THYME INHALATION TREATMENT

Inhalation treatments such as this will help to alleviate coughing and bronchial pain.

2 tablespoons dried
camomile leaves
2 tablespoons dried
thyme leaves
3-4 litres (5½-7 pints) water

Place the herbs in a heatproof bowl. Boil the water and pour over the herbs. Leave to infuse for 10 minutes. Drape a towel over your head and the bowl and inhale the steam.

FRUIT ELIXIR

Inula root loosens phlegm, stems coughing and may ease bronchitis.

15g (½oz) dried bilberries
15g (½oz) dried rosehips
15g (½oz) cress seeds
1 litre (1¾ pints) dry
white wine
40g (1½oz) dried inula root

Place the fruits and seeds in a saucepan with the wine. Boil the liquid for 5 minutes and strain it through a fine sieve into a bowl. Add the inula root and leave to infuse for a day.

Strain the liquid again, pour it into a bottle and seal. Take 1 teaspoonful three times a day, for three weeks.

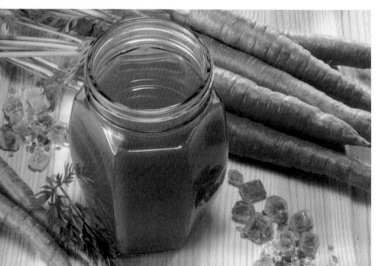

Cough medicine Carrot syrup is simple and quick to make. Pour it into a sterilised jar and seal; it will keep for several weeks.

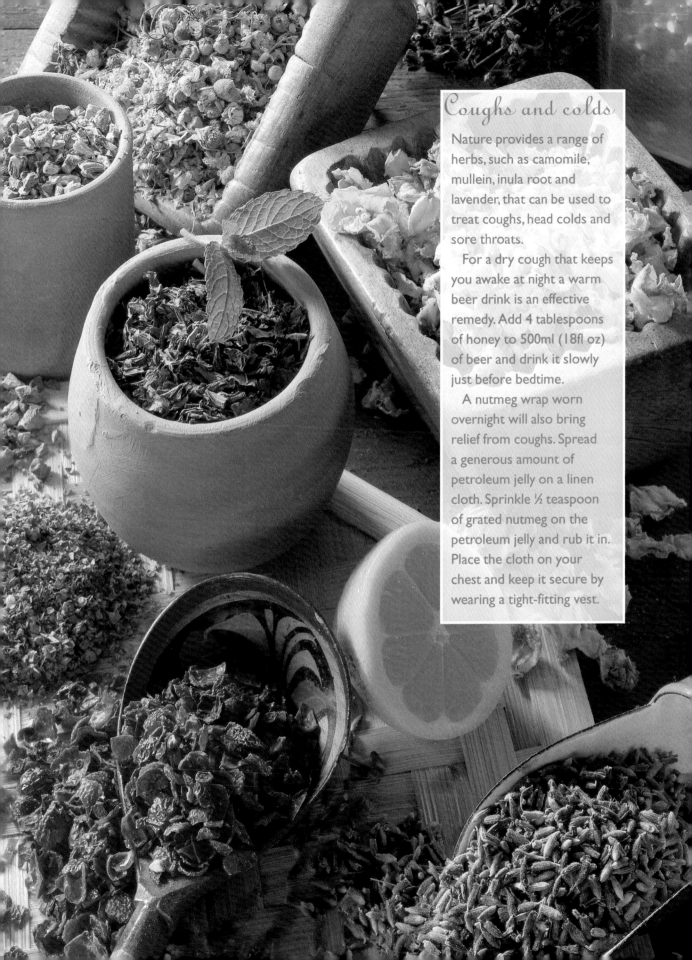

Coughs and colds

Nature provides a range of herbs, such as camomile, mullein, inula root and lavender, that can be used to treat coughs, head colds and sore throats.

For a dry cough that keeps you awake at night a warm beer drink is an effective remedy. Add 4 tablespoons of honey to 500ml (18fl oz) of beer and drink it slowly just before bedtime.

A nutmeg wrap worn overnight will also bring relief from coughs. Spread a generous amount of petroleum jelly on a linen cloth. Sprinkle ½ teaspoon of grated nutmeg on the petroleum jelly and rub it in. Place the cloth on your chest and keep it secure by wearing a tight-fitting vest.

Cider vinegar

This versatile traditional remedy is extremely easy to make and can bring many benefits. Why not test its manifold powers for yourself?

The medicinal use of vinegar dates back thousands of years. The Greek physician Hippocrates (regarded as the father of modern medicine) was using vinegar to treat his patients in 400 BC, and it has been used to heal wounds since Biblical times.

As well as being a natural antiseptic and antibiotic, cider vinegar contains important minerals, vitamins and essential acids. It is sometimes taken to relieve arthritis, to regulate blood pressure and to aid digestion. It can be added to bath water to soothe eczema and is used to condition hair.

In our grandparents' day, cider vinegar was made using a fruit press to squeeze the juice from apples. Today, traditional fruit presses have been replaced by electric juicers. The juice is left to ferment until it produces a sticky foam that appears on the surface. Adding yeast speeds up the process.

How to make cider vinegar
Makes 1 litre (1¾ pints)

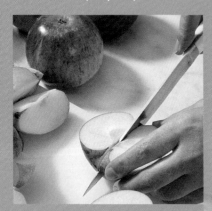

▼ Pour the juice, together with a **few pieces of the peel**, into a glass jar. Add **brewer's yeast** (see manufacturer's instructions for quantities) and seal the jar tightly with a lid. Place a cloth over the top if you wish.

▲ Wash **2kg (4lb 8oz) cooking apples**, slice them into quarters and cut out any damaged spots. Place them in a juicer and start the machine.

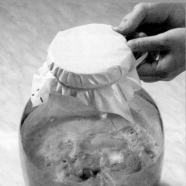

▲ Leave the mixture to infuse for four weeks, skimming off the foam and shaking the jar occasionally. Once the vinegar tastes sour, filter it through a fine sieve, transfer it to sterilised bottles and seal them with corks or caps.

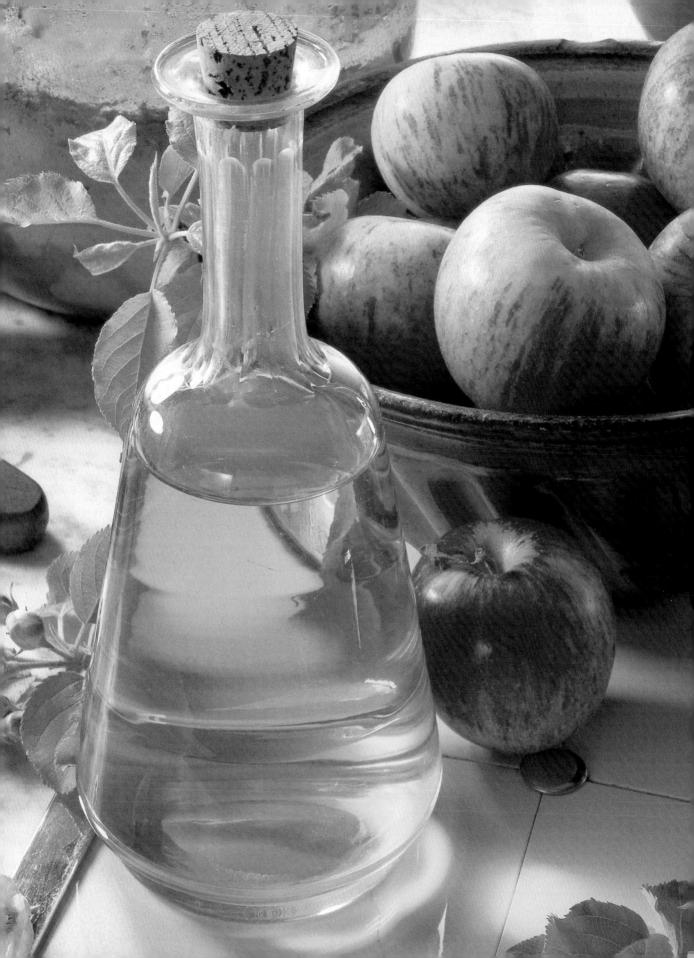

Remedies for colds

Not many people can get through the winter without catching at least one cold. If you do succumb to this common ailment, help is at hand from herbs, flowers and fruit.

A cold is caused by a virus caught from someone else and announces its onset with a runny nose and sore throat. These symptoms indicate that it is time to delve into nature's medicine cabinet, used by our forebears, in search of an effective remedy.

Once you go down with a cold, or ideally when you feel it coming on, boost your vitamin C intake to strengthen your immune system. Use citrus fruits to make hot drinks that are rich in vitamin C.

Blackcurrants, too, are an excellent source of vitamin C and can also be taken as a hot drink. Garlic is another natural ingredient that is an effective antiviral agent.

The advantage of using natural plants for healing is that they combat the symptoms of common ailments in a gentle way.

Flu is also a viral illness, but with more severe symptoms. For these, traditional home remedies can offer relief and help to speed recovery. If your symptoms persist, however, always seek advice from your doctor.

Your immune system

How susceptible you are to catching a viral infection depends on your immune system. As soon as bacteria or viruses enter your body, the immune system produces antibodies, which are part of the body's natural defence mechanism.

Unfortunately, many germs, such as the viruses that cause colds and flu, mutate extremely rapidly, so each new infection requires the production of new antibodies. If the immune system is weak, the body is unable to produce enough antibodies to fight the disease.

Keeping healthy

There are many factors that impair immunity, including poor diet, lack of regular exercise and pollution. If the body and immune system are weakened, the risk of catching an infection is higher.

Even when you have a cold you can still boost your immune system and obtain relief from the symptoms of the infection with the help of traditional remedies.

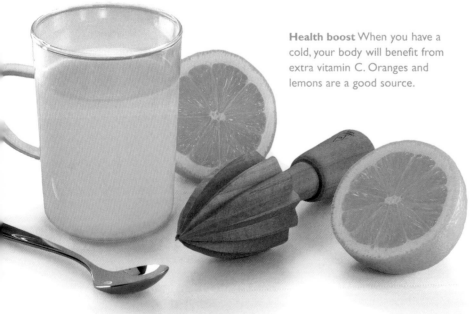

Health boost When you have a cold, your body will benefit from extra vitamin C. Oranges and lemons are a good source.

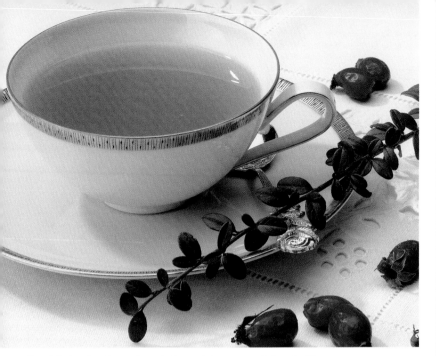

Rosehip healer Apart from being a rich source of vitamin C, rosehip tea activates the body's self-healing process.

Special properties of healing plants

Native Americans used coneflowers (*Echinacea purpurea*) to treat wounds. The active substances contained in this plant (normally taken as a tincture or a tablet) also help to stimulate the immune system and protect the body from infections. Camomile flowers, rosehips and lemon balm leaves also help to prevent colds.

HOT LEMON DRINK

The vitamin C in citrus fruit is essential to keep our immune system working effectively.

juice of I lemon
250ml (9fl oz) water
honey to sweeten

Place the lemon juice in a large mug. Boil the water and pour it into the mug. Sweeten the drink with the honey as required.

ROSEHIP TEA

Weight for weight, rosehips from dog roses contain 20 times more vitamin C than an orange.

25g (1oz) fresh rosehips
250ml (9fl oz) water
I teaspoon lemon juice
I teaspoon honey

Cut the rosehips in half, put in a saucepan and pour the water over them. Bring to the boil, remove from the heat and leave to infuse for 10 minutes. Strain the liquid through a fine sieve, then add the lemon juice and honey.

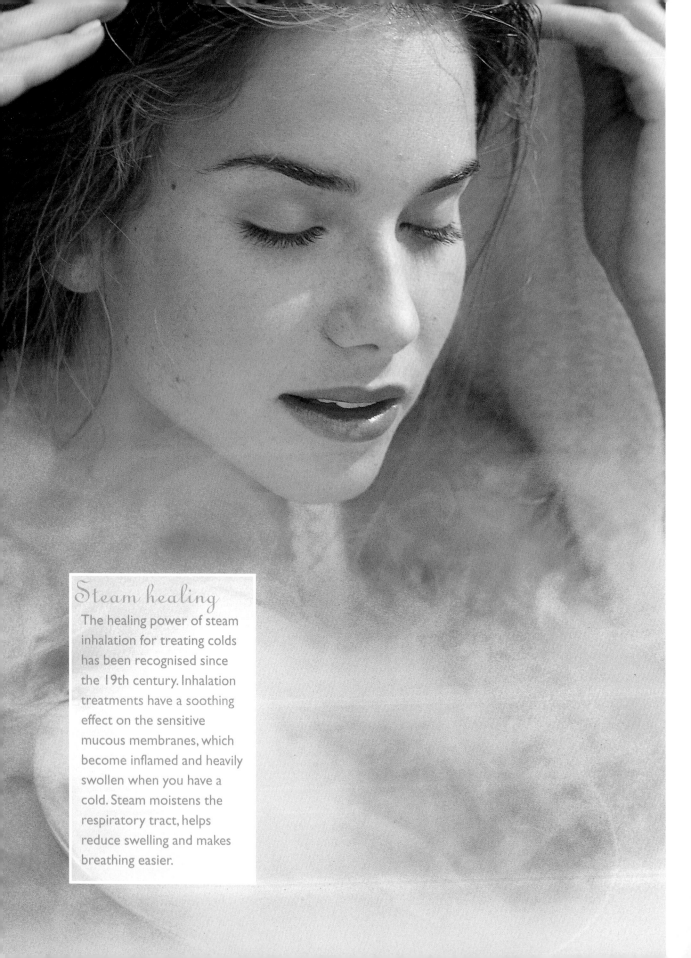

Steam healing

The healing power of steam inhalation for treating colds has been recognised since the 19th century. Inhalation treatments have a soothing effect on the sensitive mucous membranes, which become inflamed and heavily swollen when you have a cold. Steam moistens the respiratory tract, helps reduce swelling and makes breathing easier.

HOREHOUND ELIXIR

Horehound, native to Europe and Asia, is an ancient cough remedy.

**15g (½oz) dried horehound leaves
25g (1oz) fennel seeds
15g (½oz) dried coneflower leaves
1 litre (1¾ pints) white wine
honey to sweeten**

Mix the herbs together and place 3 tablespoonfuls with the wine in a pan. Boil for 4-5 minutes, strain and sweeten. Drink warm, taking 50ml (2fl oz) three times a day.

THYME AND LEMON DRINK

Thyme can relieve coughing and make breathing easier.

**15g (½oz) dried thyme leaves
25g (1oz) dried lemon tree leaves
1 litre (1¾ pints) water**

Place the herbs in a heatproof bowl. Boil the water and pour it over them. Leave the brew to cool, then strain. Drink it three times a day.

Medicinal sweating and influenza

Colds are often accompanied by high fever, so don't worry if your temperature rises temporarily. It is a sign that your body is fighting the germs. Fever overheats the body, which boosts the immune system. The higher-than-usual temperature kills many germs that are heat sensitive.

Traditionally, sweating was prescribed for fever in order to strengthen the body. Nature's medicine cabinet contains many remedies that gently help to induce sweating and get rid of toxic substances without suppressing a fever. However, this is an unsuitable remedy for people with cardiovascular complaints.

A fever becomes critical (especially for children and older people) if it does not subside, or if it rises to above 39°C (102°F). In either instance a doctor should be consulted without delay.

If coughing and a head cold are accompanied by fever and pains in the limbs, you probably have flu. Take a herbal tea to help to ease the symptoms and stay in bed.

SUNFLOWER TINCTURE

Sunflower leaves, not seeds, are used for this fever remedy.

**1 teaspoon dried sunflower leaves
50ml (2fl oz) vodka**

Place the leaves in a bottle and pour on the alcohol. Leave to infuse for ten days. Strain the liquid. Take 20 drops in a glass of water three times a day.

YARROW AND MINT TEA

For best results, take this remedy during the initial stages of flu.

**15g (½oz) dried yarrow tops
15g (½oz) dried mint leaves
15g (½oz) dried lemon balm leaves
15g (½oz) dried elderflowers
250ml (9fl oz) water**

Mix the herbs together and place 1 tablespoonful in a heatproof bowl. Boil the water and pour it over the herbs. Leave to infuse for 10 minutes, then strain the liquid through a fine sieve. Drink cups of this tea throughout the day when required.

Flower power The healing power of sunflower leaves can help to combat fever.

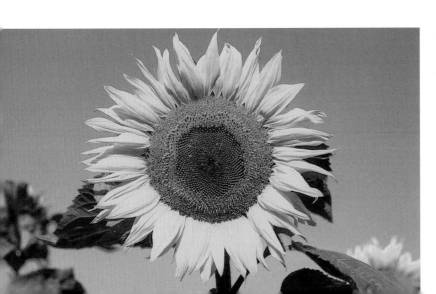

Strengthening and

There are many natural ways to boost the health of your heart and help to prevent a number of potentially life-threatening disorders.

The heart is the body's engine. It is a muscular pump which keeps the blood constantly flowing, ensuring that your body receives sufficient supplies of nutrients from the blood, as well as fresh oxygen from the lungs. The heart also enables waste products to be carried away from the tissues. A regular heartbeat is your signal that the heart is working properly.

It has long been known that, like all muscles, the heart can be trained to be healthy, specifically by exercise. Equally, lack of exercise can sometimes cause the heart to beat irregularly, especially if you are stressed. Although it may not be possible to restore an 'old' heart to youthful vitality, you can certainly improve its vigour.

Good blood circulation is also vital to health. Problems with blood vessels can give rise to unpleasant conditions, such as varicose veins and haemorrhoids, and can contribute to high blood pressure. You can use a variety of natural remedies to avoid such serious cardiovascular disorders.

GALANGAL SOUP

In ancient China, the root of the galangal plant was used to treat heart palpitations.

½ teaspoon galangal powder
1 teaspoon dried marjoram leaves
1 teaspoon ground celery seed
¼ teaspoon white pepper
200g (7oz) honey

Blend the ingredients in a small saucepan and boil the mixture. Let it cool then boil again, stirring until it achieves a thick consistency. During a four to six week treatment, take ½ teaspoonful three times a day.

Cucumber cure The juice of a cucumber can help to reduce high blood pressure. The vitamins and other substances in fresh vegetables can also boost heart health.

relaxing your heart

LEMON BALM TEA

This mixture will help those who suffer from minor or irregular heart disorders when they are under stress.

25g (1oz) dried lemon
  balm leaves
25g (1oz) caraway seeds
25g (1oz) dried valerian root
250ml (9fl oz) water

Mix the herbs together and place 2 teaspoonfuls in a heatproof bowl. Boil the water and pour over the herbs. Leave to infuse for 5-10 minutes. Strain the liquid and drink a cup of this tea every day.

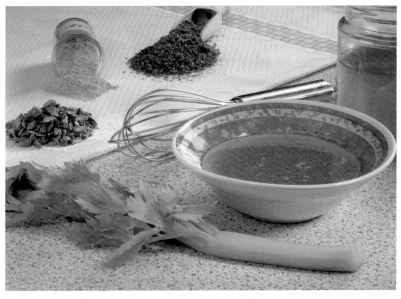

Healing plant The aromatic galangal plant has medicinal properties that have been recognised for centuries. It grows in eastern Asia, where it is also used as a seasoning for food.

RELAXATION TEA

When your heartbeat is racing, this remedy will help to slow it down.

40g (1½oz) dried motherwort
  leaves
25g (1oz) dried greater
  burnet root
25g (1oz) dried tormentil
  root
25g (1oz) dried rue leaves
25g (1oz) dried angelica root
250ml (9fl oz) water

Mix the herbs together and place 2 teaspoonfuls in a heatproof bowl. Boil the water and pour over the herbs. Leave to infuse for 10 minutes, then strain. Drink a cup of this tea when required.

HEART-STRENGTHENING TEA

This mixture of flowers and leaves should improve your circulation.

40g (1½oz) dried hawthorn
  flowers
15g (½oz) dried motherwort
  leaves
15g (½oz) dried lemon
  balm leaves
250ml (9fl oz) water

Mix the herbs together and place 2 teaspoonfuls in a heatproof bowl. Boil the water and pour over the herbs. Leave to infuse for 10 minutes, then strain through a fine sieve. Drink a cup of this tea every day.

VALERIAN WINE

This pleasant de-stressing drink will make you feel relaxed.

15g (½oz) dried valerian root
peel of an unwaxed orange
1 sprig rosemary
1 clove
1 litre (1¾ pints) white wine

Place the ingredients in a bottle and seal with a cork or screw-top cap. Leave to infuse for four weeks. Strain the liquid into a pan and boil for 1 minute. Pour the wine into a 1 litre (1¾ pint) bottle or jar and seal. Drink a liqueur glass (45ml) of the wine three times a day.

Tried & Trusted
Care for the heart

- Warm, relaxing baths with valerian root or lemon balm leaves added help to soothe the heart.

- Exercising for 20 minutes a day in the fresh air strengthens the heart and oxygenates the blood.

- If you have cardiac problems, avoid coffee, nicotine and alcohol. The caffeine they contain puts extra strain on the heart.

- Treat cardiac palpitations by drinking a glass of water containing 2 tablespoons of sugar and a dash of lemon juice.

High blood pressure

- If you have high blood pressure, avoid becoming overweight. Eat plenty of fresh fruit and vegetables, reduce your meat intake and increase the wholemeal products in your diet.

- Garlic is regarded as a cure-all by many herbalists and naturopaths. It has long been used to help to keep blood vessels from becoming clogged up and to reduce high blood pressure.

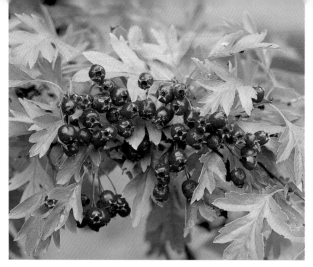

Hawthorn for hearts The flowers, leaves and berries of the hawthorn contain substances that can help to strengthen the heart of an older person.

Alleviating high blood pressure

Many people suffer from high blood pressure, which is a danger to health and must be treated. Also known as hypertension, high blood pressure is often the result of obesity and poor diet. If this disorder is coupled with diabetes and a high level of cholesterol, there is considerable risk of a heart attack or stroke.

ROSEMARY WINE

Rosemary not only flavours food, but stimulates circulation too.

15g (½oz) dried rosemary leaves
750ml (1 pint 7fl oz) white wine

Place the rosemary in a bottle and pour the wine over it. Seal with a cork or screw-top cap and leave to infuse for five days. Strain the liquid through a fine sieve into another bottle and seal. Drink a liqueur glass (45ml) of the wine at lunch and dinner.

NERVE-SOOTHING TEA

This tea can help to lower high blood pressure.

40g (1½oz) dried speedwell leaves
40g (1½oz) holy thistle seeds
25g (1oz) dried St John's wort flowers
25g (1oz) dried lemon balm leaves
25g (1oz) dried hawthorn flowers
250ml (9fl oz) water
honey to sweeten

Mix the herbs together and place 2 teaspoonfuls into a heatproof bowl. Boil the water and pour over the herbs. Leave to infuse for 15 minutes. Strain the liquid through a fine sieve. Sweeten it with honey. Drink the tea throughout the day.

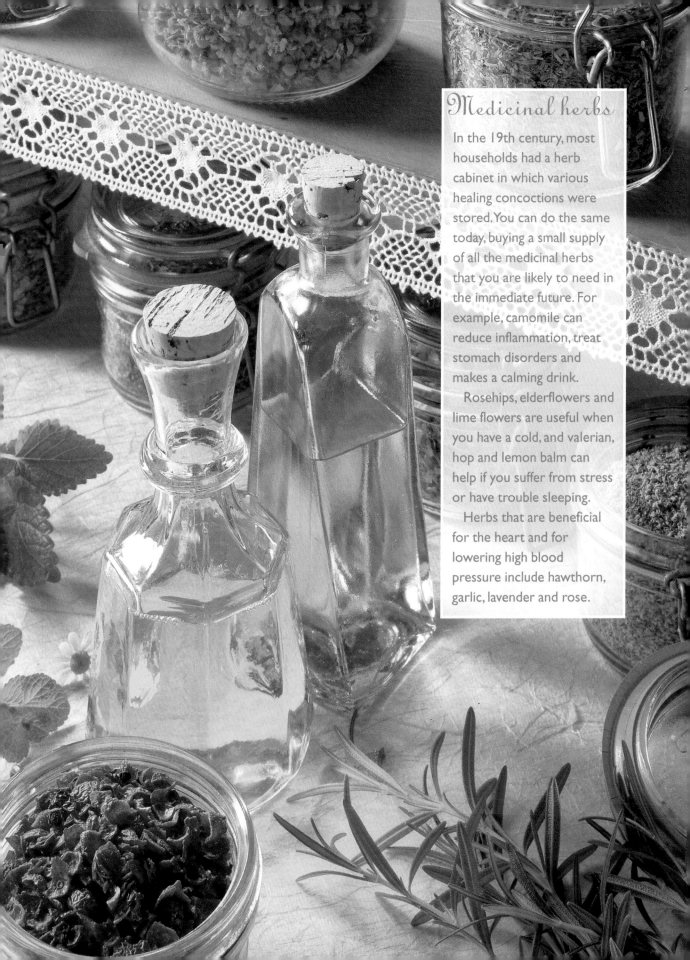

Medicinal herbs

In the 19th century, most households had a herb cabinet in which various healing concoctions were stored. You can do the same today, buying a small supply of all the medicinal herbs that you are likely to need in the immediate future. For example, camomile can reduce inflammation, treat stomach disorders and makes a calming drink.

Rosehips, elderflowers and lime flowers are useful when you have a cold, and valerian, hop and lemon balm can help if you suffer from stress or have trouble sleeping.

Herbs that are beneficial for the heart and for lowering high blood pressure include hawthorn, garlic, lavender and rose.

Maintaining healthy blood circulation

Throughout the body there is a network of blood vessels which ensures that blood is transported to every organ, and that all cells receive sufficient nutrients and oxygen. Like other body systems, circulation is susceptible to disorders. The flow of blood through a vein or artery can be hindered by fatty deposits, for instance, or the muscles in the wall of a vessel may be weakened.

Taking regular exercise is the way to prevent poor circulation. A diet low in saturated fats, such as those in meat and dairy foods, will also help to keep blood vessels in good health. If you suffer from poor circulation, you can also try some of these traditional treatments.

Treat for feet The leaves and fruit of the horse chestnut tree are the main ingredients in a footbath that helps the circulation. Dry your feet thoroughly afterwards and keep them warm.

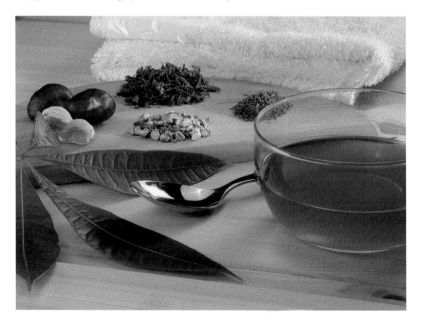

TEA FOR CIRCULATION

This tea may help to improve your circulation.

15g (½oz) dried peppermint leaves
15g (½oz) dried camomile flowers
15g (½oz) dried valerian root
15g (½oz) dried rue leaves
15g (½oz) dried silverweed leaves
250ml (9fl oz) water
honey to sweeten

Mix the herbs together and place 1 teaspoonful in a heatproof bowl. Boil the water and pour it over the herbs. Leave to infuse for 10 minutes. Strain the liquid and sweeten it with honey. Drink 1-2 cups each day.

Pestle & mortar

It is worth having a pestle and mortar to hand for preparing herbal teas. This equipment is ideal for crushing seeds and hard plant stems, and for turning dried leaves and flowers into powder.

CHESTNUT FOOTBATH

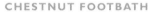

The active substances in horse chestnuts help to strengthen the blood vessels.

15g (½oz) dried horse chestnut leaves and fruit
2 teaspoons dried thyme leaves
2 teaspoons dried stinging nettle leaves
500ml (18fl oz) water

Mix the herbs, leaves and fruit together and place 2 teaspoonfuls in a heatproof bowl. Boil the water and pour it over the mixture. Leave to infuse, then strain. Add 12 tablespoonfuls of it to 4 litres (7 pints) of footbath water.

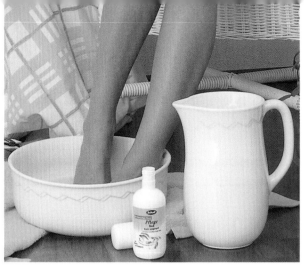

Circulation booster A foot-bath made with rosemary or eucalyptus helps blood circulation. Fill a bowl with lukewarm water, add the herbs and gradually raise the temperature by adding hot water.

Hardening of the arteries

Healthy blood vessels are elastic and can easily accommodate the changes associated with the normal day-to-day blood flow.

However, age and poor health can lead to the blood vessels becoming clogged and arteriosclerosis, or hardening of the artery walls, can result. Like earlier generations, we too can use herbal remedies to protect ourselves from these disorders.

Varicose veins

The enlarged veins we know as varicose veins are not a modern disorder; generations before us were equally afflicted and weak veins can be hereditary.

Varicose veins are caused by weakened valves in the veins which lead to a poor flow of blood back to the heart. Blood accumulates in the veins which then become bulging, twisted and painful.

Constipation can be the cause of pressure on the veins of the abdomen, preventing them from receiving blood from the legs. Weak veins can also cause painful and itchy haemorrhoids.

TEA FOR VARICOSE VEINS

Drink this to ease tired, swollen legs and strengthen the veins.

**55g (2oz) fresh horsetail 'needles' and stem
250ml (9fl oz) water**

Chop the horsetail and place 1-2 teaspoonfuls in a pan. Pour the water over the herb and leave to infuse overnight. Bring the mixture to the boil, then filter through a filter paper. Drink 2-3 cups a day for several weeks.

SOOTHING OIL BATH

Relieve the pain of haemorrhoids with soothing oils.

**6 drops each cypress oil and camomile oil
3 drops peppermint oil
20 drops vegetable oil**

Run a shallow bath. Add 2 drops each of cypress and camomile oil and 1 drop of peppermint oil to the water. Bathe for 5-10 minutes. Mix the remaining oils and rub them on the affected area.

Tried & Trusted
Good circulation

- **Putting your feet alternately in footbaths that contain hot and cold water will exercise the blood vessels. This is a popular way of treating poor blood circulation.**

- **Foot massages with rosemary oil can help to improve the flow of blood around your body. Do not use rosemary oil if you are pregnant, suffer from high blood pressure or are epileptic.**

- **Fresh garlic can help to reduce the amount of cholesterol in the blood (as can onions and ginger), which may reduce the risk of arteriosclerosis.**

Ease varicose veins

- **Strengthen your veins by taking exercise, such as swimming, cycling or running. Avoid sitting or standing for long periods.**

- **To alleviate the itching of haemorrhoids, bathe the affected area in cold water, then dry and smear over some petroleum jelly to soothe and protect.**

- **Dab 1-2 drops of camomile oil on painful haemorrhoids every day to help them to reduce in size.**

How to stay active

Keeping physically fit is vital for good health. Whenever painful joints, aching muscles or strains are a problem, you can turn to home remedies for welcome relief.

Unless the joints and muscles work efficiently, it is impossible to move without feeling pain. Together the skeleton and muscles support the body and its internal organs and enable us to walk in an upright position. They also enable every kind of movement, from strenuous running and swimming to precise actions such as writing or playing a musical instrument.

Sprains and strains can occur at any age, whatever your level of fitness, but with advancing years painful joint disorders, such as arthritis or gout are increasingly likely to become a problem.

A range of long-used natural treatments including herbs, plants and natural oils may soothe such complaints and alleviate pain.

Natural treatments can be part of a regime that helps to keep you mobile throughout your life, maintaining your freedom and independence into old age.

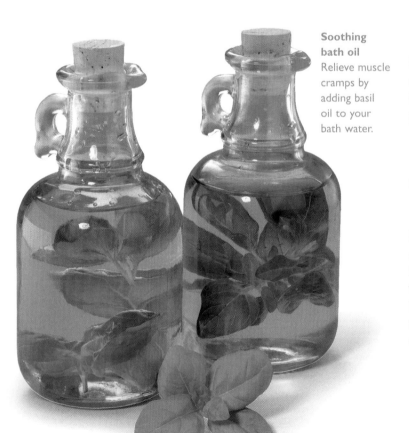

Soothing bath oil
Relieve muscle cramps by adding basil oil to your bath water.

ROSEMARY SPIRIT

Rosemary, a medicinal herb originating from southern Europe, helps to alleviate muscle aches and pains and rheumatism.

100g (3½oz) fresh rosemary leaves
500ml (18fl oz) isopropyl alcohol

Put the rosemary into a bottle. Add the alcohol and leave to infuse for ten days. Pour into a jug. Filter the liquid through a fine sieve back into the bottle. Seal the bottle with a cap or cork. Rub on the painful area as required.

all your life

Reducing the effects of cramps and pains

Muscle or joint pains, whether caused by a sport's injury or the result of a clumsy movement, are painful and frustrating. They can cause misery when they restrict our basic movements.

Cramps in the arms and legs are sudden and acutely painful contractions of the muscles. These sometimes set in during or after vigorous exercise. Taking part in any kind of work-out or sport without first doing warm-up exercises can cause injury because the muscles have not been properly prepared for strenuous activity.

Repetitive movement, such as working at a computer keyboard all day, is another cause of cramp and can also damage muscles, joints and tendons. Painful night-time cramps in the calves may indicate a mineral deficiency.

Over-exertion or an awkward movement can lead to inflammation of a joint, such as the elbow or knee, causing what is commonly known as tennis elbow and housemaid's knee. It can also damage the sheath surrounding the tendons – strong bundles of tissue that link muscles with the bone.

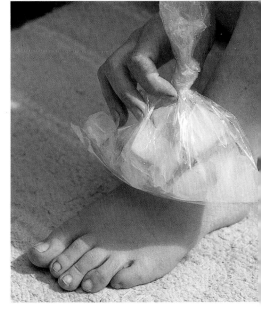

First aid Treat sprains with an ice compress to prevent serious swelling. Apply the compress as soon as possible after the injury has occurred.

CRAMP-RELIEVING BATH OIL

Use this bath treatment to relieve cramps in your arms or legs. The combination of active oils and the warmth of the water will stimulate your circulation and alleviate pain.

4 drops basil oil
4 drops marjoram oil
2 drops lemongrass oil

Add the oils to your running bath water. While bathing, gently massage the painful muscles.

TENNIS-ELBOW COMPRESSES

Painful tendons may be soothed using an easy-to-prepare compress.

1 tablespoon vinegar
1 glass water
  or
3-4 tablespoons horseradish
  or
3-4 tablespoons quark

Mix the vinegar and water, soak a cloth in the liquid and wrap it around your elbow. Alternatively, spread a generous amount of either horseradish or quark on the painful area and leave it for 20 minutes before washing off.

Warming pan

Heated bricks and copper hot-water bottles were traditionally used for heat treatments to alleviate painful torn ligaments and damaged tendons. Even today, a hot-water bottle is soothing and comforting.

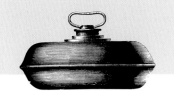

Rheumatism and gout

The term 'rheumatism' covers a whole range of medical conditions. Rheumatic fever is one of these, as are rheumatoid arthritis (inflammation of the joint) and osteoarthritis (a wearing out of the joint surfaces). Gout, on the other hand, is a metabolic disease. Large quantities of uric acid accumulate in the joints, resulting in swellings of toes and fingers.

There are, however, numerous traditional remedies that can help to alleviate the pain of these conditions. The herbs and plants that are needed for these cures can be freshly grown in your garden (see Garden herbs, pages 326–331). Alternatively they can be purchased in dried or powdered form from a herbalist.

Prehistoric perennial Horsetail is a herb that has grown on earth for millions of years. It can be used to ease the pain of joint disorders.

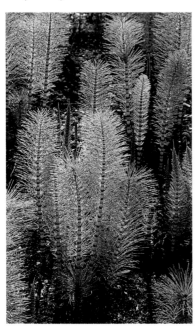

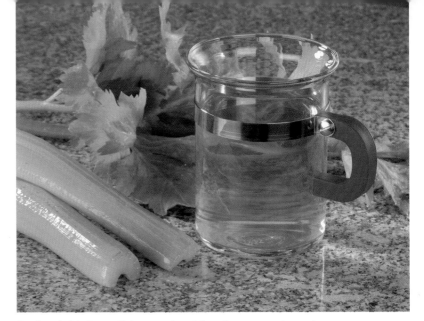

Anti-arthritis brew Celery tea is quick and easy to make, and helps to alleviate the joint pain of arthritis.

HORSETAIL BATH

Horsetail contains silica which often relieves rheumatic pain.

**1 litre (1¾ pints) water
100g (3½oz) fresh horsetail 'needles' and stems**

Place the ingredients in a bowl and leave to infuse for an hour. Strain the liquid and add the brew to your bath water.

GARLIC OIL

This oil can bring relief from the pain of swollen joints.

**3-4 tablespoons vegetable oil
2-3 tablespoons lard
3-4 cloves garlic**

Blend the oil and lard in a small bowl. Crush the garlic to a rough pulp and stir it into the fats. Gently but firmly massage this mixture into your painful joints.

Take care

Horsetail is a herb that is best used when fresh. However, if you choose to dry it, take care not to damage the often brittle stems.

CELERY TEA

Celery tea can alleviate the pain of arthritis. However, do not drink it if you suffer from a kidney disorder of any kind.

**15g (½oz) fresh celery, chopped
250ml (9fl oz) water
honey to sweeten**

Place the celery and water in a pan, bring to the boil and simmer the mixture for 3 minutes. Leave to infuse for 5-10 minutes, then strain the liquid. Sweeten the tea with the honey and drink 2 cups a day.

Tried & Trusted
Aching muscles

• **Apply arnica cream to aching muscles after performing a strenuous sport or any heavy, physical work.**

• **If you wake up at night with a cramp in your calf muscle, massage it with olive oil and 1-2 drops of violet leaf absolute.**

• **Regular swimming and aqua-aerobic exercise will help to keep your tendons and ligaments supple.**

Soothing gout pain

• **Maintain a healthy diet to regulate your digestion and to help your kidneys to remove the waste products that sometimes cause gout. Eat plenty of fresh fruit and vegetables, as well as sufficient roughage, and reduce your intake of meat and fats.**

• **To help your body to discharge waste products more efficiently, drink at least 2 litres (3½ pints) of water during the course of the day.**

ANTI-GOUT TEA

This tea mixture of leaves and berries will help to prevent gout.

25g (1oz) dried birch leaves
15g (½oz) dried horsetail 'needles' and stems
15g (½oz) dried yarrow tops
2 teaspoons dried restharrow leaves
2 teaspoons dried elderberries
2 teaspoons dried stinging nettle leaves
250ml (9fl oz) water

Mix the ingredients together and place 2 teaspoonfuls in a heatproof bowl. Boil the water and pour it over the mixture. Leave to infuse for 5-10 minutes. Strain the liquid and drink a cup at the beginning and end of each day.

DAISY TEA

Daisy flowers and leaves have been used since the Middle Ages to alleviate numerous ailments including gout and arthritis.

250ml (9fl oz) water
2 teaspoons dried daisy flowers and leaves
honey to sweeten

Place the dried daisies in a heatproof bowl. Boil the water and pour it over them. Leave to infuse for 10 minutes, then strain the liquid. Sweeten with honey and consume 2 cups a day.

Treating sprains

Sudden movements can dislocate joints and sprain or tear the ligaments that connect bones at the joints. Such damage can prove extremely painful.

DILL SPRAIN OINTMENT

Fresh dill can help to alleviate the pain caused by a sprain.

4 tablespoons fresh dill
2 tablespoons olive oil
4 tablespoons beeswax granules

Chop the dill and mix it with the oil in a bowl. Leave to infuse for 24 hours, then press the mixture through a fine sieve. Melt the beeswax by heating it in a bowl set over a pan of simmering water. Stir sufficient wax into the oil mixture to make a smooth paste. Apply the ointment to the injury and bandage the sprain.

COMFREY EXTRACT WRAP

Treat sprains, pulled muscles and tendons with this herbal wrap.

100g (3½oz) fresh comfrey root
1 litre (1¾ pints) water

Place the comfrey root and water in a saucepan and boil for 10-15 minutes. Strain the liquid and soak a linen cloth in it. Place the cloth on your sore muscles. Do not take comfrey root internally.

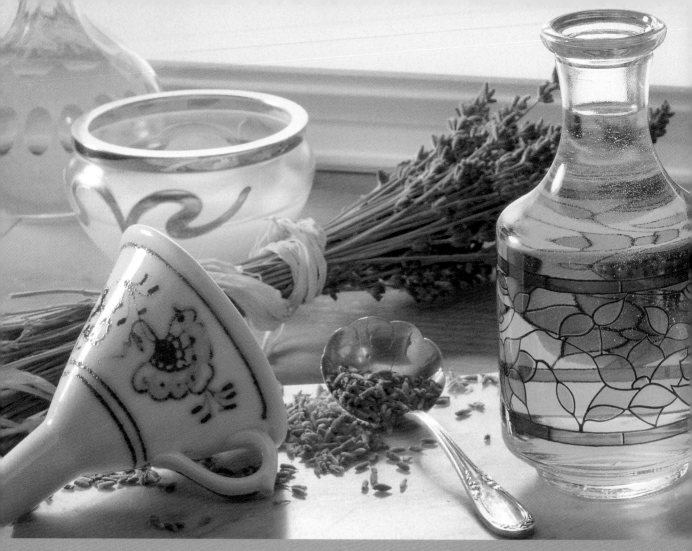

Lavender oil

Bottled in a decorative glass flacon, this freshly scented lavender oil is an ideal gift, particularly for anyone who exercises regularly.

Thanks to its fresh scent and healing properties, the lavender plant has long been used in a variety of ways. In ancient Rome, women used creams perfumed with lavender all over their bodies. The flowers reached the height of their popularity in England during the 19th century, when gentlewomen used lavender toilet water and lavender-scented ink to write letters. The plant's healing powers are now mainly obtained from the oil.

A massage with the oil after bathing makes skin silky. For those who regularly take part in sport, a lavender massage before and after exercise helps to reduce muscle ache.

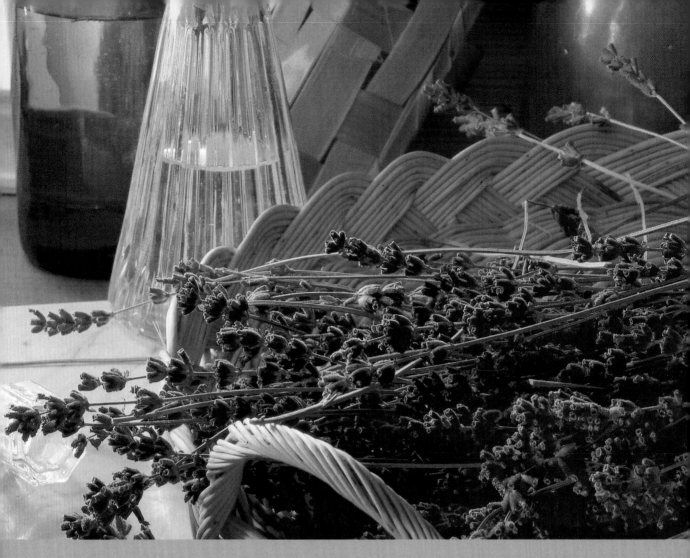

How to make lavender oil
Makes one 600ml (1 pint) bottle

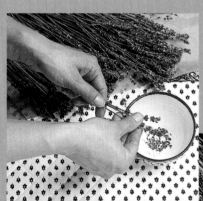

▼ Add **500ml (18fl oz) olive** or **sweet almond oil** and allow the mixture to infuse in a warm and sunny place for three days.

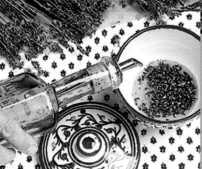

▲ Remove a handful of fresh or dried **lavender flowers** from their stalks and place them in a clean bowl.

▲ Filter the mixture into a glass bottle. To give it a stronger perfume, repeat the process using the filtered oil and a new supply of fresh or dried flowers.

A healthy digestion

Most people have occasional stomach upsets and
one in three suffer from chronic digestive problems.
A variety of herbal remedies – some used for
centuries – can bring relief.

Our digestive organs –
including the liver and gall bladder
– break down the food we eat and
ensure that the various nutrients it
contains are transported to the
right places in our bodies and that
toxic wastes are disposed of.

Digestive disorders caused by
stress, poor eating habits, lack of
exercise or a combination of all
three are commonplace. The
symptoms often include
heartburn, nausea, stomach
cramps and constipation.

To have a digestive system that
functions well, it is essential to
develop a healthy lifestyle and
eat a well-balanced diet.

The causes of an upset stomach

If you have a busy lifestyle, it is
easy to lose the habit of regular,
relaxed eating and to rush meals or
miss them altogether. This can lead
to a poor diet heavy in fatty or
refined convenience foods. Such a
diet will lack roughage and be low
in essential vitamins and minerals.

Eating one large meal a day,
rather than several smaller meals,
can also lead to problems by
overloading the digestive system. It
is much better to provide the body
with a more regular flow of food.

Without a change of lifestyle, or
at least the will to establish a new
eating regime, minor digestive
problems can develop into chronic
disorders. Add to this any undue
stress or tension and more serious
chronic conditions such as irritable
bowel syndrome and stomach
ulcers may well result.

At the first sign of a stomach
complaint try one of these
suggested herbal remedies. Such
natural treatments can also help to
combat a loss of appetite.

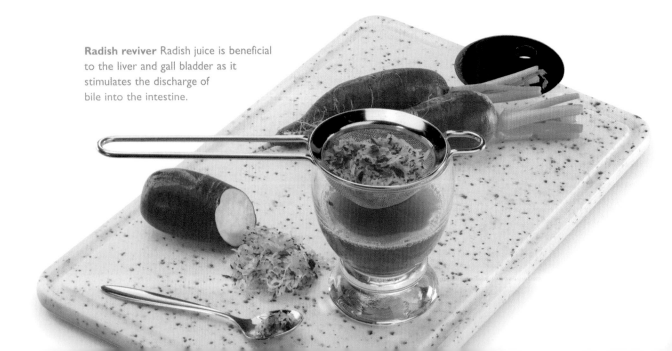

Radish reviver Radish juice is beneficial
to the liver and gall bladder as it
stimulates the discharge of
bile into the intestine.

MIXED HERB TEA

This brew is made from traditional medicinal herbs and is said to help the digestion.

25g (1oz) dried camomile flowers
25g (1oz) dried peppermint leaves
15g (½oz) dried yarrow tops
15g (½oz) dried centaury leaves
15g (½oz) dried gentian root
250ml (9fl oz) water

Mix the herbs together and place 2 teaspoonfuls in a heatproof bowl. Boil the water and pour it over the herbs. Leave to infuse for 10-15 minutes. Strain the liquid and drink a cup after meals.

BITTER ORANGE TEA

The peel of bitter Seville oranges from the Mediterranean can help to restore your appetite.

25g (1oz) Seville orange peel
25g (1oz) fresh rosehips
25g (1oz) fresh centaury leaves
250ml (9fl oz) water

Mix together the Seville orange peel and herbs and place 2 teaspoonfuls in a heatproof bowl. Boil the water and pour it over the mixture. Leave to infuse for 5 minutes. Strain the liquid and drink a cup of warm tea 30 minutes before mealtimes.

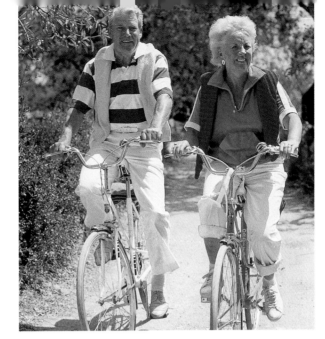

A healthy appetite Fresh air and plenty of exercise will stimulate your appetite and strengthen your immune system.

PEPPERMINT TEA

This aromatic, antiseptic tea is a classic remedy for nausea and vomiting.

55g (2oz) dried peppermint leaves
250ml (9fl oz) water

Place 1-2 teaspoons of the peppermint in a heatproof bowl. Boil the water and pour over the herb. Leave to infuse for 10 minutes. Strain the liquid and drink 1-2 cups as needed, taking small sips.

ELDERBERRY TEA

Elderberries help to combat acid heartburn after eating fatty foods.

1 teaspoon crushed fresh elderberries
250ml (9fl oz) water

Prepare and strain the tea as for Peppermint Tea, above. Drink it after heavy meals.

Problems with digestion

The body's response to invasion by viruses or bacteria may be vomiting or diarrhoea, both of which help rid it of harmful substances. Soothing herbs can often bring relief.

CARAWAY TEA

Caraway seeds help to reduce bloating and prevent wind.

15g (½oz) crushed caraway seeds
15g (½oz) crushed fennel seeds
15g (½oz) crushed aniseed
250ml (9fl oz) water

Mix the seeds together and place 2 teaspoonfuls in a heatproof bowl. Boil the water and pour over the seeds. Leave to infuse for 10 minutes. Strain the liquid through a fine sieve and drink a cup as required.

41

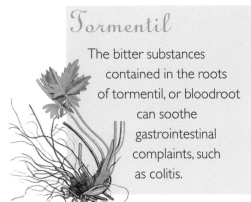

Tormentil

The bitter substances contained in the roots of tormentil, or bloodroot can soothe gastrointestinal complaints, such as colitis.

TORMENTIL TEA

Tormentil has a high tannin content and has traditionally been used to treat diarrhoea and colic cramps.

250ml (9fl oz) water
25g (1oz) dried tormentil root

Boil the water in a pan. Add the tormentil and boil for 10 minutes. Strain the liquid through a fine sieve and drink 2-3 cups a day.

PASSIONFLOWER TEA

This fragrant drink can help to soothe cramp-like colic.

25g (1oz) dried passionflower flowers and leaves
25g (1oz) dried camomile flowers
1 litre (1¾ pints) water

Place the flowers and leaves in a heatproof bowl. Boil the water and pour it over them. Leave to infuse for 10 minutes. Strain the liquid and drink a cup immediately.

SENNA TEA

Senna is one of the most effective plant laxatives, but this tea should be used only once a fortnight. If more regular help is needed, seek medical advice.

25g (1oz) dried senna pods
250ml (9fl oz) cold water

Place 1 teaspoon of senna pods in a bowl. Pour the water over them and leave to infuse for 24 hours, stirring the mixture several times. Strain the liquid and drink a small cup before bedtime.

PRUNES AND FIGS

Keep a supply of these dried fruits in the house for their effective laxative properties.

4-5 dried prunes
1-2 dried figs
250ml (9fl oz) water

Leave the fruit to soak in the water overnight. Next morning, drink the water and eat the fruit.

Liver disorders

The liver plays a vital role in digestion. It is also crucial to a healthy metabolism. But liver function can be impaired by eating too many fatty foods, drinking alcohol to excess and by smoking.

DAISY AND NETTLE TEA FOR THE LIVER

Daisy-based concoctions were used in the Middle Ages to promote healthy digestion.

25g (1oz) dried daisy flowers and leaves
25g (1oz) dried stinging nettle leaves
250ml (9fl oz) water

Mix the herbs together and place 2 teaspoonfuls in a heatproof bowl. Boil the water and pour it over the herbs. Leave to infuse for 10 minutes. Strain the liquid and drink 2-3 cups a day.

Added roughage
The fruit of the fig tree can be eaten fresh or dried. Either way, figs are tasty, aromatic and act as a mild laxative.

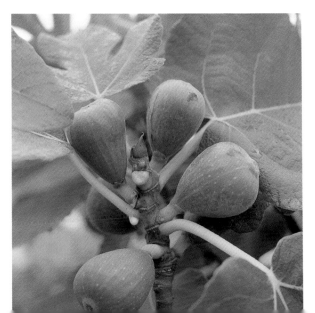

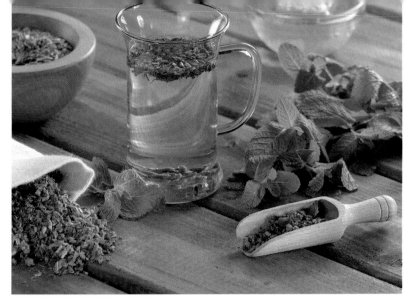

Lion's teeth The jagged tooth-like leaves, the root and the flower of the dandelion can all be used safely in large quantities for medicinal brews to aid digestion.

SORREL TEA

This remedy stimulates liver and gall-bladder activity.

15g (½oz) dried sorrel leaves
15g (½oz) dried bogbean
  leaves
250ml (9fl oz) water

Mix the herbs together and place 2 teaspoonfuls in a heatproof bowl. Boil the water and pour it over the herbs. Leave to infuse for 10 minutes. Strain the liquid and drink 1-2 cups a day.

HOLY THISTLE, HOREHOUND AND DANDELION TEA

The active ingredients contained in this mixture protect the liver and improve bile flow.

25g (1oz) holy thistle seeds
15g (½oz) dried black
  horehound leaves
15g (½oz) dried dandelion
  root and leaves
15g (½oz) dried peppermint
  leaves
250ml (9fl oz) water
honey to sweeten

Mix the seeds and herbs together and place 2 teaspoonfuls in a heatproof bowl. Boil the water and pour it over the herb mixture. Leave to infuse for 10 minutes, then strain the liquid through a fine sieve. Sweeten the tea with honey and drink 2-3 cups a day.

Take care

If you wish to serve your herbal teas from a teapot, keep one specially for this purpose. Avoid using your everyday pot, as it might be stained with tannin, an astringent substance in tea that could affect the purity of your herbal drink.

Wine with herbs

Wine has been used throughout the centuries to promote health. Try this delicious wine infused with herbs.

Paul the Apostle wrote in a letter to St Timothy: 'Do not drink water alone, but drink wine as well, for the sake of your stomach and because you are often ill.'

Consumed in small quantities, red wine has a positive effect on the heart and cardiovascular system. Therefore, it is sometimes recommended for people with circulatory disorders.

A little wine with a meal is also known to aid digestion, and the benefits of drinking wine can be further enhanced by introducing herbs and plants that contain medicinal properties into the alcohol.

Herbal wines can be invigorating as well as being good *apéritifs* or *digestifs*. For this herb wine recipe, either red or white wine can be used.

How to make herb wine
Makes one bottle

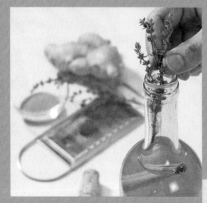

▲ Take a **bottle of wine** and pour away a glassful to make room for the herbs.
Add **1 sprig of thyme**, **½ teaspoon grated nutmeg**, **¼ teaspoon grated ginger**, **1 stick of cinnamon** and **8 large sultanas**.

▼ Seal the bottle with a cork or cap and leave to infuse for two weeks. Sieve the wine into a jug to remove the pieces of thyme and ginger.

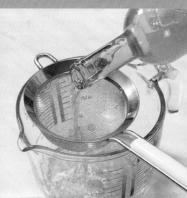

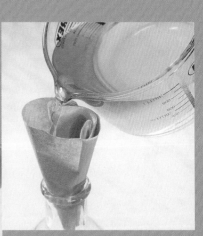

▲ Filter the wine back into the bottle and seal it again. Drink half a glass of herb wine a day. The wine can also be diluted with water for a longer drink.

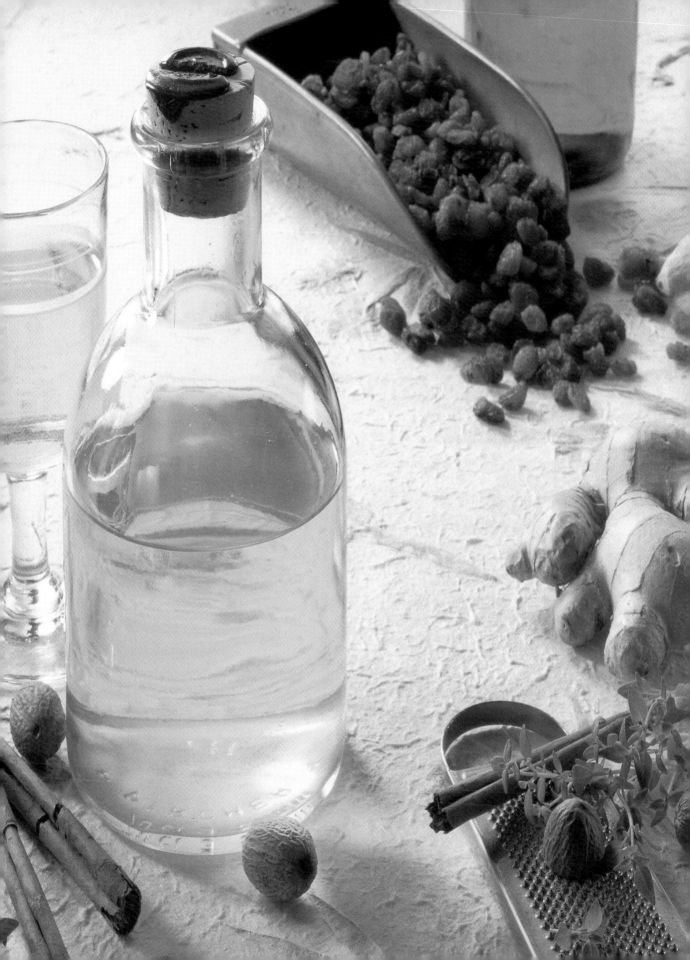

Remedies for men

Certain ailments are specific to either men or to women. There are special tailor-made natural remedies to help in each case, many of them used for centuries.

Throughout life men and women face different ailments and problems, related directly to the fact of their sexuality.

Ailments specific to men or women can affect people in their youth as well as in old age, but hormones – or the lack of them – are generally the underlying cause. Hormones control the development of the body, from when life starts as a foetus in the womb right through to old age.

The menopause, for example, sets in when the body stops or reduces its production of certain hormones.

Being responsive to the needs of our bodies and dealing with these changes in a positive way means we can adjust to each new phase in our lives. But when minor ailments occur both men and women can turn to age-old natural remedies to bring relief.

Female complaints

For most women, menstruation is a fact of life that causes few problems. For some, however, it can be a time of real suffering, particularly for those who experience exceptionally heavy bleeding and painful cramps in the lower abdomen.

Natural relief

A woman's monthly cycle is extremely variable, so there is no need to be concerned about mild irregularities. Associated complaints, such as abdominal pain, depression and headaches, are usually relatively easy to treat.

Taking a series of increasingly hot footbaths may help with stomach cramps, and a hot-water bottle held on the abdomen is comforting. Herbal teas may help women cope with mood swings.

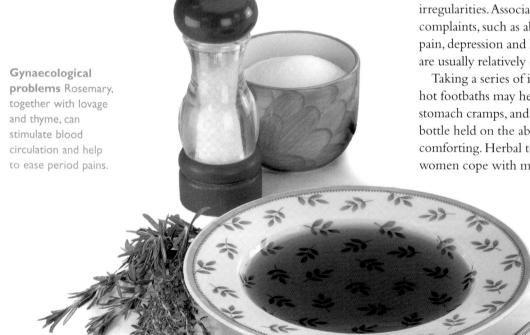

Gynaecological problems Rosemary, together with lovage and thyme, can stimulate blood circulation and help to ease period pains.

and women

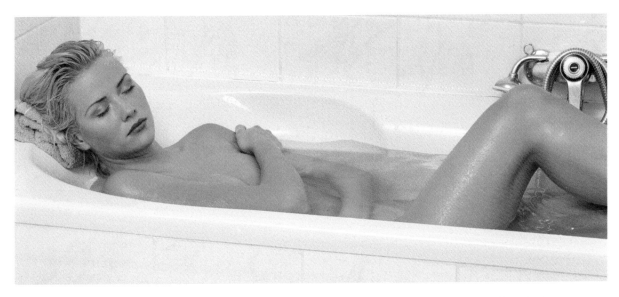

Time to relax A hot bath before bedtime can help to stimulate menstrual bleeding.

Vaginal discharge

The mucous membrane in the vagina produces an acidic secretion that inhibits the growth of germs. Drinking certain herbal teas helps to stimulate this secretion.

If the secretion is excessive or changes in any way, it is always best to consult a doctor. It is not advisable to use any natural or self-help treatments while pregnant.

The menopause

The natural changes that take place in a woman's body during the menopause can produce a range of unpleasant symptoms such as hot flushes and night sweats. Taking herbal remedies can help to relieve much of the discomfort. But the most important thing is to approach these hormonal changes with a positive mental attitude.

WARM HERBAL SOUP

This herbal broth can help to bring on a late period and to give relief from premenstrual bloating.

1 litre (1¾ pints) water
1 sprig rosemary
2 sprigs thyme
15g (½oz) dried lovage leaves
25g (1oz) dried parsley leaves
15g (½oz) dried ribwort leaves
2 teaspoons salt
2 teaspoons honey
½ teaspoon lemon juice

Place the cold water in a pan and sprinkle the herbs into it. Add the salt, honey and lemon juice and simmer for an hour. Strain the liquid through a fine sieve. Consume the soup several times a day for three days.

Lovage

The seed, leaf and root of lovage can all be used in herbal treatments. It should not be used during pregnancy or by those with kidney problems.

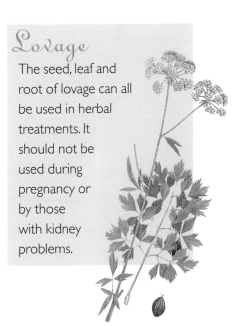

47

VALERIAN AND CAMOMILE FLOWER TEA

Valerian root is a proven help with menstrual pain. Use this tea only at the start of a period.

25g (1oz) dried valerian root
25g (1oz) dried camomile flowers
25g (1oz) dried peppermint leaves
250ml (9fl oz) water

Mix the herbs together and place 2 teaspoonfuls in a heatproof bowl. Boil the water and pour it over the herbs. Leave to infuse for 5 minutes. Strain the liquid and sweeten it with honey. Drink 1-2 cups, taking sips each time.

HYSSOP AND THYME TEA

Hyssop is a medicinal herb that helps to relieve menstrual cramps.

25g (1oz) dried hyssop flower tops
25g (1oz) dried thyme leaves
25g (1oz) dried white horehound leaves
25g (1oz) dried St John's wort flowers
250ml (9fl oz) water

Place 2 teaspoons of the mixed herbs in a heatproof bowl. Pour boiling water over the mixture and leave to infuse for 5 minutes. Strain the liquid through a fine sieve and drink a cup of the tea twice a day.

Take care

Valerian can be used as a quick and potent antiseptic. However, do not take it internally for more than ten days as it can damage the body's nervous system.

RUE TEA

This tea can help to ease painful periods and stem excessive bleeding.

25g (1oz) dried rue leaves
25g (1oz) dried yarrow tops
250ml (9fl oz) water

Mix the herbs together and place 1-2 teaspoonfuls in a saucepan. Pour on the water and simmer for 5 minutes. Strain the liquid through a fine sieve. Drink a cup three times a day.

CRAMP-RELIEVING TEA

Drink this tea to help to ease cramps in the lower abdomen.

25g (1oz) dried yarrow tops
15g (½oz) dried lemon balm leaves
15g (½oz) dried camomile flowers
15g (½oz) fennel seeds
15g (½oz) apple skin
500ml (18fl oz) water

Make this tea in the same way as for the Hyssop and Thyme Tea (see above). Drink a cup of the cramp-relieving tea three times a day.

Traditional practice

In times past, what did a pregnant woman do when her baby's due date had passed and the baby refused to be born? Nowadays, medicines are used to induce labour, but before these drugs were invented, natural methods were employed.

Our rural ancestors considered egg water to be a simple but effective method of inducing labour. In many cultures, the egg is regarded as a symbol of fertility, and it was logical to presume that it would make childbirth easier.

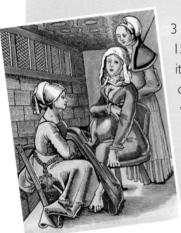

Egg water was prepared by boiling 3 eggs in 1 litre (1¾ pints) of water for 15 minutes. Once the water had cooled, it was given to the pregnant woman to drink, the assumption being that the water contained the ingredient that caused eggs to hatch. This substance, it was thought, was transmitted to the child in the womb, telling it that the time to be born had arrived.

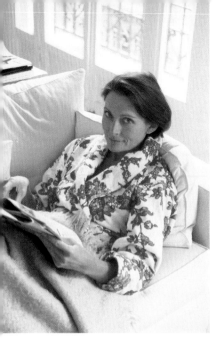

Take it easy If you suffer from pain during menstruation, physical exertion may make it worse. If so, put your feet up and take plenty of rest.

TANSY DRINK

This pleasant, sweetened milk drink helps to alleviate the discomfort of menstrual cramps.

100g (3½oz) dried tansy leaves
55g (2oz) dried marigold
  leaves
55g (2oz) dried lady's mantle
  leaves
250ml (9fl oz) milk
1 teaspoon butter
2 teaspoons honey
pinch of cinnamon

Mix the herbs together and place 1 tablespoonful in a saucepan with the milk. Warm the mixture and leave to infuse for 5 minutes. Strain the milk through a fine sieve, then add the butter, honey and cinnamon. Drink the herbal milk three times a day.

DOGWOOD BARK AND WOODRUFF TEA

Both dogwood bark and woodruff are considered to provide effective relief from migraines, melancholy and the effects of the menopause.

25g (1oz) dried dogwood
  bark
25g (1oz) dried yarrow tops
25g (1oz) dried woodruff
  leaves
25g (1oz) dried senna pods
25g (1oz) dried couchgrass
  root
250ml (9fl oz) water

Mix the herbs together and place 2 teaspoonfuls in a heatproof bowl. Boil the water and pour it over the herbs. Leave to infuse for 10 minutes. Strain the liquid through a fine sieve. Drink a cup after getting up in the morning and another cup before bedtime.

ROSEMARY TEA

Rosemary is a herb that alleviates a range of complaints associated with the menopause.

1 teaspoon dried rosemary
  leaves
250ml (9fl oz) water

Place the rosemary in a heatproof bowl. Boil the water and pour it over the herb. Leave to infuse for 10 minutes. Strain the liquid. Drink 3 cups twice a day.

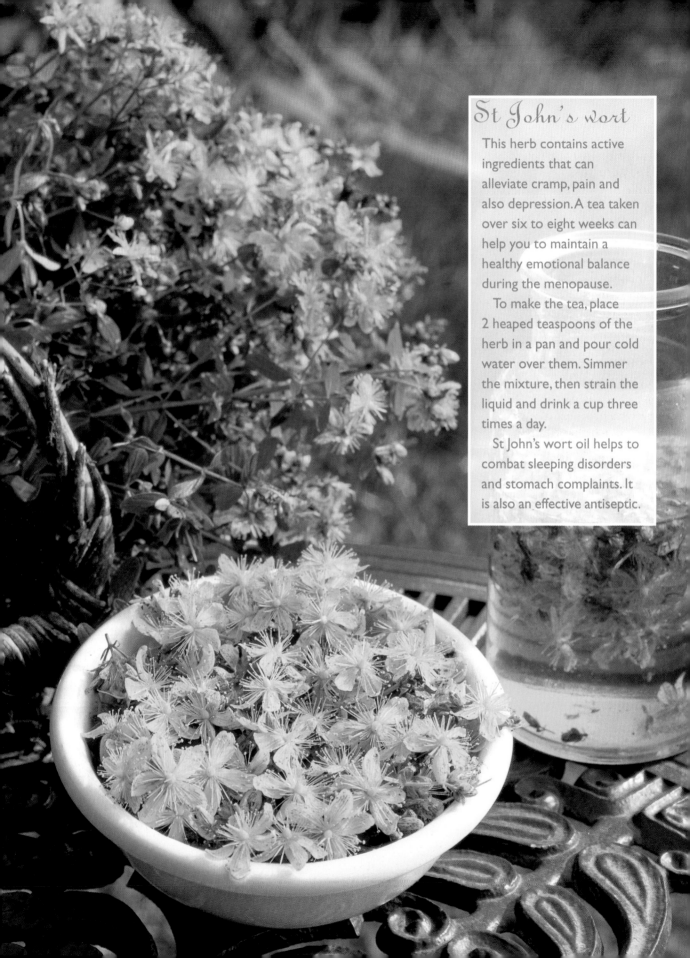

St John's wort

This herb contains active ingredients that can alleviate cramp, pain and also depression. A tea taken over six to eight weeks can help you to maintain a healthy emotional balance during the menopause.

To make the tea, place 2 heaped teaspoons of the herb in a pan and pour cold water over them. Simmer the mixture, then strain the liquid and drink a cup three times a day.

St John's wort oil helps to combat sleeping disorders and stomach complaints. It is also an effective antiseptic.

Ailments that affect a man's well-being

Young men seldom have to deal with impotence, but when it occurs, it is usually an indication of a mental or emotional problem.

From the age of 40, however, a whole range of physical conditions can lead to male impotence, including diabetes and high blood pressure, especially if coupled with an unhealthy lifestyle.

For centuries a range of foods and substances, from asparagus and celery to rhinoceros horn and oysters, have been said to have a positive effect on sexual stamina and performance. Most usually, however, attention to overall health and treatment of any specific problem will do more to help men out of this predicament.

Other common causes for concern in older men are prostate and urinary problems. Many herbal remedies provide help with these complaints, but always consult a doctor if the discomfort is persistent, prolonged or severe.

GOLDEN ROD TEA

The active ingredients in this herb can help to combat inflammation of the urinary tract.

2 teaspoons dried golden
  rod leaves
250ml (9fl oz) water

Place the golden rod in a heatproof bowl. Boil the water and pour it over the herb. Leave to infuse for 10 minutes. Strain the liquid through a fine sieve. Drink 2 cups of the tea a day.

ROSEBAY TEA

As rosebay is a diuretic, this tea makes it easier for men with prostate complaints to urinate.

25g (1oz) dried rosebay
  leaves
25g (1oz) dried stinging
  nettles
15g (½oz) dried birch leaves
15g (½oz) dried horsetail
  'needles' and stems
250ml (9fl oz) water

Mix the herbs together and place 2 teaspoonfuls in a heatproof bowl. Boil the water and pour it over the herbs. Leave to infuse for 10 minutes. Strain the liquid through a fine sieve. Drink 2-3 cups a day over a three-week period.

CELERY SOUP FOR MEN

This soup, made with celery, may help men suffering from impotence.

1 celery heart
50ml (2fl oz) double cream
250ml (9fl oz) bouillon or
  chicken stock
garnish of cress, pumpkin
  seeds, alfalfa sprouts,
  lovage leaves and fresh
  tarragon

Braise the celery in the oven at 180°C (350°F, gas mark 4) for 45 minutes or until soft. Mash with the cream. Stir in the bouillon or stock and heat the soup in a bain-marie to just simmering. Garnish and serve immediately.

Tried & Trusted
A good sex life

• Improved blood circulation around the abdomen can often help to combat impotence. Bear's garlic is said to be effective. Pour 500ml (18fl oz) of white wine over a handful of bear's garlic leaves and heat the mixture until it is just about to simmer. Leave to infuse for a week. Strain the liquid through a fine sieve. Store the herbal wine in a cool, dark place. Drink 250ml (9fl oz) every evening.

• Essential oils are believed to help stimulate sexuality. Mix 2 drops each of ginger and black pepper oils with jojoba oil and massage into the lower back, buttocks and insides of the thighs. Take great care to avoid the genital area.

Prostate problems

• Pumpkin seeds are good as a preventive treatment for prostate disorders. Chew and eat ten seeds several times a day. This remedy should be taken over several months.

• A change in diet has often proved helpful for men with prostate problems. Reduce your intake of animal fats, drink as much water as possible (until late in the afternoon) and eat plenty of roughage.

Look after your skin

Healthy skin is a valuable asset to anyone's appearance, whatever their age. Traditional herbal remedies can help you to preserve a clear, youthful complexion.

First impressions of a person make a lasting impact, and among the first things we notice about people are their face and skin.

For thousands of years women, especially, have been using lotions and creams to keep their skin silky-smooth. And today, new and costly products are being developed all the time, offering the promise of a more beautiful and, above all, more youthful skin.

Often, however, proprietary skin treatments contain a variety of chemicals that can irritate sensitive skin or cause allergic reactions.

Less expensive and equally effective alternatives are the recipes that your grandmother might have used.

Natural ingredients are gentle on the skin. You will also find that these remedies give you the best results if you combine them with a nutritionally balanced diet of proteins and vitamins, drink plenty of water and ensure that you take regular physical exercise and get a good night's sleep. Make these activities a part of your daily routine and your skin will be the beneficiary.

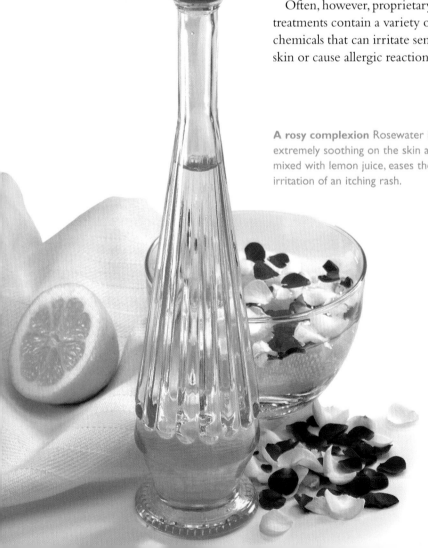

A rosy complexion Rosewater is extremely soothing on the skin and, mixed with lemon juice, eases the irritation of an itching rash.

Skin blemishes

Among the most prevalent skin problems are spots and acne. Teenagers are the ones most often afflicted with the tell-tale oily skin, blackheads and pimples. Hormonal changes are probably to blame for these skin blemishes, but acne can also be caused by medication, cosmetics or even vitamin pills.

Boils are a more painful skin problem. These red, raised lumps appear when bacteria cause hair follicles to become inflamed and pus-filled abscesses develop. Boils need medical attention and sometimes need to be lanced under local anaesthetic.

Remedies for acne

Extreme cases of acne need to be treated both for cosmetic and medical reasons. Whatever the cause, the rule with acne is never to squeeze a pustule with your fingers. Instead, clean it with a gentle tincture.

You can also treat acne with steam inhalation treatments and compresses containing natural substances. Neat lemon juice can be effective, too, as it has antibacterial properties.

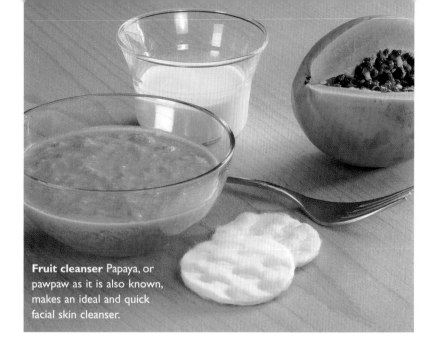

Fruit cleanser Papaya, or pawpaw as it is also known, makes an ideal and quick facial skin cleanser.

ANTI-ACNE TONIC

This treatment can be taken internally as a drink, or used externally as a face wash. Heartsease is a good skin cleanser for people with eczema or stubborn acne, while Iceland lichen relieves irritations and horsetail promotes the healing process.

25g (1oz) dried heartsease leaves
25g (1oz) dried eyebright leaves
15g (½oz) dried Iceland lichen
15g (½oz) dried horsetail 'needles' and stems
500ml (18fl oz) water

Mix the herbs together and place 2 teaspoonfuls in a heatproof bowl. Boil the water and pour it over the herbs. Leave to infuse for 10 minutes. Strain off the liquid and drink a cup three times a day. Alternatively, soak a cotton-wool pad in the tonic and gently dab it onto your skin.

LAVENDER VINEGAR

This traditional treatment is a reliable remedy for acne.

25g (1oz) dried lavender flowers
15g (½oz) dried arnica flowers
750ml (1 pint 7fl oz) cider vinegar

Mix the ingredients in a jug and pour into a bottle. Seal tightly. Leave to infuse for two weeks, shaking the bottle regularly. Filter the solution and add it to water when you wash your face.

LAVENDER OIL

Soothing lavender protects and cares for irritated skin.

5 drops lavender oil
5 drops almond oil

Mix the oils in a bowl. Dip a cotton-wool pad into the oil and apply to your skin. Repeat twice a day.

PAPAYA MASK

Papaya flesh makes an effective treatment for blackheads.

1 ripe papaya
2-3 tablespoons single cream

Remove the skin and seeds from the fruit. Place the flesh in a bowl and mash it with a fork. Mix in the cream. Apply the mask to your skin using your fingers. Leave it on for 30 minutes, then rinse off thoroughly.

TRIGONELLA COMPRESS

Use this compress on painful boils that may need to be lanced.

1 tablespoon trigonella seeds
1 tablespoon boiling water

Grind the seeds using a pestle and mortar. Add the water and mix it to a paste. Spread the paste onto a gauze cloth and, while it is still hot, apply the compress to the boil. Repeat this several times.

Skin rashes and other dermatological problems

Among the most common skin complaints of modern times are minor ailments such as dry, inflamed skin and unsightly rashes, as well as more serious conditions, such as eczema. Allergies are often to blame, but trying to pinpoint the cause of a dermatological complaint can be very difficult and frustrating.

Another extremely unpleasant skin problem is psoriasis, a disorder in which skin cells proliferate too quickly, leaving flaking scaly patches. While no cure has yet been found, the symptoms can be soothed with compresses and medicinal teas.

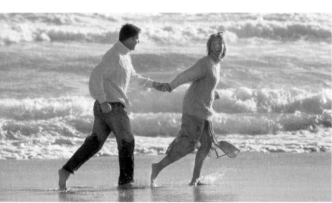

Gentle therapies

Most skin ailments can be treated using natural remedies. External applications, such as baths, creams, ointments and compresses, can help, as can a range of teas. Such treatments alleviate pain and irritation, while also providing good skin care. Even if you are receiving medical treatment, traditional homemade remedies can be an ideal supplement.

COMPRESS FOR SORE SKIN

This compress has good anti-inflammatory properties.

25g (1oz) dried lady's mantle leaves
25g (1oz) dried daisy flowers and leaves
25g (1oz) dried woundwort leaves
250ml (9fl oz) water

Make an infusion as for Blackthorn and Lemon Balm Tea (right). Leave the solution until it is lukewarm. Soak a cotton-wool pad in it and place it on your skin.

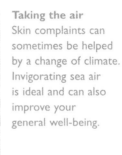

Taking the air
Skin complaints can sometimes be helped by a change of climate. Invigorating sea air is ideal and can also improve your general well-being.

OAK BARK WASH

Oak bark washes are an old anti-inflammatory remedy.

1 litre (1¾ pints) water
3 tablespoons dried oak bark

Boil the water in a pan, then add the oak bark. Boil it for 30 minutes. Strain the liquid, then use when washing your face.

BLACKTHORN AND LEMON BALM TEA

This tea can bring relief from itchy skin rashes.

25g (1oz) dried blackthorn flowers and leaves
15g (½oz) dried lemon balm leaves
25g (1oz) dried yarrow tops
25g (1oz) dried stinging nettle leaves
15g (½oz) dried sage leaves
15g (½oz) dried horsetail 'needles' and stems
250ml (9fl oz) water

Mix the herbs together and place 2 teaspoonfuls in a heatproof bowl. Boil the water and pour it over the herbs. Leave to infuse for 10 minutes. Strain the liquid through a fine sieve and drink 2 cups three times a day.

SOOTHING COMPRESS

Both mallow and camomile contain substances that soothe the skin, especially after exposure to the sun.

25g (1oz) dried mallow flowers
25g (1oz) dried camomile flowers
250ml (9fl oz) water

Mix the herbs in a heatproof bowl. Boil the water and pour it over the herbs. Leave to infuse until cold. Dip a cotton-wool pad into the solution and dab it on your skin.

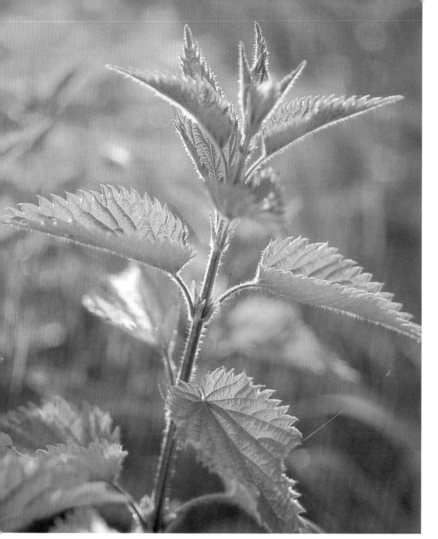

Stinging nettles The astringent young leaves of stinging nettles are rich in vitamins and minerals. They can be used to make steam facials and soothing bath mixtures that invigorate the skin.

Getting rid of warts the natural way

Although warts are not normally painful, they can be extremely unpleasant. They are often caused by viruses and are quite contagious. Young children are particularly susceptible to warts, which usually appear in areas such as the hands, face, knees or scalp. Fortunately, there are natural remedies that will help to get rid of them, so we do not need to rely on witchcraft as our forebears sometimes did.

ANTI-WART REMEDY

Pleurisy contains alkaloids that poison warts.

**55g (2oz) dried pleurisy root
glycerine**

Finely grate the root and press it through a muslin cloth, squeezing the juice into a bowl. Mix the juice with an equal amount of glycerine. Apply it to the warts every day for three weeks.

Tried & Trusted
Corn treatment

• To remove callused skin from your feet, bathe them in warm water and pat them dry. Halve one or more sultanas and place the cut side on each corn. Hold it in place with a plaster. Repeat this treatment until the corn can easily be removed.

Athlete's foot

• Dog's mercury can help to alleviate athlete's foot. Pour 1.2 litres (2 pints) of water over a handful of dog's mercury leaves in a large pan. Boil for 1 minute. Strain the liquid through a sieve and pour into a small bowl. Bathe your feet in this solution for 10 minutes. Repeat regularly.

• A lavender-oil footbath also helps to soothe athlete's foot. Add 2 drops of the oil to a bowl of warm water and bathe your feet in it for 10 minutes.

• Combat sweaty feet and help to prevent athlete's foot with a paste made from baking soda and lukewarm water. Spread it over your feet, leave it on for a few minutes, then rinse it off. Carefully dry your feet.

Treating common foot complaints

Athlete's foot is caused by a fungus and, like warts, it is contagious and easily transmitted in places where people walk barefoot, such as swimming pools.

The first signs of athlete's foot are itchy feet and cracked or peeling skin between the toes. If these symptoms are not treated, the disease will spread to your toenails, which will become brittle and crack. The people most prone to athlete's foot are those whose feet perspire a lot.

Corns are areas of thickened skin caused by ill-fitting shoes and can cause great discomfort.

Both complaints need to be treated at the first sign of the problem. Recurrences are common and the treatment often long-term.

COMFREY AND ROSEMARY FOOT BALSAM

For generations, people have used this remedy to treat athlete's foot.

25g (1oz) dried comfrey root
15g (½oz) dried rosemary leaves
750ml (1 pint 7fl oz) olive oil
40g (1½oz) beeswax

Mix the herbs and oil in a bowl. Heat the mixture in a bain-marie for 30 minutes, then allow to cool. Filter the oil and leave to stand overnight. Melt the wax in a bowl placed in a saucepan of simmering water. Gradually add the oil until you achieve the consistency of double cream. Massage your feet gently with the ointment.

ONION AND LEMON CORN MIXTURE

This is a simple, tried-and-proven remedy for the treatment of stubborn corns.

dash of lemon juice
1 onion slice
pinch of salt

Drip the lemon juice onto the onion slice and sprinkle it with salt. Place the onion on the corn and hold in place with a plaster. Leave it on overnight. Repeat this procedure about eight times, after which the corn and its root should be easy to remove.

A perfect pair of feet Keep foot problems at bay with remedies, such as herbal ointments and footbaths.

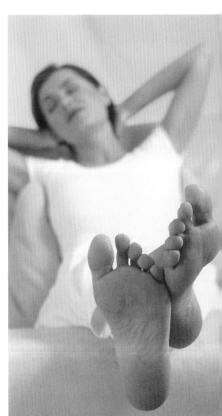

Irritating summertime ailments

While we eagerly await the arrival of warm weather each year, summer is the time when insect bites and sunburn can be a problem. In our grandparents' day, a pale skin was considered attractive. Today, the increasing evidence linking over-exposure to the sun with serious skin conditions makes it all the more important to adopt a sensible approach, by covering up and using high protection sun creams.

ONION OR LEMON COMPRESS

Onions and lemons have a cooling and disinfecting effect and reduce the swelling caused by insect bites.

1 slice of lemon
or
1 onion slice

Place the slice of lemon or onion on the insect bite or sting and hold it in place with a plaster.

QUARK AND BUTTERMILK SUNBURN WRAP

This wrap will cool the skin and alleviate the pain of sunburn.

55g (2oz) quark
or
55g (2oz) yoghurt
1 tablespoon buttermilk

Mix the two ingredients in a bowl. Spread them on a small cotton cloth and place it on sunburnt skin until the mixture is no longer cool. Repeat two to three times a day.

ST JOHN'S WORT OIL

Use this soothing oil to ease sunburn and keep the skin cool.

250ml (9fl oz) olive oil
125ml (4fl oz) white wine
150g (5½oz) fresh St John's wort flowers

Mix the oil and wine in a bowl, add the St John's wort and leave the mixture to infuse for four days, stirring it occasionally.

Simmer the mixture for 3 hours in a bain-marie and press it through a sieve. Pour the oil into a small, dark-coloured bottle, seal tightly and store in a cool, dark place. Dab the oil onto sunburnt skin when needed.

MARIGOLD BUTTER

Small cuts and open wounds will heal quickly with this remedy.

70g (2½oz) fresh marigold flowers
100g (3½oz) butter

Crush the flowers in a bowl. Melt the butter and pour it over them. Place the bowl over a pan of simmering water and heat the mixture to 70°C (158°F). Leave to infuse for 20 minutes, stirring several times. Filter the butter and allow it to cool. Apply the ointment to the wound.

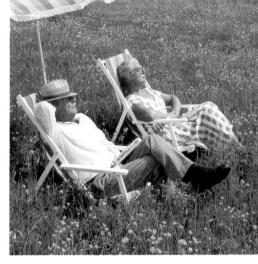

Sunbathing safely To avoid sunburn, apply a high-factor sun lotion and wear protective clothing. Spend the hottest part of the day in the shade.

YARROW WRAP

The essential oil found in yarrow helps to disinfect and heal wounds.

25g (1oz) dried yarrow tops
250ml (9fl oz) red wine

Boil the yarrow with a little water until soft. Wash the wound with the wine and cover it with a sterile cloth. Spread the yarrow over the cloth and hold it in place with a bandage. Repeat this three to five times a day.

PLANTAIN-LEAF COMPRESS

Plantain leaves can help to soothe insect bites and significantly reduce swelling. Apply this treatment to the sting or bite immediately.

fresh plantain leaves

Crush the plantain leaves and immediately spread them on the sore spot. Hold them in place with a plaster and keep the area cool. You can use dock leaves as an alternative to plantain.

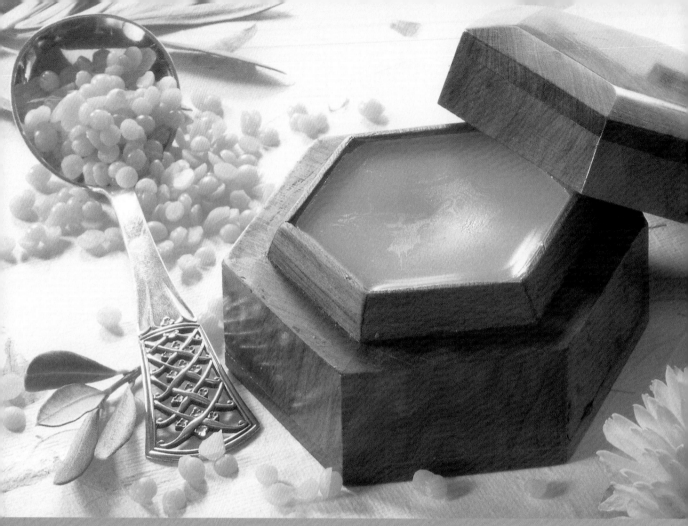

Calendula ointment

Use marigold flowers to make a healing salve
to treat skin disorders and to provide soothing
care for cuts and grazes.

Marigold, or *Calendula officinalis*,
its scientific name, has been cultivated in
European gardens since the 12th century,
although it originally came from Egypt.

This medicinal herb is suitable for both
internal treatments and external applications.
Nowadays, it is mostly used for treating cuts
and sprains, or menstrual pain.

Marigolds are easy to grow yourself among
summer flowers in your garden borders, or
in pots on the patio. When you harvest the
flowers, use only the open yellow ones as
they will be ripe and contain the most
medicinal properties. Before making the
ointment you will need to dry the flowers
by hanging them in a warm, airy place.

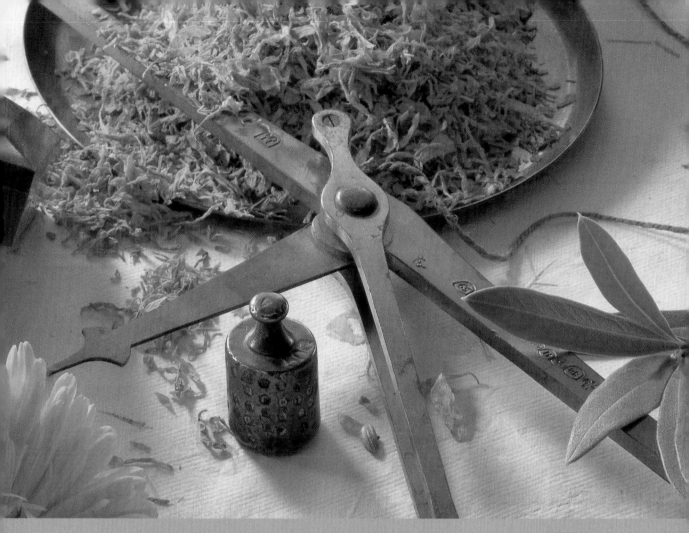

How to make calendula ointment
Makes one 650ml (1 pint 2fl oz) jar

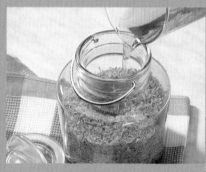

▼ Strain the oil into a pan and heat it until it is almost boiling. Add **40g (1½oz) cocoa butter** and **40g (1½oz) beeswax granules**.

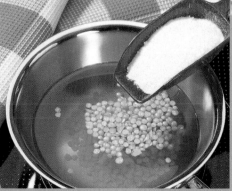

▲ Pour **500ml (18fl oz) peanut** or **olive oil** over **55g (2oz) dried marigold flowers** in a jar. Seal the jar tightly with the lid and leave the mixture to infuse in a warm place for three weeks.

▲ When all the ingredients have melted, remove the pan from the heat and stir the contents thoroughly. Leave the mixture to cool. When it starts to set, transfer it to a dark-coloured, sealable jar or decorative pot and secure the lid tightly.

A new lease of life

Whether you've had a hectic day, or feel that life is getting on top of you, there are many old-fashioned restorative and comforting herbal remedies that can perk you up.

Most of us are able to cope mentally and emotionally with occasional difficult situations. But as daily life becomes ever more hectic, stress, tiredness, anxiety and exhaustion are on the increase. If these problems are not resolved, they can have a detrimental effect on your general physical health as well as your mental fitness.

There are many pharmaceutical remedies available that can help us to cope with this type of problem, but the drawback is that such medication often produces unpleasant side effects if taken over long periods. For this reason, many people are turning to the healing remedies of past generations to combat depression and stress.

Homemade treatments can help to restore mental equilibrium, combat anxiety, promote sleep, restore optimism and give you new vitality. Take advantage of these simple alternatives to prescription pills and try the remedies, but be sure to see a doctor if the problem persists.

RELAXATION TEA

This mixture of herbs has a relaxing effect and can help to calm anxiety.

- 15g (½oz) dried lemon balm leaves
- 15g (½oz) dried peppermint leaves
- 15g (½oz) dried valerian root
- 25g (1oz) dried orange blossom
- 15g (½oz) crushed aniseed
- 25g (1oz) dried passionflower leaves
- 250ml (9fl oz) water

Mix the herbs together and place 2 teaspoonfuls in a heatproof bowl. Boil the water and pour it over the herbs. Leave to infuse for 15 minutes. Strain the liquid. Drink 3 cups a day, one late in the evening, for a minimum of a month.

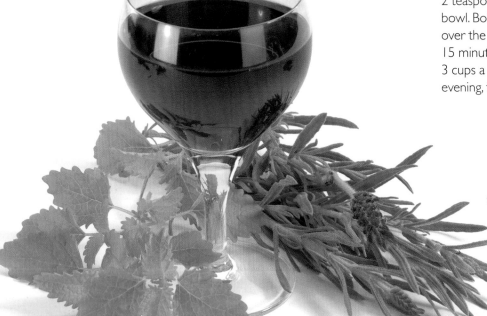

Sweet dreams A glass of red wine, containing hops, lavender and other herbs, can help you to sleep well.

HAWTHORN AND PLUM TEA

Hawthorn has restorative and relaxing properties. At the same time, it also has a positive effect on all cardiac functions. While it can take some time for the benefits of this remedy to work, it is worth waiting for its soothing results.

55g (2oz) dried hawthorn
   flowers
1 plum
1 litre (1¾ pints) water

Place the hawthorn flowers and plum in a large heatproof bowl. Boil the water and pour it over them. Leave to infuse for 15 minutes. Strain the liquid through a fine sieve. Drink 3 cups a day, one late in the evening, for a month.

GOODNIGHT TEA

This bedtime drink will help people who have trouble falling asleep.

25g (1oz) dried hop flowers
25g (1oz) dried elderflowers
25g (1oz) dried primrose
   flowers
55g (2oz) dried oat straw
   flower tops
250ml (9fl oz) water

Mix the herbs together and place 3 tablespoonfuls in a heatproof bowl. Boil the water and pour it over the herbs. Leave to infuse for 10 minutes. Strain the liquid through a fine sieve and drink the tea just before bedtime.

SLEEP-INDUCING WINE

This traditional sleeping draught is gentle and easily digestible.

25g (1oz) dried St John's
   wort flowers
25g (1oz) dried lemon
   balm leaves
15g (½oz) dried lavender
   flowers
15g (½oz) dried hop flowers
1 litre (1¾ pints) red wine

Mix the herbs in a bowl and pour the wine over them. Cover and leave to infuse for one week. Strain the liquid and pour it into a sterilised bottle. Take 1-3 tablespoonfuls at bedtime.

SLEEPING CUSHION

The fragrant aromas of these herbs will be inhaled during sleep, helping to ensure a restful night.

55g (2oz) dried hop flowers
55g (2oz) dried St John's
   wort flowers
25g (1oz) dried lavender
   flowers
25g (1oz) dried valerian root

Put the herbs in a small linen bag and place it under your pillow.

Tried & Trusted
Calming anxiety

• A lime blossom bath can help to relieve the symptoms of everyday stress. Pour 3 litres (5¼ pints) of boiling water over 200g (7oz) of lime blossoms. Leave to infuse for 20 minutes, strain the liquid, then add it to your bath water.

• Carrot juice can give you a boost if your nerves are frayed. Drink two glasses of juice a day.

• Sugared milk can be effective against bouts of anxiety. Milk contains substances that soothe and relax the brain. The sugar helps to accelerate their effects.

• Lavender, rosemary and mint make a soothing bath lotion. Boil 150g (5½oz) of each herb in 3 litres (5¼ pints) of water. Leave to infuse for 20 minutes, then strain the liquid. Add it to your bath water.

• Valerian is a balm used to combat stress. Add valerian root to any tea or to your bath water to soothe your nerves.

• If you're having trouble getting off to sleep, a mustard footbath before going to bed can help you to nod off (see Headache self-help, page 11).

Healthy children,

All children get their share of childhood diseases and ailments as they grow up. You can help them through these uncomfortable times with soothing herbal remedies.

When we have children, we take on the responsibility for their health and well-being. During the course of their childhood they will suffer ailments ranging from teething discomfort and bed-wetting to serious diseases such as chickenpox.

During their early years, before their immune systems have developed sufficient antibodies, children are also prone to minor infections such as coughs, colds and stomach upsets.

Many parents question the safety of pills, syrups and ointments prescribed by doctors. It is not surprising, therefore, that old herbal remedies are being rediscovered, since they contain no artificial or genetically modified substances. These recipes draw on the healing powers of natural ingredients, which also help to strengthen a child's immunity to disease.

However, a child with a fever, in pain or with persistent symptoms should always be seen by a doctor.

HERBAL SQUASH

This aromatic drink tastes delicious and will encourage your child's appetite. The mixture will keep longer if stored in an airtight bottle. Be sure to sterilise the bottle, including the seal, before use.

- 1 teaspoon each ground ginger, cardamom and coriander
- 15g (½oz) caraway seeds
- 15g (½oz) star anise
- 15g (½oz) dried dandelion flowers
- 15g (½oz) dried lemon balm leaves
- 100g (3½oz) honey
- 1 litre (1¾ pints) apple juice

Place all the ingredients in a saucepan and bring to the boil. Remove the pan from the heat and allow the mixture to cool. Repeat this process twice more. Strain the liquid through a fine sieve. Pour the squash into a sterilised bottle and seal it. Give your child 100ml (3½fl oz) a day.

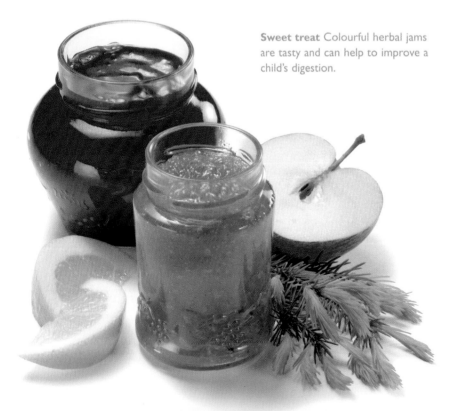

Sweet treat Colourful herbal jams are tasty and can help to improve a child's digestion.

happy parents

ROSEHIP AND SLOE JAM

This jam will stimulate your child's appetite and digestion.

150g (5½oz) fresh rosehips
300g (10½oz) fresh sloes
250ml (9fl oz) sea buckthorn juice
1kg (2lb 4oz) jam sugar

Cut the rosehips in half, wash the fruit thoroughly and leave it to soak in the sea buckthorn juice for 8 hours. Heat the mixture in a bain-marie, then press it through a sieve into a pan.

Add the sugar to the liquid and boil it until a setting consistency is reached. Pour the jam into sterilised jars. Give your child a spoonful before breakfast, or spread it on bread or toast.

Rosehips

Hips from the dog rose appear in hedgerows between August and October. Freshly harvested rosehips contain a high level of fruit acid that can stimulate the appetite.

Star quality
Star anise is a tropical spice from southern China and south-east Asia. It contains a large amount of essential oil that tastes sweet and helps to strengthen the gastric system.

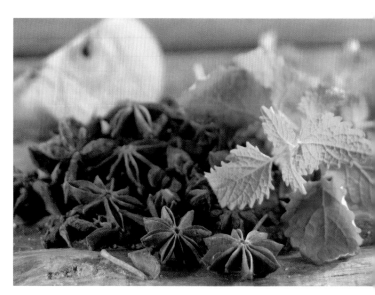

SLUMBER TEA

When children have trouble dropping off to sleep, this tried-and-proven remedy can help.

25g (1oz) dried valerian root
15g (½oz) dried lemon balm leaves
15g (½oz) dried camomile leaves
15g (½oz) dried orange blossom
15g (½oz) dried rosehips
250ml (9fl oz) water
honey to sweeten

Mix the herbs together and place 2 teaspoonfuls in a bowl. Boil the water and pour it over the herbs. Leave to infuse for 10 minutes, then strain the liquid. Sweeten the tea with honey and give it to your child 30 minutes before bedtime.

STINGING NETTLE TEA

Stinging nettles can help to combat a weak bladder and bed-wetting.

25g (1oz) dried stinging nettle leaves
250ml (9fl oz) water

Place the nettles in a heatproof bowl. Boil the water and pour it over the nettles. Leave to infuse for 10 minutes, then strain the liquid through a fine sieve. Give your child small sips of nettle tea throughout the day, but not in the evening.

Tried & Trusted

A good night's sleep

• Help your children to fall asleep quickly by keeping to a strict bedtime routine. A story in bed will calm them down and encourage them to settle quietly. Alternatively, a bedside chat will help to release the tensions of the day's excitement.

Stop bed-wetting

• Children generally wet their beds because they are sleeping too soundly to get up and go to the toilet. Another reason could be that they are afraid of the dark. If so, place a night light in the child's bedroom or just outside the room.

• To help to stop bed-wetting, tie a hand towel around a child's waist, binding it with a thick knot at the back. Most children wet their bed lying on their backs and the knot should wake them up as soon as they roll over.

Improving appetite

• If children have a poor appetite, check that they are not consuming sweets or sweet drinks before mealtimes. Some soft drinks contain levels of sugar equal to 40 cubes per 1.5 litres (2¾ pints) of liquid.

Boosting immunity

• There are various herbs, such as eyebright, watercress and plantain, that can help to strengthen a child's immune system. This is especially important during times of change, for example, when a child starts school. Consult a medical herbalist for the correct proportions of herbs in each mixture.

Help for colds

In winter, children barely recover from one cold before the next one is on its way. Once children go to school, where colds spread like wildfire, they are even more prone to catching such infections.

Effective help is at hand in the form of herbal recipes. These can help to prevent a cold or may be used to treat one when it arrives.

Reducing fevers

If your child has a cold accompanied by fever, do not immediately try to reduce it, as the fever helps to fight the germs in your child's body. Consult a doctor if your child's temperature exceeds 39°C (102°F) or is persistent.

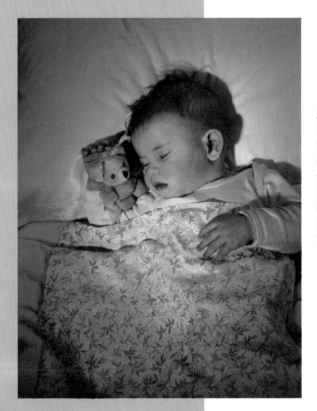

A peaceful night
Babies are less likely to wake at night if they are warm and cosy. For a very young baby, keep the bedroom at a temperature of 16-20°C (61-68°F).

CAMOMILE AND ROSEHIP TEA

This tea is a good preventive remedy, as well as a treatment when your child is starting a cold.

15g (½oz) dried camomile
   flowers
15g (½oz) dried rosehips
250ml (9fl oz) water
honey to sweeten

Mix the herbs in a heatproof bowl. Boil the water and pour it over the herbs. Leave to infuse for 15 minutes. Strain the liquid through a fine sieve and sweeten it with honey. Give the tea to your child up to three times a day.

PRIMROSE AND HEARTSEASE FEVER TEA

This traditional herbal drink should give a feverish child some relief.

25g (1oz) dried primrose
   flowers
25g (1oz) dried heartsease
   flowers
25g (1oz) dried white willow
   leaves
25g (1oz) dried watercress
25g (1oz) dried coneflower
   root
1 litre (1¾ pints) water

Mix the herbs together and place 3 tablespoonfuls in a heatproof bowl. Boil the water and pour it over the herbs. Leave to infuse for 10 minutes. Strain the liquid through a fine sieve. Give a beaker of tea to your child every hour.

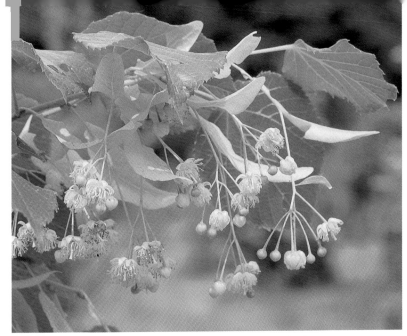

Natural healer An infusion of lime blossom is a relaxing drink that helps to activate the body's immune system.

RADISH AND HONEY JUICE

Soothing for coughs, this remedy is quick and easy to make.

1 black radish
3 teaspoons honey

Hollow out the radish and make a small hole in the bottom. Place it on top of a heatproof glass or a mug, spoon the honey inside and place the glass on a heated surface. Give your child the juice that collects in the glass, up to four times a day.

Take care

When making an infusion with rosehips, make sure that you sieve the tea before giving it to a child. Rosehips contain tiny seeds covered in spiky hairs which could severely irritate a child's digestive tract.

LIME AND CAMOMILE TEA

This tea can help if your child has a cold accompanied by a sore throat. Its active ingredients will soothe inflammation and loosen phlegm.

25g (1oz) dried lime blossom
25g (1oz) dried camomile
   flowers
250ml (9fl oz) water
honey to sweeten

Mix the herbs together and place 1 teaspoonful in a heatproof bowl. Boil the water and pour it over the herbs. Leave the mixture to infuse for 5 minutes. Strain the liquid through a fine sieve and sweeten it with honey.

Give your child a cup of lukewarm tea each day as needed. If they have a sore throat it will be easier to drink the tea in small sips.

CATMINT SYRUP

Try this age-old recipe to help to relax stomach cramps.

25g (1oz) dried catmint
  shoot tips
granulated sugar
250ml (9fl oz) water

Place the catmint in a heatproof bowl. Boil the water and pour it over the herb. Leave to infuse for 5 minutes. Strain the liquid, then add sufficient sugar to achieve a syrupy consistency. Give your child 3 teaspoonfuls a day.

BORAGE AND HONEY TEA

This tea can help children to recover their strength when recuperating from an illness.

25g (1oz) dried borage flowers
3 teaspoons honey
1 litre (1¾ pints) water

Place the flowers in a heatproof bowl. Boil the water and pour it over them. Leave to infuse for 30 minutes. Strain the liquid and sweeten it with honey. Give your child a cup every 2 hours.

Aromatic herb
When dried, catmint leaves develop a sharp balsam-like taste. As a herbal infusion it will ease headaches, upset stomachs and muscle cramps.

ELDERFLOWER TEA

Use this tea to restore energy after a bout of coughing.

25g (1oz) dried elderflowers
25g (1oz) dried sweet
  violet flowers
25g (1oz) dried ribwort leaves
25g (1oz) dried sundew leaves
250ml (9fl oz) water

Mix the herbs in a heatproof bowl. Boil the water and pour it over the herbs. Leave to infuse for 1 minute. Strain the liquid. Give your child a cup three times a day.

Measles and chickenpox

Although measles is a highly contagious viral disease, thanks to immunisation it is now quite rare. If the illness takes its normal course, traditional remedies can help to alleviate a child's discomfort. If, however, complications, such as earache, arise consult your doctor at once.

Chickenpox is a common childhood disease whose symptoms can also be eased with natural remedies.

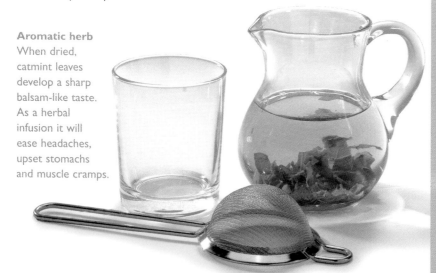

Tried & Trusted
Soothing rashes

• **Help to stop a measles rash from spreading by washing your child's body with lukewarm salt water once a day. Make this by dissolving 1 teaspoon of salt in 250ml (9fl oz) of water. After washing, dry the skin gently but thoroughly with a towel.**

• **Chickenpox rashes are extremely itchy. To stop children scratching, use a sponge to dab a solution of elderflowers on the affected areas.**

• **Children suffering from chickenpox need to drink plenty of fluids, ideally fruit juices that contain high levels of vitamin C. A particularly good concoction is a mixture of watercress juice and carrot juice.**

Help for teething

• **Cool inflamed gums by applying a moist cloth. A chilled teething ring is another good way to fight inflammation of the gums. Cool the ring by placing it in the refrigerator for an hour before use.**

• **Give a teething baby something to chew on, for example, a piece of crust. This exercise should make it easier for the teeth to break through the gums.**

Teething pain

Teething often causes infants a lot of suffering and also upsets parents when their babies cry uncontrollably. Not only do babies suffer from swollen and aching gums, but they may also get diarrhoea and become generally cranky and miserable – especially at night.

Generations before us have already developed ways of lessening the pain of the age-old problem, enabling both parents and children to get a good night's rest.

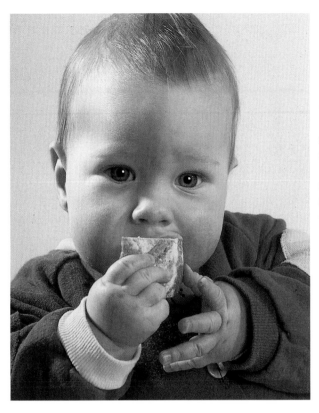

Biting hard
Bread crusts are an ideal teething aid for infants. But never leave a small child alone with the crust as he may easily choke.

SAFFRON AND HONEY MASSAGE BALSAM

Alleviate teething pains with this sweet-tasting balsam.

1 teaspoon honey
pinch of saffron

Mix the honey and saffron, dip your finger into the mixture and gently massage it over your baby's gums. Repeat this process three times a day.

Take care

Diarrhoea in infants can be extremely serious if it doesn't clear up within 24 hours as babies can quickly become dehydrated. If you are at all worried about your baby's diarrhoea, seek medical help immediately.

BILBERRY TEA

Many infants are prone to diarrhoea when they teethe. Bilberries can help to bring the diarrhoea under control.

1 tablespoon dried
bilberries
250ml (9fl oz) water

Place the bilberries in a pan. Pour the water over the berries and boil for 10 minutes. Strain the liquid through a fine sieve. Either add 2 teaspoonfuls to your baby's bottle three to five times a day, or dispense it on a plastic spoon. Store any leftover tea in the refrigerator and prepare a fresh infusion every other day.

ANISEED AND FENNEL TEA

Aniseed and fennel are invaluable herbs when children have uncomfortable wind or diarrhoea.

25g (1oz) aniseed
25g (1oz) fennel seeds
250ml (9fl oz) water

Crush the aniseed and fennel seeds using a pestle and mortar. Boil the water and pour it over the seeds. Leave to infuse for 10 minutes, then strain the liquid. Either add 2 teaspoonfuls to your baby's bottle three to five times a day, or dispense it on a plastic spoon. Refrigerate any leftover tea and discard after two days.

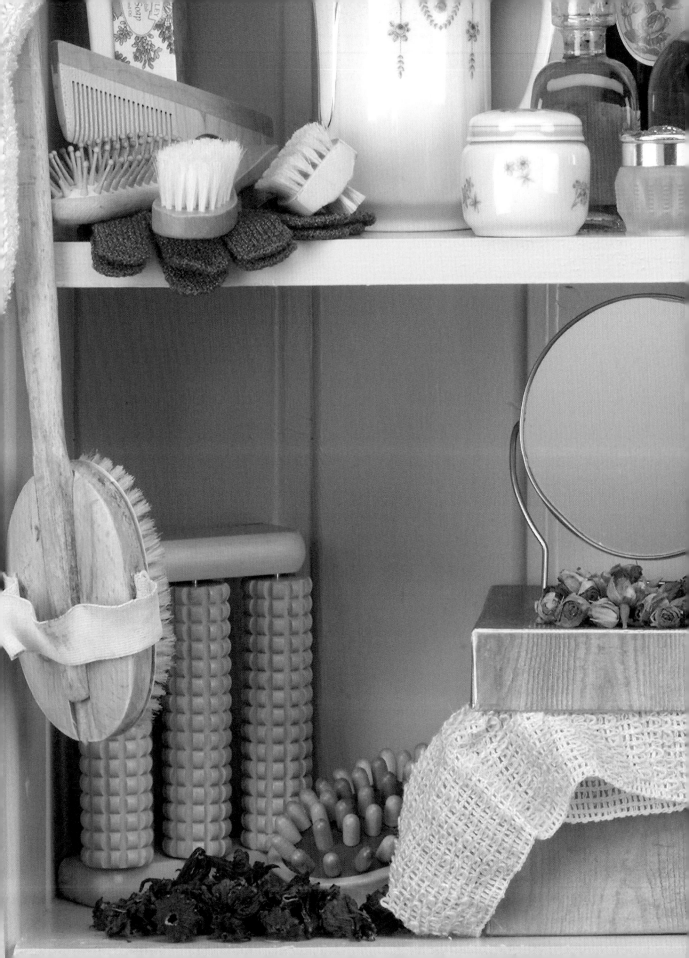

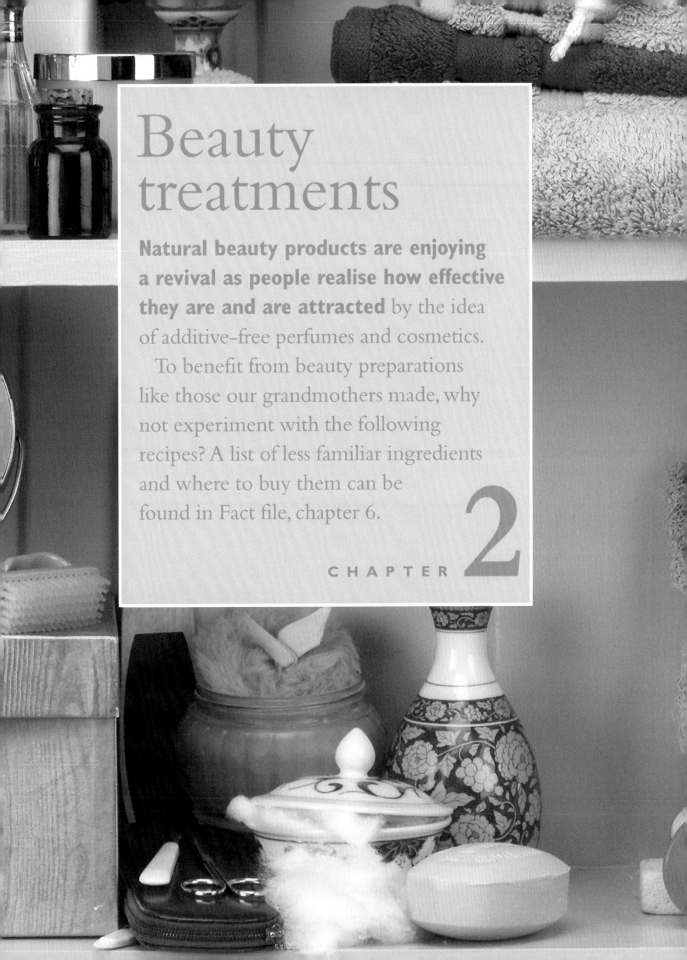

Beauty treatments

Natural beauty products are enjoying a revival as people realise how effective they are and are attracted by the idea of additive-free perfumes and cosmetics.

To benefit from beauty preparations like those our grandmothers made, why not experiment with the following recipes? A list of less familiar ingredients and where to buy them can be found in Fact file, chapter 6.

CHAPTER 2

Natural hair care

Glossy, well-conditioned hair can greatly enhance your appearance. Natural shampoos and herbal rinses will help you to preserve its lustre and protect it from the damaging effects of styling and pollution.

Most children have lovely healthy hair, but as we grow older our hair needs care and attention to maintain its natural beauty. Exposure to sun, wind and atmospheric pollution as well as the use of colours, perms, sprays and gels all take their toll.

There are a huge number of commercial preparations designed to produce glossy hair, but many people are suspicious of their chemical ingredients, some of which may irritate the scalp or cause allergic reactions.

Our grandmothers made their own hair treatments using natural ingredients. A range of herbs, flowers and oils can protect healthy hair and provide remedies for dandruff, dry or greasy, fine or dull hair.

For the following recipes you can use dried herbs and flowers available from herbalists or grow fresh ones yourself. To select the correct variety see Garden herbs, pages 326-331. Some recipes specify the use of 'purified' (distilled) water, which is available from chemists.

Normal hair care

Hair colour and type – curly, straight, thin or thick – are hereditary. With luck you will be blessed with strong, well-balanced hair – not too dry or too greasy – that is easy to style. But in order to keep that natural balance, even such 'normal' hair needs a special daily hair-care programme.

So make rinses, conditioners and revitalising treatments an integral part of your cleansing routine. Equally, prepare them from herbal ingredients that have been used for centuries to enhance the natural beauty of hair.

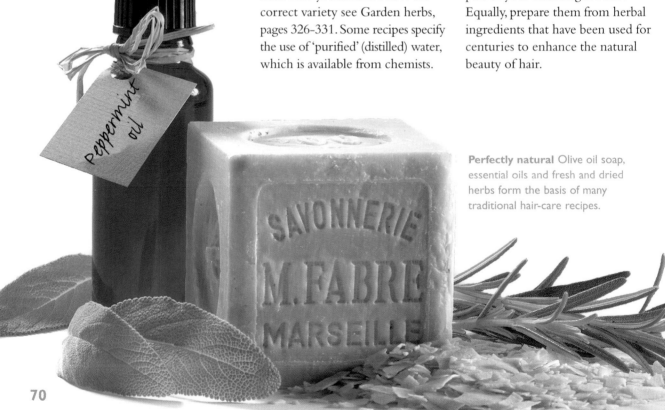

Perfectly natural Olive oil soap, essential oils and fresh and dried herbs form the basis of many traditional hair-care recipes.

HERBAL SHAMPOO

You can make a gentle shampoo with the French olive oil soap, *savon de Marseille*, which contains only olive oil and other natural ingredients. It is available in health shops. This recipe is for fair hair. If you have dark hair, use sage instead of camomile.

8 tablespoons dried
    camomile flowers
1 tablespoon dried
    peppermint leaves
2 tablespoons dried
    rosemary leaves
600ml (1 pint) water
55g (2oz) grated olive oil soap
    or
55g (2oz) soap flakes
3 drops peppermint oil
    or
3 drops eucalyptus oil
2 tablespoons vodka

Put the herbs and water in a pan, bring to the boil and simmer for 10 minutes. Remove from the heat and leave to infuse for 30 minutes. Strain the liquid through a fine sieve and pour it into another pan.
   Add the soap and set the pan over a low heat, stirring continuously until the soap has dissolved. Remove from the heat and leave to cool. Mix the essential oil with the vodka, then add it to the soapy mixture. Pour the shampoo into a screw-top jar and leave in a warm place for three to four days before using.

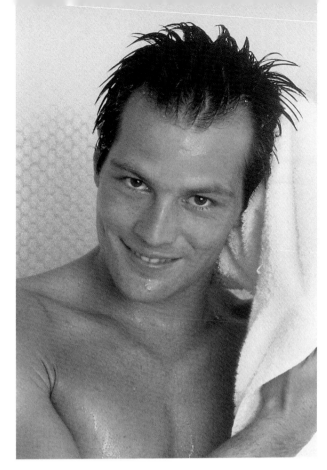

Back to basics
The essence of hair care starts with gentle cleansing. A shampoo based on olive oil soap is ideal.

BASIC SHAMPOO

This shampoo is also based on *savon de Marseille*. It has a pleasant fragrance and creamy consistency. It will produce no side effects.

1 tablespoon olive oil soap
    or
1 tablespoon soap flakes
100ml (3½fl oz) water
herbal extract of your choice
    or
essential oil of your choice

Grate the olive oil soap, if using. Boil the water in a pan, then turn down the heat and add the soap to the water, stirring continuously until it has dissolved. Remove from the heat and leave to cool. Stir in a few drops of your chosen herbal extract or essential oil.

Take care

If you have sensitive skin or are prone to allergies, always test the individual ingredients separately on your scalp before making up and using a shampoo, rinse or treatment.
   This allows you to isolate any intolerances and avoids the discomfort caused by a full-scale allergic reaction.

71

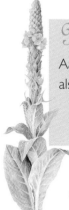

Mullein

Aaron's rod, as mullein is also known, can be made into a strong infusion to brighten fair hair.

COMFREY SHAMPOO

This shampoo will cleanse and condition your hair.

15g (½oz) dried comfrey root
100ml (3½fl oz) water
2 egg yolks
4 teaspoons isopropyl alcohol

Put the comfrey root in a pan. Pour the water over it and leave to infuse for 3 hours. Bring to the boil, stirring continuously. Cover and leave to cool. Strain the liquid, then stir in the egg yolks and alcohol. Massage half the shampoo into wet hair and rinse. Repeat twice.

Complementary ingredients The egg yolks in comfrey shampoo make your hair soft, while the comfrey root reduces inflammation of the scalp.

CAMOMILE CONDITIONER

You can modify this recipe to suit your hair colour. Add dried camomile for fair hair and walnut shells if you have dark hair. If using walnut shells, crush to a powder using a pestle and mortar or coffee grinder.

100ml (3½fl oz) water
1 tablespoon dried
   camomile flowers
   or
1 tablespoon walnut shells,
   crushed
6 tablespoons lemon juice
   or
6 tablespoons fruit vinegar

Boil the water and pour it over the camomile flowers or shells. Leave to infuse for 10 minutes. Strain the liquid, then mix in the lemon juice or vinegar; leave to cool slightly. After washing your hair, work the conditioner through the damp hair. Do not rinse out.

MILD HERBAL CONDITIONER

The horsetail in this conditioner will make dull hair shine again.

500ml (18fl oz) water
1 teaspoon dried stinging
   nettle leaves
1 teaspoon dried mullein
   flowers
1 teaspoon dried horsetail
   'needles' and stems

Boil the water and pour it over the herbs. Leave to infuse for 10 minutes, then strain the liquid. When cool, massage into the scalp. Leave for 3 minutes, then rinse.

BIRCH LEAF CONDITIONER

This invigorating conditioner is suitable for all hair types.

1 teaspoon dried lavender
   flowers
1 teaspoon dried birch leaves
1 litre (1¾ pints) fruit vinegar
few drops lavender oil

Put the flowers, leaves and fruit vinegar in a bottle, seal and leave to infuse for seven days. Strain the liquid, then add the lavender oil. To use, dilute 1 part conditioner with 2 parts water, massage into the scalp and comb through the hair. Do not rinse out.

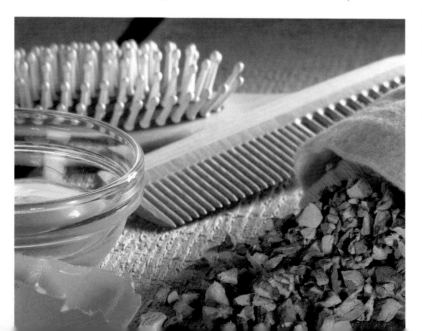

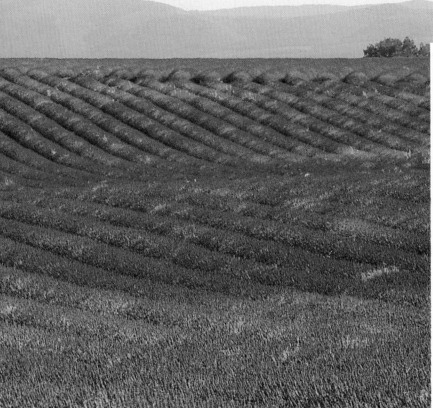

Lovely lavender

An intoxicating fragrance emanates from the lavender fields of Provence, in the south of France. It is a scent that can be found in many skin-care products.

The blue-purple flowers and their essential oil can also be used in hair-care preparations. If you add a few drops of lavender oil to the last rinse, or use a homemade lavender conditioner, your hair will smell beautifully fresh. Lavender has a relaxing effect and is suitable for all hair and skin types.

FRAGRANT HAIR TREATMENT

This nourishing treatment gives normal hair a healthy shine.

50ml (2fl oz) almond oil
2 teaspoons jojoba oil
20-30 drops fragrant essential oil of your choice

Mix the oils and massage them thoroughly into your scalp. Wrap a towel around your head and leave for 30-60 minutes. Shampoo and rinse thoroughly.

SETTING LOTION

Forget those expensive styling products and make your own setting lotion using this old recipe.

250ml (9fl oz) purified water
1 teaspoon honey
dash of vinegar
essential oil of your choice

Warm the purified water and honey in a pan, then add the vinegar. Add up to 30 drops of essential oil, according to preference. Wash your hair, then apply the setting lotion to the damp hair and style.

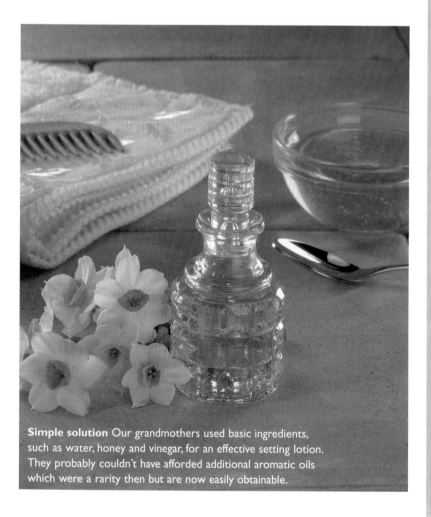

Simple solution Our grandmothers used basic ingredients, such as water, honey and vinegar, for an effective setting lotion. They probably couldn't have afforded additional aromatic oils which were a rarity then but are now easily obtainable.

Tried & Trusted
Normal hair

- **Hair should be brushed frequently to keep it healthy. Brushing stimulates the scalp and aids circulation.**

- **For soft, silky hair dab 125ml (4fl oz) of full-cream milk onto the hair with a flannel. Leave on for 15 minutes, then rinse out.**

- **Fair hair acquires a silky shine if 2 tablespoons of lemon juice are added to the shampoo.**

- **Beer makes a good setting lotion. Pour 50-85ml (2-3fl oz) into a spray bottle and spray onto your hair. Don't worry about the smell; it will disappear once the hair is dry.**

Greasy hair

- **Don't brush greasy hair too much, as this stimulates the sebaceous glands into producing more sebum. When blow-drying, brush upwards to create volume.**

- **To keep your hair as grease-free as possible, stick to a healthy diet with plenty of fruit, vegetables and wholemeal products. Avoid sweets and processed and fatty foods.**

Treating greasy hair

If your hair gets greasy and limp soon after shampooing, it's because the sebaceous glands in the hair follicles are producing too much sebum (the hair's lubricating oil). As a result, the hair needs washing more frequently.

Harsh shampoos also increase the need for washing, as they strip the nutrients from your hair. This alters the hair's natural balance and makes it become greasy more quickly. To prevent this, you need a shampoo that regulates the production of sebum. Herbs that can help to prevent hair from becoming too greasy include calendula, horsetail, southernwood and yarrow.

Cosmetic companies add specific chemicals to their products to combat greasy hair. However, before these brands were available people looked at the problem more holistically. Too many spicy foods, fats and sugars can make the hair greasy, as can stress, hormonal change and lack of sleep.

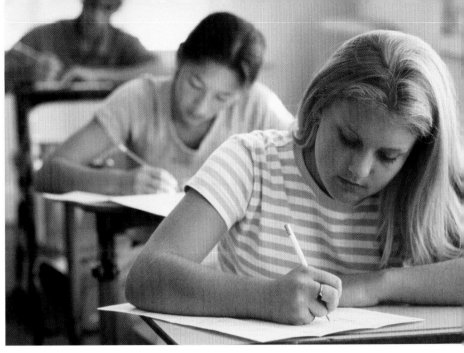

Difficult times Hormones and stress can have an effect on the hair, as teenagers well know. Use a herbal rinse to counteract greasy hair and to help restore the hair's natural balance.

DRY SHAMPOO

When you're short of time, try this remedy to revitalise your hair.

2 tablespoons orris root powder
2 tablespoons cornflour

Mix the ingredients together in a small dish. Using a comb, part your hair in narrow bands and sprinkle the shampoo along each row. Leave for 10 minutes, then brush your hair vigorously.

HERBAL CONDITIONER FOR FINE GREASY HAIR

Fine hair tends to get greasy more quickly because there are more hair follicles producing sebum.

1 teaspoon dried rosemary leaves
1 teaspoon dried camomile flowers
1 teaspoon dried stinging nettle leaves
100ml (3½fl oz) water
1 tablespoon fruit vinegar

Put the herbs in a bowl, boil the water and pour it on the herbs. Add the vinegar and leave to infuse for 10 minutes before straining the liquid through a fine sieve.

After washing your hair, apply this conditioner to the damp hair. Don't rinse out.

This conditioner can also be made with equal quantities of thyme and horsetail.

Hair lotion

Hair lotions, available at chemists in the 1920s, were among the first commercially produced cosmetics. Apart from colouring and perfumes, they also contained various conditioning agents.

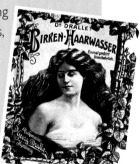

Take care

Try to avoid getting any herbal hair remedy in your eyes. If you do, rinse your eyes immediately with cold water.

Nourishing treatments for dry hair

Dry hair does not produce much sebum and consequently tends to be coarse and brittle – a condition that worsens with age. Sun, sea water, chemical hair dyes and perms cause further damage and result in split ends. Trimming the damaged hair is sometimes the only remedy.

But hair need not become too dry. With the right conditioning treatment, even dry, straw-like hair can become manageable again.

Apply repair treatments regularly to tone your hair and to prevent the strands from becoming brittle and tangled. The weaker the hair, the more important this is. You can make your own natural products based on traditional recipes.

EGG SHAMPOO

This shampoo will protect dry hair. Products containing egg are most effective when used immediately.

1 egg white
2 egg yolks
1 teaspoon honey
1 tablespoon olive oil
juice of 1 lemon

Whisk the egg white and fold in the yolks. Stir in the honey, olive oil and lemon juice. Massage the shampoo into the scalp and thoroughly coat the hair. Leave for a few minutes and rinse the hair, using plenty of water, until all the shampoo has gone.

Culinary remedy If you have dry hair, all the ingredients for an egg shampoo can be found in the kitchen.

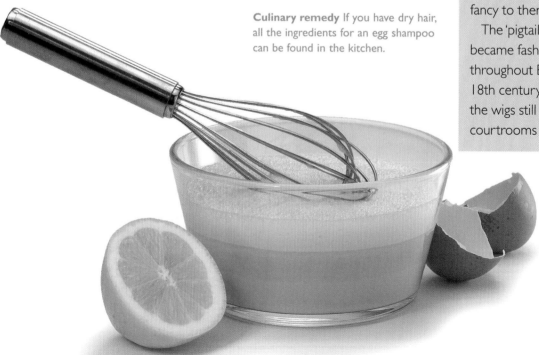

Wigs

The idea of wearing false hair as a fashion accessory is a very old one. The ancient Egyptians and Babylonians wore wigs as a sign of rank. Women favoured wigs in

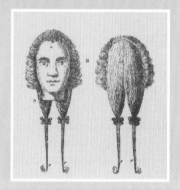

ancient Rome, but it was not until the 1620s, during the reign of Louis XIII of France that men took a fancy to them.

The 'pigtail' wig (above) became fashionable throughout Europe in the 18th century and these are the wigs still worn in British courtrooms today.

PAMPER YOUR HAIR

If you want to give your hair a treat now and then, try this recipe. It will make it light and silky.

1 egg yolk
2 tablespoons olive oil

Slowly stir the yolk into the oil. Massage immediately into dry hair, wrap a towel around your head and leave for 30 minutes to get the most out of the treatment. Shampoo, then rinse afterwards.

ROSEMARY, THYME AND NETTLE TREATMENT

This remedy works on brittle hair and split ends. A weekly application will help to guarantee success.

40ml (1½fl oz) castor oil
5 teaspoons olive oil
15g (½oz) dried thyme leaves
15g (½oz) dried rosemary leaves
15g (½oz) dried stinging nettle leaves

Mix the oils. Put the herbs in a bottle, pour in the oils and seal with a stopper or cap. Leave to infuse for two days, then strain the liquid through a fine sieve. Massage the oil into the scalp and hair. Cover with kitchen foil, then wrap a towel around it. Leave for at least 2 hours, then shampoo as usual.

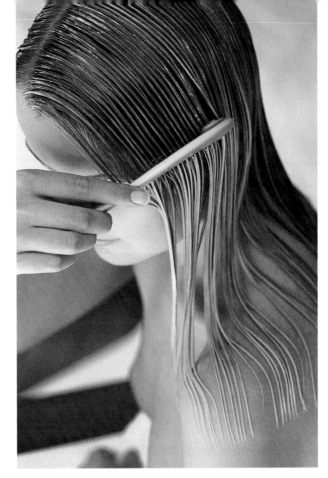

Methodical hair care Treatments have to be worked in carefully, covering the hair's entire length from the roots to the tips. That way, all the important nutrients can be absorbed.

TREATMENT WITH HENNA AND AVOCADO OIL

Henna leaves, harvested in spring, contain little colour, but a lot of tanning material. Neutral henna leaf powder makes hair easy to style but won't colour the hair.

1 tablespoon dried henna leaf powder
1 tablespoon avocado oil
1 egg yolk

Mix the henna, avocado oil and egg yolk into a paste, then thoroughly coat wet hair. Leave for 30-60 minutes, then rinse out.

FIVE OILS LOTION

Treat dry hair to this nourishing hair treatment once a month.

50ml (2fl oz) almond oil
30ml (1fl oz) sunflower oil
30ml (1fl oz) walnut oil
30ml (1fl oz) castor oil
1 teaspoon attar of roses

Pour the ingredients into a bottle and leave to infuse for two days in a cool place. Massage the lotion into your scalp and comb it through your hair. Wrap a towel around your head and allow the treatment to work overnight. Use a mild shampoo to wash your hair the next morning. Rinse thoroughly with plenty of water.

Floral hair lotion

Pamper your hair every now and then with a conditioning treatment made from nourishing plant extracts.

Not so long ago, cosmetics using natural ingredients from the kitchen and garden were dismissed as cranky. Attitudes have changed, however, as the damaging effects of chemicals have become apparent.

Today, many people find that they have allergic reactions to chemical substances in cosmetics, and doctors are often unable to pinpoint the exact cause.

You can reduce the risk of irritation by making your own cosmetics from tried-and-tested ingredients. Cider vinegar and nettles boost the circulation in the scalp, while marigold and rosemary moisturise it.

Propolis (bee-glue) tincture, comes from the beekeeper's treasure-trove and is a natural antibiotic. Avocado oil nourishes the hair, increasing shine.

How to make floral hair lotion
Makes one 375ml (13fl oz) bottle

▼ Next, pour **30 drops of propolis tincture**, **20 drops of rosemary tincture** and **1 tablespoon of avocado oil** into the bottle. Seal the bottle and shake again.

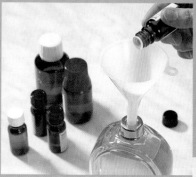

▲ Using a small funnel, pour **300ml (½ pint) cider vinegar**, **20 drops of marigold tincture** and **10 drops of stinging nettle tincture** into a bottle. Seal the bottle and shake well.

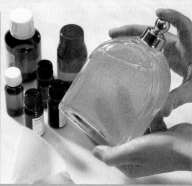

▲ Wash your hair as normal. Moisten a cotton-wool pad with the lotion and dab your wet scalp with it. Leave to dry naturally if possible.

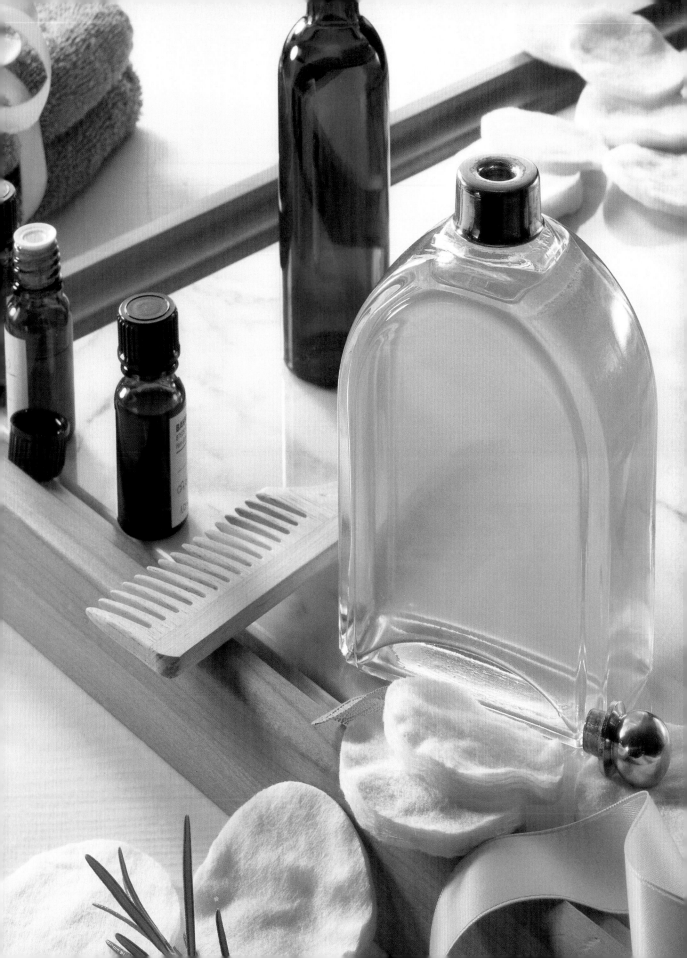

Bring new life to lacklustre hair

If hair looks lifeless, it may be due to a residue of shampoo and conditioner left on after washing. Or perhaps you have damaged your hair with styling lotions.

Revive your hair's radiance with a conditioner made from nourishing ingredients. The following shampoos, rinses and conditioners all protect the hair without the use of harsh chemicals.

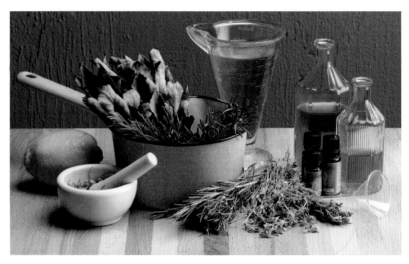

Perfect rinse With ingredients such as lemon, herbs, fruit vinegar and essential oils, you can make an instant hair rinse.

TREATMENT FOR DULL HAIR

Nourish your hair once a week with this quick treatment.

30ml (1fl oz) olive oil
30ml (1fl oz) lemon juice

Warm the oil and stir in the lemon juice. Dampen your hair, massage the mixture into your scalp and comb it through your hair. Wrap a towel around your head and leave for an hour. Shampoo and rinse.

CORNFLOWERS FOR GREY HAIR

This rinse adds fresh shine and delicate blue radiance to dull hair.

2 handfuls dried cornflowers
500ml (18fl oz) water
few drops lemon juice

Put the cornflowers in a heatproof bowl. Boil the water and pour it over them. Leave to infuse for 3 hours. Strain the liquid, then add the lemon juice. Comb into towel-dried hair. Do not rinse out.

HAIR RINSE WITH SAGE

Apply this rinse every three days to enhance your hair's shine and prevent it from becoming brittle.

250g (9oz) dried sage leaves
1 litre (1¾ pints) water
250ml (9fl oz) vodka

Put the sage leaves and water in a pan and bring to the boil. Simmer for 15 minutes. When cool, pour into a glass bottle and leave to infuse for 48 hours, shaking occasionally. Strain the liquid through a fine sieve, add the alcohol and return to the bottle. Seal with a stopper.

SOAPWORT SHAMPOO

Soapwort cleans and strengthens the hair; lemon adds radiance.

1 tablespoon dried
**   soapwort leaves**
250ml (9fl oz) water
1 tablespoon lemon juice
1 egg yolk
1 drop lemon oil

Place the soapwort and water in a pan and bring to the boil. Stir in the other ingredients and leave to infuse for 10 minutes. Pour into a bottle and seal.

Soapwort

Rub the leaves and stems of the herb *Saponaria officinalis* and they will make a lather – hence its common name.

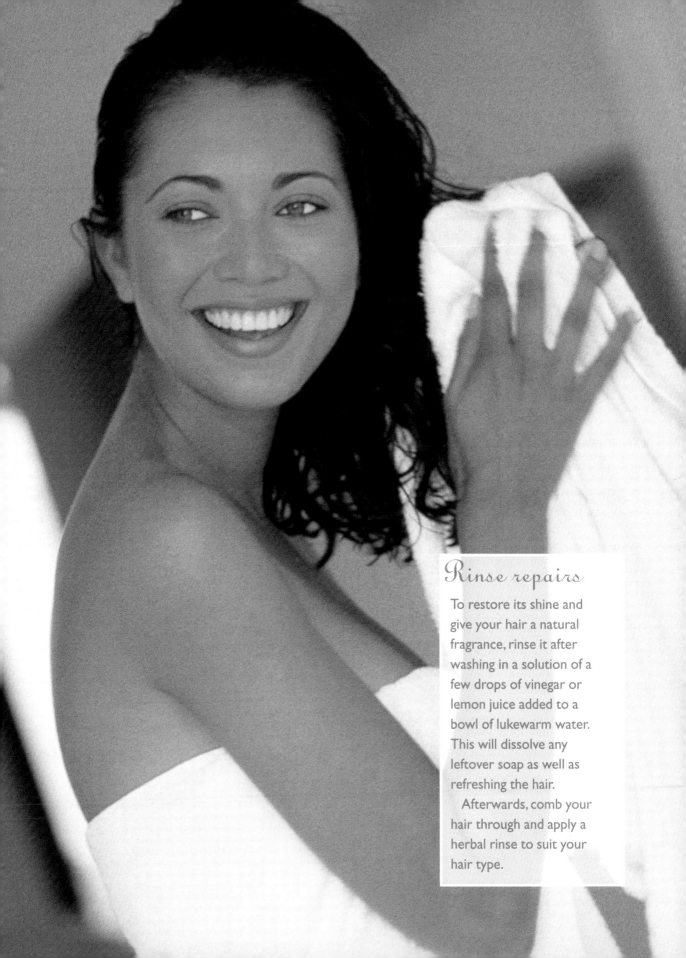

Rinse repairs

To restore its shine and give your hair a natural fragrance, rinse it after washing in a solution of a few drops of vinegar or lemon juice added to a bowl of lukewarm water. This will dissolve any leftover soap as well as refreshing the hair.

Afterwards, comb your hair through and apply a herbal rinse to suit your hair type.

Fighting the irritating problem of dandruff

You don't always have to use extreme measures, such as tar products, to combat the production of dead skin cells that we know as dandruff. In most instances it can be dealt with successfully using gentle, traditional methods.

Serious cases of infection and a very itchy scalp are sometimes diagnosed as the chronic skin condition seborrhoeic dermatitis. But before you seek medical advice, it is worth trying natural methods that are kind to the skin. If these remedies do not work, consult a specialist.

HERBAL HAIR RINSE

This herbal rinse reduces the production of sebum and soothes inflammation of the scalp.

1 teaspoon dried horsetail
   'needles' and stems
1 teaspoon dried
   rosemary leaves
1 teaspoon dried thyme leaves
100ml (3½fl oz) water
1 tablespoon fruit vinegar

Mix the herbs in a heatproof bowl. Boil the water and pour it over the herbs. Add the vinegar and leave to infuse for 15-20 minutes. Strain the mixture and use after shampooing.

Essential oils For extra fragrance, add a few drops of your favourite essence to a rinse or conditioner.

Take care

When using cedarwood oil, try to buy Atlas oil rather than the oil from the Texas or Virginian cedarwood, as it is the least harsh of the three. While all cedarwood oils have a powerful aroma, the Atlas oil has a sweet balsamic scent, whereas the Texas variety has a smoky tar-like odour.

ESSENTIAL OIL TREATMENT FOR DANDRUFF

Cedarwood oil, used in Tibet as a temple incense, is good for getting rid of dandruff. But as this treatment contains rosemary oil, do not use it if you are pregnant or suffer from high blood pressure or epilepsy.

1 tablespoon wheatgerm oil
3 drops cedarwood oil
2 drops rosemary oil
2 drops lemon oil

Blend the oils together. Massage the mixture into your scalp and leave to work for 2 hours. Wash your hair and rinse thoroughly.

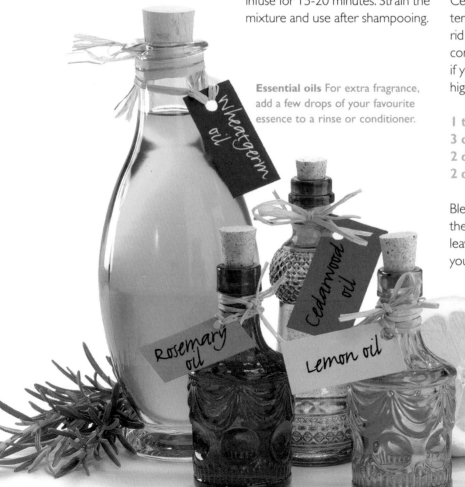

HAIR TONIC WITH OAK AND WHITE POPLAR BARK

A perfect anti-dandruff tonic.

25g (1oz) oak bark powder
25g (1oz) white poplar bark
   powder
1 litre (1¾ pints) water

Place the ingredients in a pan, bring to the boil and simmer for 20 minutes. Strain the liquid through a fine sieve. Pour into a glass bottle and seal. Massage the hair tonic into your scalp every day.

NETTLE TONIC

Stinging nettles can make a very effective dandruff remedy.

40g (1½oz) stinging nettle
   tincture
½ teaspoon arnica tincture
50ml (2fl oz) witch hazel

Mix the ingredients in a glass bottle with a dropper and shake. Massage 8-10 drops into your scalp.

Take care

Essential oils, when undiluted by carrier oils (see Main ingredients, pages 332-339), are highly concentrated and should be handled with care. When using a new oil, dilute 1 drop of essential oil in 1 teaspoon of carrier oil and test it on your skin for irritation. With the exception of lavender and tea tree oils, pure essential oils should not be applied undiluted to the skin.

Preventing hair loss

Thinning hair can spark panic in both men and women. There are many reasons for hair to fall out or thin. The reason may be hereditary, it might be the result of illness, or it might be caused by a hormonal disorder and stress.

NASTURTIUM HAIR LOTION

Nasturtiums contain sulphur which can help to prevent hair loss.

55g (2oz) dried nasturtium
   seeds and leaves
55g (2oz) dried thyme leaves
   and flowers
1 litre (1¾ pints) vodka

Place the herbs and alcohol in a bowl, cover and leave to infuse for ten days. Strain the liquid and store in a glass bottle with a cap. Massage the lotion into your scalp once a day.

WATERCRESS RINSE

This rinse will give a boost to thinning, brittle hair.

1 handful fresh watercress
   leaves
1 tablespoon fruit vinegar
500ml (18fl oz) purified water

Chop the watercress leaves and place them in a bowl. Mix the fruit vinegar and the water in a separate bowl. Pour this liquid over the watercress. Leave to infuse overnight, then strain the liquid. After shampooing, slowly pour the rinse over your hair and dry.

Often, thinning hair and baldness are also due to a lack of vitamins and minerals, such as iron.

   Women do not usually go bald, but after the menopause some find that their hair becomes wispy and thin in patches.

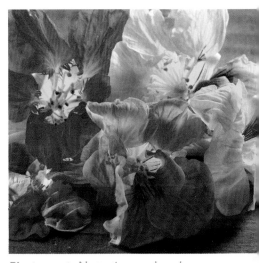

Plant secrets Nasturtium seeds and leaves may help to stimulate hair growth.

STIMULATING HAIR LOTION

Rosemary oil stimulates the roots of the hair, but do not use it if you are pregnant or suffer from high blood pressure or epilepsy.

3 drops rosemary oil
3 drops ylang ylang oil
30ml (1fl oz) vodka
1 tablespoon orange floral
   water

Dissolve the essential oils in the alcohol and dilute the mixture with the floral water. Pour the lotion into a glass bottle and seal. Massage a few drops into your scalp daily.

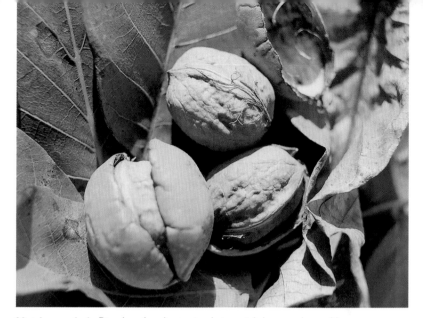

Nut-brown hair Powdered walnuts give hair a rich brown sheen. Always test a natural dye on a few strands of hair first to judge the effectiveness of the colouring and to estimate how long it should be left on.

Using herbal hair colourings

Nature provides us with a rich palette of hair colours, from cool blonde to fiery red, warm brown and mysterious black. Pure vegetable dyes colour and condition the hair without damaging it. Be daring, experiment and have fun.

CAMOMILE COLOUR RINSE

Increase the amount of camomile flowers if you have long hair.

115-140g (4-5oz) dried
   camomile flowers
500ml (18fl oz) water
dash of lemon juice

Put the flowers and water in a pan, bring to the boil, then cover and simmer for 20 minutes. Strain the liquid then add the lemon juice. Apply the rinse to your hair after washing it, then dry.

WALNUT BROWN

Natural dyes do not last as long as commercial products. This colour will rinse out after three washes.

225-350g (8-12oz) walnut
   shells
dash of vegetable oil
dash of fruit vinegar
little hot water

Grind the shells to a very fine powder using a pestle and mortar or coffee grinder. Blend with the oil, vinegar and sufficient hot water to form a creamy paste. Leave for 15 minutes.

Wash and dry your hair. Add more hot water to the paste to make it spreadable. Paint the paste onto your hair with a pastry brush. Cover with a plastic shower cap and sit in a warm room while the dye soaks in. Regularly check your hair until it is the shade you want. Shampoo and condition afterwards.

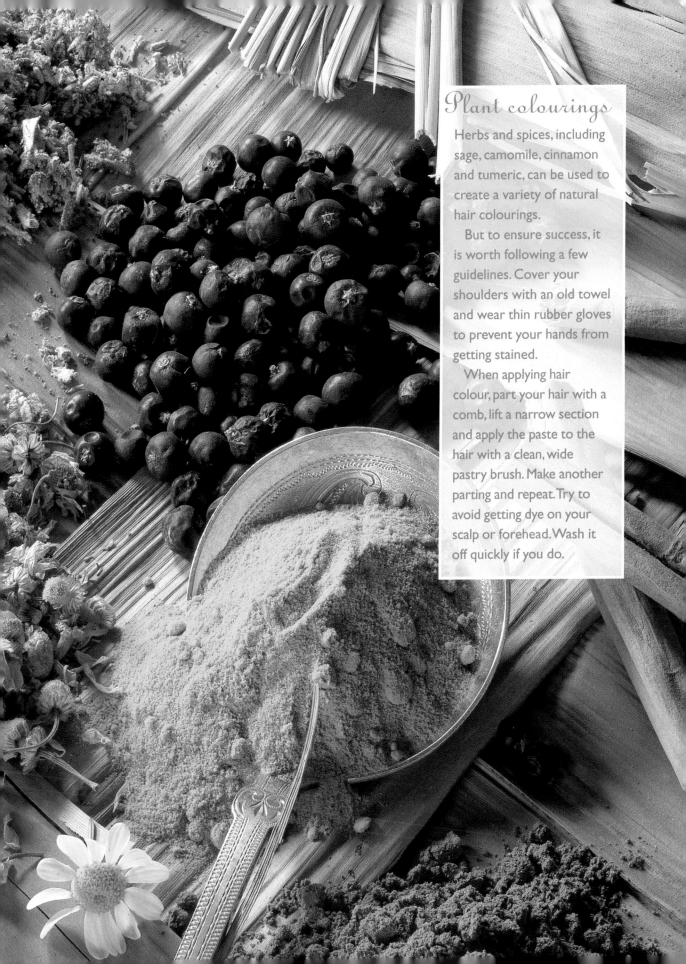

Plant colourings

Herbs and spices, including sage, camomile, cinnamon and tumeric, can be used to create a variety of natural hair colourings.

But to ensure success, it is worth following a few guidelines. Cover your shoulders with an old towel and wear thin rubber gloves to prevent your hands from getting stained.

When applying hair colour, part your hair with a comb, lift a narrow section and apply the paste to the hair with a clean, wide pastry brush. Make another parting and repeat. Try to avoid getting dye on your scalp or forehead. Wash it off quickly if you do.

Dazzlingly beautiful

Whatever your skin type, you can benefit from a wide range of wholesome, traditional skin-care recipes to keep your complexion looking radiant and fresh.

Today's shops offer an overwhelming choice of attractively packaged skin-care products. But long before beauty had been commercialised, women knew how to enhance their appearance and care for their looks.

For natural face-care products, we need look no further than our grandmothers' dressing tables. They knew how to keep their skin looking fresh and youthful, and how to protect it from harsh conditions using surprisingly simple preparations.

The needs of different skin types have long been understood by most women. There were recipes for wrinkles and fine lines, imperfections and redness of the cheek, as well as protective treatments for sensitive areas around the eyes and lips.

The creams on an Edwardian dressing table contained some of the best ingredients that nature could provide.

Which skin type?

To be able to care for your skin properly, you first need to establish your skin type. To do this, press a piece of tissue paper onto your face 3-4 hours after washing. Normal or dry skin leaves almost no trace of grease, whereas oily skin will mark the paper all over.

Combination skin will leave traces of grease around the forehead, nose and chin. If you tend towards this skin type, treat the more sensitive, dry areas around the cheeks and eyes with remedies for dry skin. Care for the oily zones with lotions designed for oily skin.

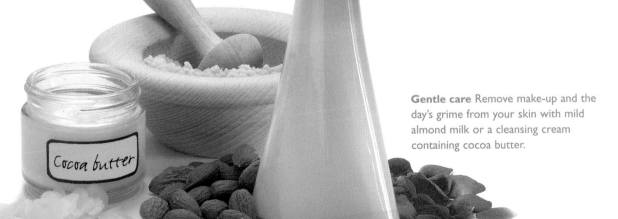

Gentle care Remove make-up and the day's grime from your skin with mild almond milk or a cleansing cream containing cocoa butter.

face and neck

Normal skin

Firm, smooth and unblemished natural skin also has a fine texture and small pores. It produces a balanced amount of sebum and moisture and has good circulation. You are lucky if your skin is this type, but you should still make sure that you look after it.

CLEANSING CREAM WITH COCOA BUTTER

This gentle cleanser will remove most types of make-up. Apply it to your face and neck and leave on for 5 minutes before removing. Wash your face with warm water and finish with a toner.

I teaspoon white
   beeswax granules
25g (1oz) lanolin
I teaspoon cocoa butter
40ml (1½fl oz) olive oil
40ml (1½fl oz) rosewater

Melt the wax in a bowl set over a pan of boiling water, then add the lanolin and cocoa butter. When the mixture has liquefied, add the oil and heat to 65°C (149°F). Warm the rosewater in a heatproof dish to the same temperature.
   Take the wax mixture off the heat and blend in the rosewater, using an electric hand-mixer on a low setting, until the cream is cold and thick. Transfer to a jar, seal and store in a cool place.

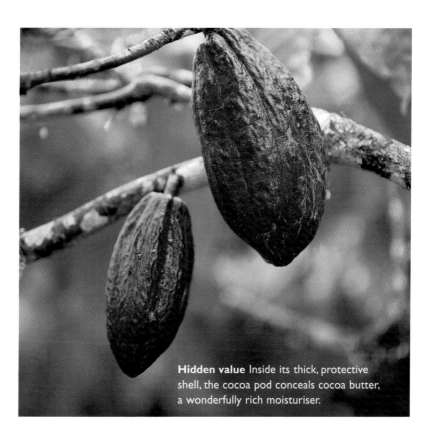

Hidden value Inside its thick, protective shell, the cocoa pod conceals cocoa butter, a wonderfully rich moisturiser.

ALMOND MILK

This natural cleansing milk suits all skin types.

55g (2oz) almonds
200ml (7fl oz) rosewater
¼ teaspoon dried masterwort
   leaves

Pound the almonds to a paste with a little of the rosewater using a pestle and mortar. Slowly stir in the remaining rosewater. Powder the masterwort leaves, then add them to the mixture. Transfer to a bottle, seal and use for cleansing your face.

Rosewater

Fragrant rosewater is a by-product made during the steam distillation of the essential oil known as attar of roses. Rosewater forms the basis of many cosmetic products.

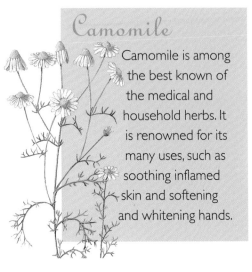

Camomile

Camomile is among the best known of the medical and household herbs. It is renowned for its many uses, such as soothing inflamed skin and softening and whitening hands.

FLOUR SKIN SCRUB

Treat your skin with this gentle scrub once a week.

115g (4oz) cornflour
55g (2oz) wheat flour
115g (4oz) dried milk powder

Mix all the ingredients and store in an airtight container. After washing, blend a little of the mixture with warm water to make a paste and massage your face with the scrub for a few minutes. Rinse off.

Versatile ingredients Rosewater and camomile tincture will soothe and refresh your skin. Mixed with witch hazel and honey, they make a revitalising toner.

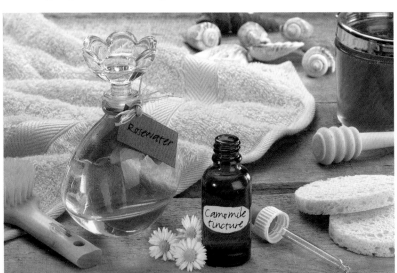

TONER WITH ROSEWATER AND WITCH HAZEL

This refreshing, fragrant toner will suit all skin types.

50ml (2fl oz) rosewater
½ teaspoon honey
50ml (2fl oz) witch hazel
10 drops camomile tincture

Warm the rosewater and dissolve the honey in it. Add the witch hazel and camomile tincture, pour into a dark glass bottle with a stopper and shake well. After washing, moisten a cotton-wool pad with the toner and wipe it gently over your face and neck.

Take care

Homemade skin-care products will not keep for as long as the ones you buy in the shops, which have added preservatives. All freshly made cosmetics should be stored in the fridge and used within two to four weeks.

SANDALWOOD FACE TONER

Red sandalwood bark firms the skin after cleansing.

15g (½oz) red sandalwood bark
100ml (3½fl oz) isopropyl alcohol
250ml (9fl oz) rosewater

Put the sandalwood bark into a dark glass bottle with a stopper. Pour in the alcohol and rosewater, seal and leave to infuse for two weeks. Strain the liquid through a fine sieve.

Pour it back into the bottle, replace the stopper and shake thoroughly. Add a few drops of toner to a damp cotton-wool pad and dab it onto your face.

ELDERFLOWER LOTION

The white flowers of the elder tree were traditionally picked in June and July to make a soothing toner. You can also use 25g (1oz) dried elderflowers for this recipe.

100g (3½oz) fresh elderflowers
300ml (½ pint) water
3 tablespoons eau de cologne

Crush the flowers using a pestle and mortar. Transfer them to a heatproof bowl. Boil the water, pour it over the flowers, then leave to cool. Strain the liquid through a fine sieve and stir in the eau de cologne. Store in a dark glass bottle with a stopper.

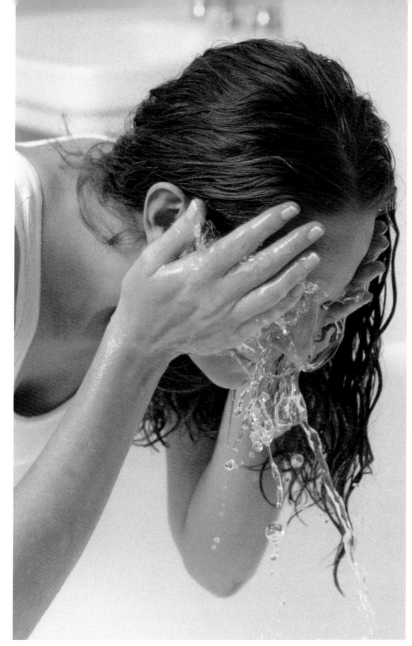

Pure and simple Use warm water to rinse your face first thing in the morning and last thing at night. Very hot or cold water can damage the blood vessels and cause unsightly red thread veins.

Establishing a daily skin-care routine

Each time you cleanse your face, rinse it with plenty of water to remove all traces of the cleanser.

Ideally, you should tone your skin after cleansing to refresh and revitalise it. Depending on your skin type and the ingredients used, toners can do even more.

They can stimulate and soothe pores, stop inflammation, improve circulation and temporarily tighten the skin.

Toners matched to the needs of your skin type should be considered a necessity for healthy skin and good looks, rather than a luxury.

COLD CREAM

A recipe for this cleansing cream was devised by the Greeks in about 300 BC. It has been used and adapted ever since.

1 tablespoon aloe vera gel
150ml (5fl oz) corn oil
1 tablespoon white
**   beeswax granules**
2 tablespoons lanolin
2 tablespoons lavender water
2-3 drops camomile oil

Whisk together the aloe vera gel and the corn oil in a bowl. Melt the beeswax and lanolin in a bowl set over a pan of simmering water. Slowly stir in the aloe vera mixture.

Remove from the heat, then add the lavender water and camomile oil. Keep stirring the mixture until it is cool and has set. Transfer the cream to a small jar with a lid and keep in the fridge.

MOISTURISING FACE GEL

This simple face gel protects the skin from drying out, and is quick and easy to prepare.

150ml (5fl oz) water
1 teaspoon gelatine
1 teaspoon attar of roses
3 teaspoons glycerine

Boil the water, then leave it to cool a little. Dissolve the gelatine in the water, stirring occasionally. Stir in the attar of roses and glycerine. Once the gel has cooled, transfer it to a small jar with a lid and store in a cool place.

ALMOND OIL CREAM

This cream has been in use for centuries and is made from ingredients with proven benefits. Apply it thinly, wait for it to be absorbed by the skin, then pat your face dry with a paper tissue.

½ teaspoon beeswax granules
1 teaspoon cocoa butter
15g (½oz) lanolin
30ml (1fl oz) almond oil
40ml (1½fl oz) rosewater
3 drops lavender oil

Melt the beeswax in a bowl set over a pan of simmering water. Add the cocoa butter and lanolin. When all the ingredients have melted, stir in the almond oil and heat to 60°C (140°F). Warm the rosewater to the same temperature.
   Remove the beeswax mixture from the heat, add the rosewater and beat using an electric hand-blender on a low setting. While the mixture is still lukewarm, add the lavender oil drop by drop and continue whisking until the cream is cold. Transfer to a ceramic jar with a lid and keep in the fridge.

HYSSOP FACE LOTION

Hyssop flowers from June to September, producing violet, pink or white blooms. Its active properties help to promote smooth, clear skin.

55g (2oz) fresh hyssop flowers
1 litre (1¾ pints) water

Put the hyssop in a heatproof bowl. Boil the water then pour it over the herb and leave to infuse for 10 minutes. Strain the liquid through a fine sieve and pour it into a bottle and seal.

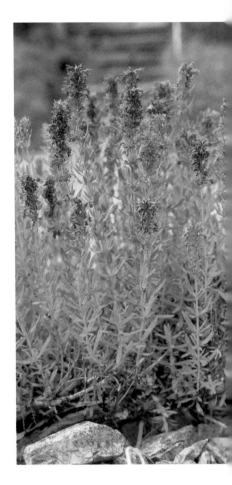

Natural cleanser
Aromatic hyssop has been used for medicinal and culinary purposes since the 1st century AD.

Cleopatra's beauty

Born in 69 BC in Alexandria, then capital of Egypt, Cleopatra was known for her beauty and for her love-affairs with Julius Caesar and Mark Antony. She became Cleopatra VII, ruler of Egypt, when she was just 18 years old.
   Whether she was beautiful in the modern sense is doubtful; historians suggest that she may have had rather coarse features and a bent nose. Nevertheless, she was a woman of her time. All ancient Egyptian women placed a huge importance on beautifying rituals. These began with cleansing and oiling the skin with fragrant oils such as frankincense and myrrh and continued with the application of make-up. Rouge was made from iron oxide and malachite was used to make green eye colour.

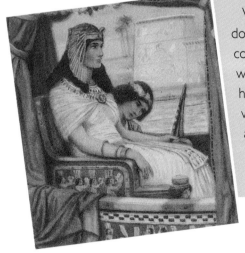

FLOWER POLLEN AND ALMOND MASK

Pollen is rich in vitamins, minerals, protein and hormone-like substances and can easily be dissolved in liquid.

25g (1oz) ground almonds
15g (½oz) flower pollen
15g (½oz) honey
4 teaspoons witch hazel
4 teaspoons almond oil

Mix all the ingredients into a creamy paste. Wash your face and neck and smooth the mask over your skin. Leave for an hour. Wash off with warm water.

CARROT AND POTATO MASK

Carrots are a good source of beta-carotene, a natural antioxidant which can combat the effects of age and help to firm your skin.

2 carrots
1 tablespoon potato flour
1 egg yolk

Finely grate the carrots, add the potato flour and egg yolk, then stir thoroughly. Wash your face and neck and immediately apply the paste. Leave for 20 minutes. Wash off with warm water and rinse with cold.

Tried & Trusted

Day and night care

- Cleanse your face morning and evening, then treat it with a moisturising cream that meets the needs of your skin type.

- Applying a protective cream to your face each morning safeguards it from sunlight and pollutants.

- Night cream has a supportive role, helping your skin to regenerate while you sleep.

Normal skin care

- Wash your face morning and evening with yarrow tea. It will leave your skin wonderfully clear and soft.

- For a natural, refreshing toner, peel a piece of cucumber, chop it up and squeeze out the juice through a clean cloth. Use immediately on your face.

Fruit facials

- Mash 1 tablespoon of strawberries and mix it with 1 tablespoon of organic natural yoghurt. Apply the mixture to your face and neck, cover with a warm cloth and leave for a few minutes. Rinse off with cold water. This is not suitable if you are prone to allergies.

- To make a nourishing face pack for radiant skin, finely grate two apples, add a little lemon juice and apply it thinly to your face. Leave for 10 minutes, then wash off.

- When applying a mask, avoid the eye and lip areas.

More beauty tips

- Remember that a balanced diet, including plenty of water, regular exercise, fresh air and sufficient sleep are just as important as your external skin-care routine.

- Sleeping on your back and using soft sheets are said to prevent wrinkles on the face and neck.

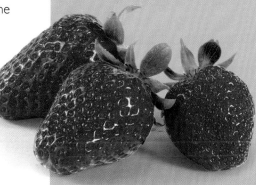

Edible goodness Apply a thin layer of homemade organic strawberry yoghurt to cool and soothe sore skin (see Fruit facials, above).

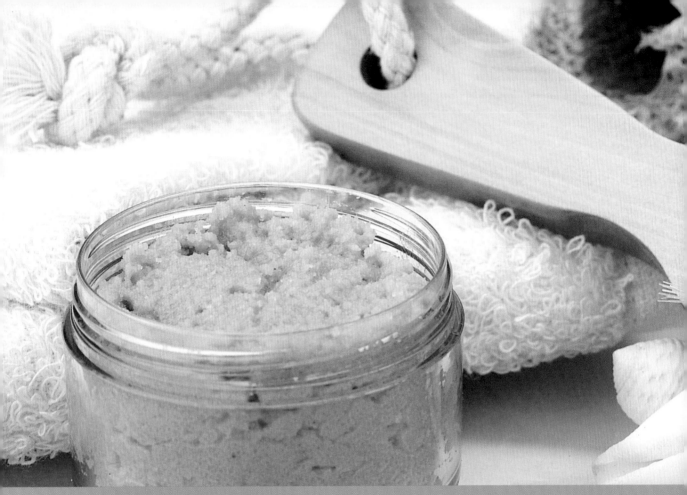

Exfoliating scrub

Include regular exfoliating – the removal of dead skin cells – in your beauty routine to encourage cell renewal and develop a better skin tone. This scrub is full of natural goodness.

It is easy to forget that regular use of soap and water has a drying effect on the face. In order to soften and refresh the skin, you should use a facial exfoliating scrub once or twice a week.

Making your own scrub minimises the risk of unwanted reactions to synthetic or highly perfumed products.

Exfoliation takes away the top layer of dead skin cells and stimulates the lymphatic drainage system, helping to remove toxins and promoting circulation in your face.

The result is a healthy, glowing appearance and a clear improvement in the condition of the skin. This scrub will last for up to two months if stored in an airtight jar.

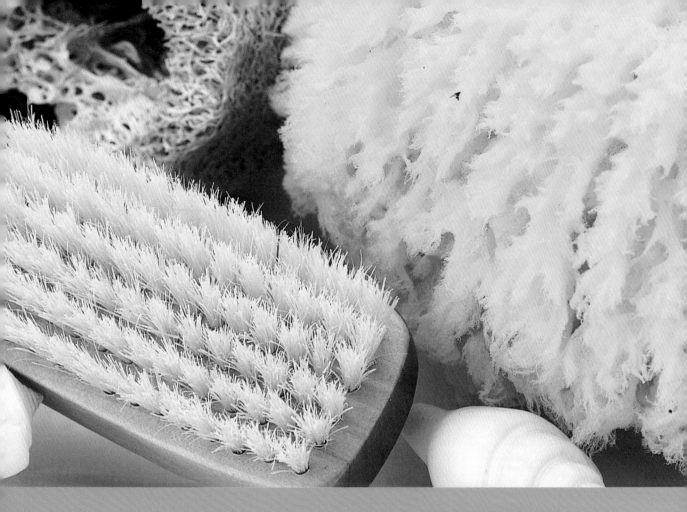

How to make an exfoliating scrub
Makes one 40g (1½oz) jar

▼ Grind **1 tablespoon of kaolin** and **2 tablespoons of ground rice** to a fine powder using a pestle and mortar.

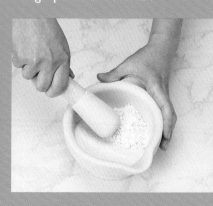

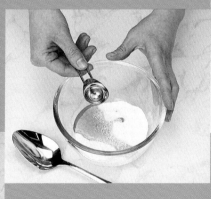

▲ Warm **1 tablespoon of clear honey**, then add it to the kaolin mixture together with **1 teaspoon of orange floral water**. Blend thoroughly with a metal spoon.

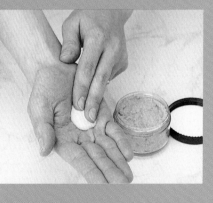

▲ Add **1 drop each of geranium oil** and **juniper oil**. Mix the scrub with a few drops of water in the palm of your hand and massage it into the skin using circular movements. Rinse afterwards.

Cleansing and toning greasy, problem skin

Oily skin is characteristically shiny and thick with large pores that tend to become clogged due to over-production of sebum. This frequently causes skin blemishes such as blackheads and spots.

Well chosen skin-care products can help to tighten pores and regulate sebum production. Frequent cleansing and toning are important if you have oily skin. Equally, use only gentle products that will not stimulate the excess production of sebum.

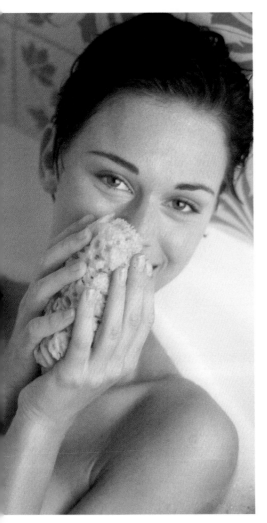

SAGE TONER

Rosemary helps to clean blocked pores, while the sage acts as an antiseptic to protect the skin.

4 drops rosemary oil
4 teaspoons sage tincture
75ml (2½fl oz) witch hazel

Mix the rosemary oil with the sage tincture, then add the witch hazel. Store the toner in a dark glass bottle with a stopper. Pour a few drops of the toner onto a moistened cotton-wool pad and gently wipe it over your face.

FACE CREAM WITH YARROW

Yarrow is a strong antiseptic which helps reduce spots and blackheads. Orange floral water can regulate the production of sebum.

100ml (3½fl oz) water
15g (½oz) dried yarrow tops
30ml (1fl oz) orange floral water
100g (3½oz) cream base

Heat the water and yarrow in a pan and boil for 3 minutes. Cover and leave to cool. Strain the liquid, mix with the orange floral water and slowly fold in the cream base. Transfer to a pot with a lid and store in a cool place.

Careful cleansing Always wash around your nose and mouth with a sponge or face flannel as these areas quickly become greasy.

ALMOND CLEANSING MILK

Cleanse your face with this paste every night to remove make-up, grime and dust particles.

115g (4oz) ground almonds
125ml (4fl oz) full-fat milk
1 tablespoon almond oil

Blend all the ingredients and apply the lotion immediately, avoiding the sensitive eye area. Massage over the face in a circular motion and rinse with lukewarm water.

PEPPERMINT FACE LOTION

Peppermint improves circulation and cleans and tightens the pores.

250ml (9fl oz) water
25g (1oz) dried peppermint flowers and leaves
50ml (2fl oz) witch hazel

Place the water and peppermint in a pan and simmer for 15 minutes. When cool, strain the liquid. Stir in the witch hazel and pour the lotion into a dark bottle. Seal, shake and store in a cool place.

Take care

Do not use rosemary essential oil if you are pregnant, have high blood pressure or suffer from epilepsy. Essential oils are potent substances and can be harmful. Consult a qualified aromatherapist for advice.

Tried & Trusted

Toning oily skin

- Oily skin with enlarged pores benefits from being rubbed with a slice of lemon, but no more than once a week. The acid tightens the pores.

- Make an effective toner for oily skin with 6 drops of bergamot oil, 4 drops of lavender oil and 50ml (2fl oz) of purified water.

Masks galore

- For enlarged pores, you can also try a mask made from 3 tablespoons of wheatgerm and 3 tablespoons of yoghurt. Blend them together and smooth onto your face and neck. Leave to dry for about 25 minutes, then wash off with warm water.

- Peel and grate an apple. Mix it with 1 tablespoon of honey, or mix 2 tablespoons of wheatgerm with 2 tablespoons of buttermilk. Apply to the face and leave for 20 minutes.

- For a natural anti-wrinkle mask, make an infusion of 250ml (9fl oz) water and 1 tablespoon of dried mallow flowers. Leave for 30 minutes, then strain. Fold 3 tablespoons of the infusion into a stiffly beaten egg white. Apply the paste to your face and rinse after 20 minutes.

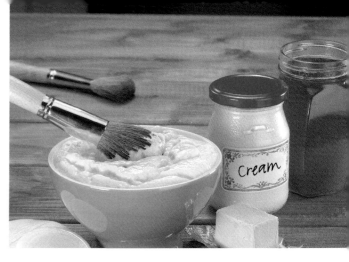

Full of nourishment
Brewer's yeast is full of B vitamins and has been used for generations to combat oily skin. Blend it with cream and honey to make a fabulous face mask.

ORANGE FACE MASK FOR OILY SKIN

Only freshly squeezed orange juice should be used.

juice of ½ orange
8 tablespoons flour

Squeeze the orange juice into a small bowl and stir in enough flour to make a thick paste. Apply the face mask with a soft brush after cleansing and leave on for 20 minutes. Wash off with plenty of warm water.

CREAM AND YEAST MASK

Use this mask to purify your skin. Yeast helps to dry the skin, while cream and honey soften it.

15g (½oz) brewer's yeast
4 teaspoons cream
2 teaspoons honey

Crumble the yeast and blend it with the cream to make a paste. Stir in the honey. Dampen your face with water, then apply the mask to your face and neck. Leave for 20 minutes and rinse off with plenty of warm water.

STEAM FACIAL

The steam opens the pores and helps to cleanse your skin.

2-3 handfuls dried peppermint leaves
5 litres (8¾ pints) water

Place the herbs in a heatproof bowl. Boil the water and pour it over them. Drape a towel over your head and bend over the bowl to soak up the steam. After 15 minutes, wipe your face with a flannel, then rinse with cold water.

HERB COMPRESS

This compress will soften, cleanse and tighten your pores.

2 litres (3½ pints) water
2 handfuls fresh rosemary flowers and leaves

Put the herbs in a heatproof bowl. Boil the water and pour it over them. Leave to infuse for 10 minutes, then strain the liquid. Dip a clean square of muslin into the liquid, squeeze out the excess and place it over your face. Leave for 5-10 minutes, then rinse.

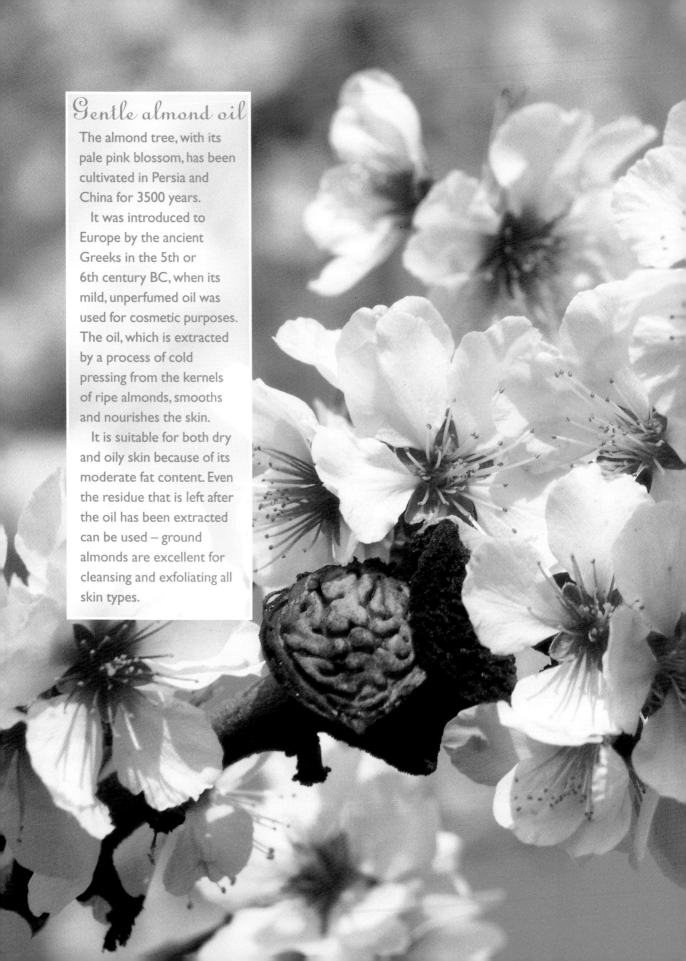

Gentle almond oil

The almond tree, with its pale pink blossom, has been cultivated in Persia and China for 3500 years.

It was introduced to Europe by the ancient Greeks in the 5th or 6th century BC, when its mild, unperfumed oil was used for cosmetic purposes. The oil, which is extracted by a process of cold pressing from the kernels of ripe almonds, smooths and nourishes the skin.

It is suitable for both dry and oily skin because of its moderate fat content. Even the residue that is left after the oil has been extracted can be used – ground almonds are excellent for cleansing and exfoliating all skin types.

Caring for and cleansing dry, sensitive skin

The sebaceous glands in dry skin do not produce enough sebum, so the skin feels tight and is prone to unsightly scaly patches.

Although thin, fine-pored skin looks fragile, it feels rough and tends to flake. It is very sensitive to weather and air pollution. It tends to age early and in later life is often ruddy and marked with burst blood vessels.

Protective barrier

Cosmetic products for dry skin aim to improve sebum production and protect and moisturise the skin. If you have dry skin, it is important to use a rich skin cream during the day and also at night when the cells are regenerating.

CAMOMILE AND GERANIUM ESSENTIAL OIL CREAM

Camomile and geranium oil will improve the texture of dry skin.

25g (1oz) lanolin
25g (1oz) petroleum jelly
3 drops camomile oil
3 drops geranium oil

Combine the lanolin and petroleum jelly in a bowl, add the oils and stir until thick and creamy. Transfer to a small pot with a lid and store in a cool place.

JOJOBA CREAM

Native Americans traditionally used oil from the seeds of the desert plant *Simmondsia chinensis* (jojoba) for medicinal purposes.

1 teaspoon beeswax granules
2 teaspoons lanolin
½ teaspoon cocoa butter
30ml (1fl oz) jojoba oil
40ml (1½fl oz) orange floral water
3 drops neroli oil

Melt the beeswax, lanolin and cocoa butter in a bowl set over a pan of simmering water. Add the jojoba oil and heat to 60°C (140°F). Heat the orange floral water in a separate pan to the same temperature, then mix it with the fats, using a hand-blender on a low setting. When hand hot, add the neroli oil and whisk until cool. Store in a sealed jar in a cool place.

TONER FOR SENSITIVE DRY SKIN

After washing, freshen your face with this stimulating toner.

85ml (3fl oz) rosewater
2 teaspoons marigold tincture

Mix the rosewater and marigold tincture in a dark glass bottle. Seal the bottle, shake well, then store in a cool place. After cleansing your skin, gently dab a little of the toner onto your face and neck with a cotton-wool pad.

ALMOND AND AVOCADO OIL CLEANSING MILK

Almond and avocado oils have a consistency similar to the skin's natural oil. They therefore make an effective cleansing treatment.

100ml (3½fl oz) rosewater
1 tablespoon honey
15g (½oz) dried milk powder
4 teaspoons almond oil
4 teaspoons avocado oil

Warm the rosewater in a pan, dissolve the honey and milk powder in it, then add the oils. Pour into a dark glass bottle, seal and shake thoroughly. Store the cleansing milk in the fridge. Massage the milk into your face and neck twice a day. Remove the residue with damp cotton wool.

CUCUMBER LOTION FOR TIRED SKIN

The combination of cool cucumber and vitamin-rich carrot juices creates a refreshing lotion.

½ cucumber
30ml (1fl oz) almond oil
50ml (2fl oz) carrot juice
juice of ½ lemon

Peel and finely grate the cucumber, then squeeze out the juice through a clean muslin cloth. Mix the ingredients, then pour them into a dark bottle with a stopper. Store in a cool place. Shake before use, then apply the lotion with a moistened cotton-wool pad.

Making the most of mature skin

The skin shows signs of ageing, just like other parts of the body. Lines develop as the tissue loses elasticity.

Mature skin needs more care than younger skin. Rich night creams are beneficial since they stimulate the natural process of regeneration. Valuable plant oils can help to make the skin smooth and elastic. Other natural and traditional treatments can make fine lines less visible and firm facial contours.

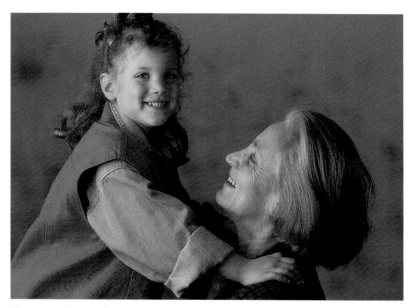

Natural radiance Beauty is not a question of age. Laughter lines, for example, can make a face more expressive and attractive.

NOURISHING OIL FOR AGEING SKIN

Wheatgerm oil is rich in vitamin E which helps guard against ageing.

50ml (2fl oz) almond oil
1 teaspoon wheatgerm oil
15 drops lavender oil
10 drops frankincense oil
3 drops neroli oil

Combine the oils in a dark glass bottle with a stopper, seal and shake. After washing, gently massage the oil into your face.

OIL COMPRESS

A weekly oil compress can regenerate slack neck skin.

3 teaspoons wheatgerm oil
3 teaspoons honey

Warm and blend the oil and honey. Paint the mixture over your neck with a soft brush. Cover with a damp towel and leave for an hour. Do not wash off.

FACE LOTION WITH HOPS

This is a real rejuvenating tonic. Hops are used in cosmetic products for stressed, inelastic skin.

25g (1oz) dried hop flowers
200ml (7fl oz) water
40ml (1½fl oz) rosewater
**30ml (1fl oz) isopropyl
    alcohol**

Simmer the hops in the water for 15 minutes. Cover and leave to cool. Strain the liquid through a fine sieve, then pour it into a dark glass bottle with a stopper. Add the other ingredients, seal and shake thoroughly. Store in a cool place.

After cleansing, pour a few drops of the lotion on a moistened cotton-wool pad and gently dab it onto your face.

CUCUMBER CLEANSING MILK

This refreshing, firming cleanser removes the day's grime from mature skin, before other creams are applied.

½ cucumber
40ml (1½fl oz) rosewater
30ml (1fl oz) glycerine

Peel and finely grate the cucumber, then squeeze the juice through a clean muslin cloth. Pour it into a dark glass bottle with the other ingredients and seal. Shake vigorously and store in a cool place. Use within a week.

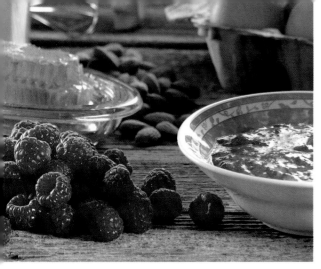

Raspberry reviver
Fresh fruits contain vitamins A and C, as well as pectin – a natural coagulant. They make a refreshing face mask that is guaranteed to revive tired skin.

- **Comfrey keeps the skin looking youthful. Put 2 teaspoons of chopped dried comfrey root in 250ml (9fl oz) of cold water, bring to the boil and simmer for 15 minutes. Strain the liquid, then add 1 tablespoon of the infusion to any face mask.**

- **For a quick moisturiser, peel and grate three raw potatoes and spread the pulp on your face. Wash off after 20 minutes.**

- **Help to prevent your neck skin from sagging by including the skin around your throat in all facial treatments. As the skin on the neck is thicker than facial skin, it responds to richer preparations.**

- **When combined with vitamin C, vitamin E fends off free radicals which damage the skin's protective coating and cause premature ageing. Ensure your diet contains sufficient vitamin E – one good source is cold-pressed wheatgerm or avocado oil.**

FIRMING RASPBERRY MASK

Slack, tired skin can become beautifully firm and smooth again with the help of this mask.

100g (3½oz) fresh raspberries
15g (½oz) ground almonds
15g (½oz) honey
1 egg yolk

Mash the fruit and mix it with the other ingredients. Smooth the paste over your face and neck and leave for at least 30 minutes. Rinse off with lukewarm water.

BORAGE COMPRESS

This compress can also be made with horsetail. It gives ageing facial skin a real boost.

2 handfuls fresh borage leaves
2 litres (3½ pints) water

Place the borage in a heatproof bowl. Boil the water and pour it over the herb. Leave to infuse for 10 minutes. Strain the liquid, then soak a piece of muslin in the warm infusion. Place the cloth on your face and relax for 5 minutes.

Exercising to keep fit

Regular exercise is now recognised as being essential to staying fit and healthy. But it was very different in our grandparents' day. Until the 1890s, when the development of the bicycle made cycling possible, women were discouraged from any form of physical activity.

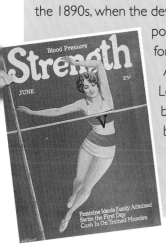

All this changed in 1930 when The Women's League of Health and Beauty was founded by Mollie Bagot Stack with the aim of bringing exercise and 'figure training' to the masses. Within three months of opening the first class in central London, the League had over a thousand members.

Don't despair of freckles

Even as late as the 1930s, most people, especially young girls, hated the freckles on their faces. Nowadays, they are not considered a blemish but some people, like our grandmothers, would still rather be without them.

The remedies on this page were designed to fade freckles and may be fun to try – they certainly won't cause any skin damage as they all use natural ingredients.

Freckles are actually deposits of a pigment called melanin. Most people, especially those with dark skin, produce adequate amounts of melanin in the surface tissues of the skin. Those with fairer, sensitive skin produce less melanin and are more at risk from the sun.

So freckles serve as a warning that you will need extra protection against the sun's harmful rays and should use a high factor sun cream.

Natural plant power Dandelions have many medicinal uses. Made into a rinse they can make the skin fairer and help freckles fade.

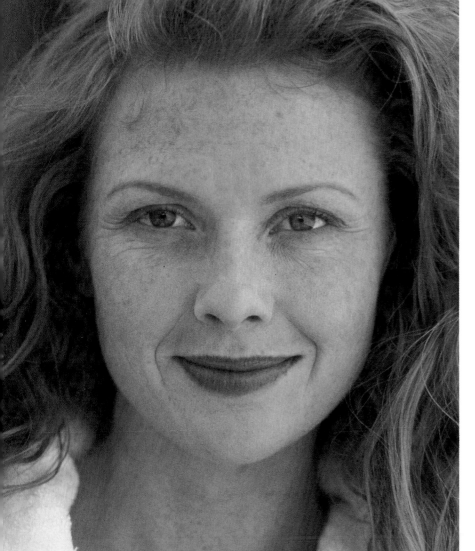

LEMON AND GLYCERINE ANTI-FRECKLE LOTION

Every night after cleansing, put a few drops of this lotion on a cotton-wool pad and dab it on your freckles.

75ml (2½fl oz) isopropyl
   alcohol
75ml (2½fl oz) glycerine
250g (9oz) honey
juice of 1 lemon

Blend the alcohol with the glycerine, then stir in the honey and freshly squeezed lemon juice. Pour the mixture into a dark bottle and seal. Shake the bottle before using the lotion.

DANDELION RINSE

Wash your face twice a day with this infusion to help freckles fade.

55g (2oz) dried dandelion
   flowers
1 litre (1¾ pints) water

Place the flowers and water in a pan, cover and simmer for 30 minutes. Strain the liquid into a dark glass bottle and seal.

Take care

Even in moderate climates, exposure to the sun damages and dries out the skin, speeding up the signs of ageing. The face, neck and hands are most at risk, because they are most exposed.

Combating spots and unsightly blackheads

Spots, pimples and blackheads occur when pores become inflamed and infected as a result of being clogged with thickened sebum. Keeping a 'spot-less' complexion depends on thorough cleansing and meticulous hygiene.

People with oily or combination skin are most susceptible to spots. Recipes for oily skin can also be used to treat blackheads, especially cleansers and toners.

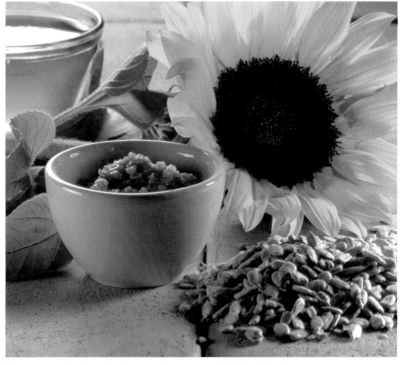

Sunny complexion You have to be patient with blemished skin. If you regularly apply a sunflower mask, your complexion should visibly improve over time.

MARIGOLD CREAM

Marigolds are easy to grow in the garden or in a window box. This cleansing cream will help to heal inflamed spots.

15g (½oz) dried marigold flowers
100ml (3½fl oz) water
4 teaspoons almond oil
100g (3½oz) cream base

Place the flowers in a heatproof bowl. Pour the water into a saucepan and bring to the boil. Pour it over the flowers. Cover the bowl with a cloth or plate and leave to infuse until cool.

Strain the liquid through a fine sieve into a clean bowl. Add the almond oil. Fold in the cream base and transfer the lotion to a small pot with a lid.

After washing, apply the cream sparingly to your skin with your fingertips or a moistened cotton-wool pad. Leave for a few minutes to soothe the inflamed skin, then wash off.

SUNFLOWER MASK

Sunflower seeds are rich in lecithin which benefits cell growth.

1 handful dried sunflower seeds
1 teaspoon honey
1 teaspoon vegetable carrier oil

Grind the seeds in a coffee grinder. Warm the honey in a bowl over a pan of boiling water. Take off the heat, then add the oil and ground seeds to make a paste. Add a little hot water if it is too solid. Wash your face, then smooth the mask evenly over your face and neck. Leave for 30 minutes, then rinse.

ORANGE-KAOLIN MASK

Kaolin promotes good circulation in the skin and destroys bacteria. Vitamin C from oranges helps to purify the pores.

3 teaspoons orange juice
2 teaspoons kaolin

Mix the freshly squeezed orange juice and kaolin in a small bowl to make a smooth paste. Wash your face, then apply the mask to the skin and leave for 15 minutes. Rinse off with lukewarm water.

Tried & Trusted
Clear skin

- To help clear blackheads, rub your face with a slice of raw potato after cleansing.

- Get rid of the odd spot by dabbing it with a little thyme oil. Repeat two to three times a day, avoiding the eyes.

- Skin blemishes heal more quickly if you dab them with a little lemon juice or a piece of freshly cut garlic.

- For a steam facial, put two handfuls of anti-inflammatory herbs, such as eucalyptus, sage or camomile, in a basin. Pour 3 litres (5¼ pints) of boiling water over the herb. Drape a towel over your head and bend over the bowl to soak up the steam. Steam your face for 10 minutes.

- Australian Aborigines have dabbed tea tree oil on infected skin for generations.

Irritated, red skin

- For gentle cleansing, moisten cotton wool with a little buttermilk and wipe it over your face and neck.

- Wash your face morning and night with anemone and horsetail infusion. To make this, infuse 140g (5oz) of each dried herb in 600ml (1 pint) boiling water. Leave for 10 minutes, then strain and add to your washing water.

Soothing sensitive and irritated skin

Sensitive skin can easily become tight due to changes in the weather, as a reaction to cosmetic products or because of stress. Small broken blood vessels and red patches often appear on the cheeks and nose.

The most important thing for patchy, irritated skin is soothing care. Applying a paste or mask will stop the irritation and have a calming effect.

CAMOMILE LOTION

If your skin develops reddish patches, perhaps because you are stressed, treat it with this toner.

250ml (9fl oz) water
25g (1oz) dried camomile flowers
5 teaspoons lemon juice
40ml (1½fl oz) rosewater

Heat the water in a pan with the flowers and simmer for 3 minutes. Cover and leave to cool. Strain the liquid through a fine sieve. Stir in the lemon juice and rosewater, then pour it into a dark glass bottle with a stopper. After washing, pour a few drops of the lotion onto a moistened cotton-wool pad and gently wipe your face and neck.

Deep clean If your skin is susceptible to blemishes, have a weekly steam facial to keep spots at bay.

WILD STRAWBERRY PASTE

Combat little dilated blood vessels around the nose and on the cheeks with an effective paste made from the fresh leaves of wild strawberries.

1 handful fresh wild strawberry leaves
few drops boiling water

Crush the leaves and blend them into a paste with a little boiling water. Apply the paste to your skin and leave for a few minutes. Rinse off with lukewarm water.

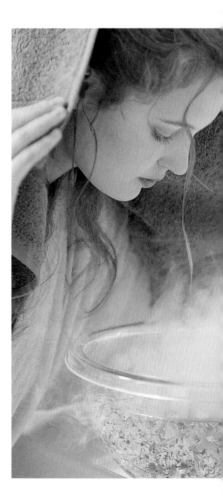

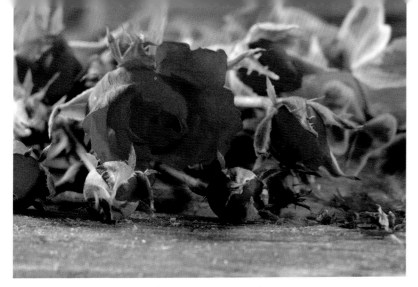

Smoothing gel Combine rosebuds, ivy leaves, cornflowers and linseed in a gentle gel for the delicate area around the eyes.

Keeping the sparkle in your eyes

For bright, youthful eyes you need a regular beauty regime coupled with plenty of sleep, fresh air and a balanced diet. Your eyes really do reflect your general state of health.

You should pay special attention to the delicate skin around your eyes. Start your eye care from an early age – don't wait for the first wrinkles to show. Regular eye treatment in the morning and evening should be part of your beauty routine.

ANTI-WRINKLE EYE CREAM

Try this simple, old-fashioned remedy for smoothing away lines and crow's feet around the eyes.

few drops almond oil
small quantity of lanolin

Blend a few drops of almond oil with a little lanolin. Apply regularly to the area beneath the eyes before going to bed.

FIRMING IVY LOTION

This mild gel firms the skin of the eye area and reduces puffiness.

25g (1oz) dried rosebuds
2 tablespoons dried ivy leaves
1 tablespoon dried cornflowers
125ml (4fl oz) water
40ml (1½fl oz) rosewater
1 tablespoon linseed

Place the rosebuds, ivy leaves and cornflowers in a heatproof bowl. Boil the water and pour it over them. Leave to infuse for 2 hours. Strain the liquid.

Meanwhile, heat the rosewater in a bowl set over a pan of boiling water. Pour it onto the linseed and leave to soak for 2 hours. Strain the liquid through a fine sieve.

Combine both mixtures and pour into a dark glass bottle with a stopper. Store in a cool place. After cleansing your face, pat the lotion on your eyelids and then apply anti-wrinkle eye cream (left).

Anti-ageing cream

Keep your skin soft and supple as the years go by. This anti-ageing cream can help to minimise advancing lines and wrinkles.

From the age of 50, most skin shows signs of the inevitable ageing process. The elastin fibres start to decline, leading to a loss of tone and eventually to sagging.

The collagen fibres that support the skin also lose strength, resulting in lines and wrinkles. A great deal of damage to the collagen fibres is due to over-exposure to ultraviolet light and free radical activity.

You can help your skin by using a protective facial sun screen, and by using moisturisers with vitamin E – an effective antioxidant.

To make the marshmallow infusion used in the recipe below, soak 25g (1oz) of chopped dried marshmallow root in 150ml (5fl oz) water for two hours. Place in a pan and simmer gently for 5 minutes. Cool, then strain the liquid.

How to make anti-ageing cream
Makes one 40g (1½oz) pot

▼ Dissolve **½ teaspoon of borax** in **2 tablespoons of marshmallow infusion** (see above).

▲ Put **1 tablespoon of avocado oil, 2 tablespoons of almond oil, 1 teaspoon of cocoa butter** and **1 teaspoon of beeswax granules** in a bowl set over a saucepan of simmering water. Heat gently until the wax melts.

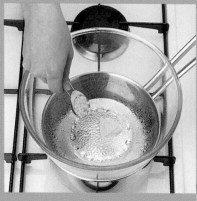

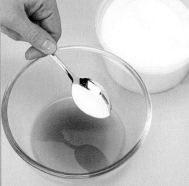

▲ Slowly add the infusion to the oils, stirring continuously. Once cooled, add **5 drops each of sandalwood oil** and **bergapten-free or rectified bergamot oil**. Store the cream in a dark glass pot in the refrigerator. It will keep for up to two months.

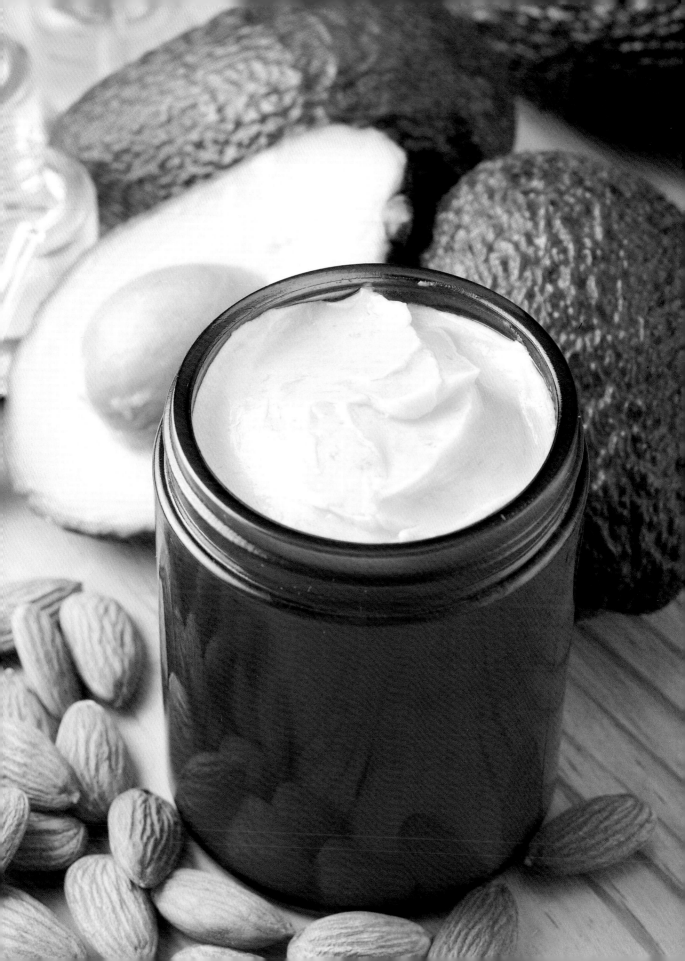

Beautiful soft lips

Good oral hygiene should be a number one priority. But you don't need to rely solely on commercial toothpastes and mouthwashes for perfect results. Mix your own natural preparations.

A radiant smile that shows soft, delicate lips and flawless, healthy teeth – plus fresh breath – are great assets to your looks.

It is essential to look after your teeth and lips as part of your daily body-care routine, both in order to look attractive and for your general well-being. Teeth problems can cause ill health throughout the body and any ailment which affects the mouth, from ulcers to cracked lips, is most unpleasant.

There are many toothpastes and mouthwashes on the market today, but traditional methods of cleaning your teeth and gums using natural ingredients can also play a positive role in achieving quality oral and dental hygiene.

Strong, healthy teeth

Most of us are blessed with healthy teeth and gums and it is up to us to keep them that way. The greatest damage to teeth is the result of tooth decay caused by bacteria and receding gums. Both can be very painful and can lead sooner or later to fillings or even the loss of one or more teeth. But it doesn't have to come to that.

Lifelong companions

With proper care and a healthy diet you can keep your own teeth well into old age. Visit the dentist twice a year. Use a toothbrush with synthetic bristles and renew it every three months.

Clean your teeth for at least 2-3 minutes after every meal, massaging the gums at the same time. Try a natural toothpaste and a herbal mouthwash for tingling clean mouth and gums.

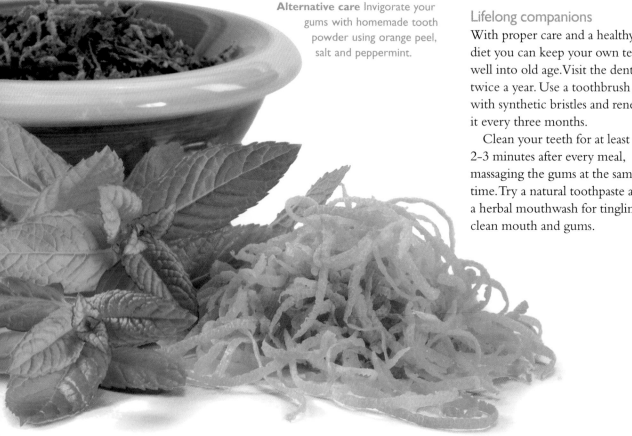

Alternative care Invigorate your gums with homemade tooth powder using orange peel, salt and peppermint.

and white teeth

Soft lips and fresh breath for a winning smile

Your lips have extremely soft skin which cannot secrete its own oil. Lips are therefore very sensitive to wind, cold and strong sunlight. Apply a natural balm several times a day to provide your lips with oil and moisture, to protect them from the weather and to make them full and smooth.

Cracked lips can be a symptom of fever or a bad cold. To avoid cracked lips at any time keep up your liquid intake. Try to drink 2 litres (3½ pints) of mineral water each day.

Healthy teeth A balanced diet with plenty of vitamin C is just as important to dental hygiene as regularly brushing.

ORANGE AND PEPPERMINT TOOTH POWDER

This effective tooth powder will strengthen your gums and is useful if they have begun to recede.

40g (1½oz) unwaxed orange peel
25g (1oz) dried peppermint leaves
2 teaspoons sea salt

Finely grate the skin of an orange and leave the peel to dry overnight. Crush the peppermint in a pestle and mortar, then add it with the salt to the peel. Put the mixture in a screw-top jar. Dampen your toothbrush, then dip it in the powder before brushing.

Earlier tooth care

Previous generations had ideas about oral hygiene that seem strange today. Ancient Egyptians used twigs to clean their teeth while the Romans used their own urine as toothpaste. The ammonia content in the urine would have acted as a bleach.

LEMON TOOTHPASTE

The combination of ingredients in this toothpaste is the result of centuries of herbal wisdom.

Lemon strengthens the gums and removes brown deposits from the teeth. Sage and cinnamon oil have an antiseptic effect. Orris root relieves pain – in the past teething babies were given it to chew.

1 lemon
1 teaspoon fresh sage leaves
1 teaspoon orris root powder
½ teaspoon cinnamon oil
1 tablespoon purified water

Mash the flesh of the lemon and chop the sage leaves. Mix them in a bowl with the orris root and cinnamon oil. Stir in the water to make a paste. Transfer to a jar and seal. This will keep for one year.

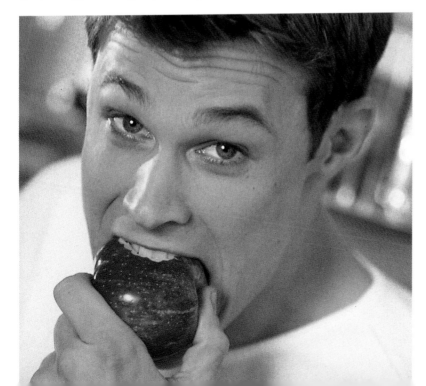

BLACKCURRANT LEAF MOUTHWASH

This mixture used to be given to children to gargle when they had a sore throat. It helps to combat mouth and throat infections.

**1 handful fresh
  blackcurrant leaves
500ml (18fl oz) water
2 teaspoons lemon juice**

Place the blackcurrant leaves and water in a pan. Boil uncovered until half the water has evaporated. Add the freshly squeezed lemon juice, then strain through a fine sieve. Add 2 teaspoons of the mixture to a glass of water and rinse your mouth.

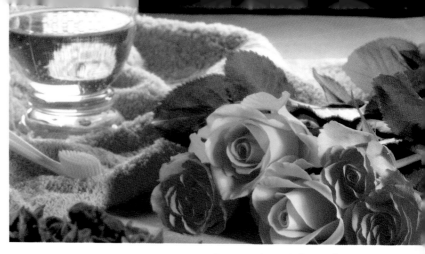

Fragrant breath A mouth rinse with rosewater and aniseed is very refreshing first thing in the morning.

SAGE MOUTHWASH

Sage helps to heal and strengthen bleeding gums.

**6 fresh sage leaves
500ml (18fl oz) water
pinch of salt**

Finely chop the sage leaves and place them in a heatproof bowl. Pour the water and salt into a pan and boil. Pour the boiling water over the sage and leave to cool. Strain the liquid through a fine sieve. After brushing your teeth, use the mouthwash as a gargle.

LIQUORICE AND WINE RINSE

This rinse will freshen bad breath caused by an upset stomach.

**100g (3½oz) dried
  liquorice root
1 litre (1¾ pints) white wine**

Cut the liquorice root into pieces, place in a bowl with the white wine and leave to infuse for ten days. Strain the liquid into a sterilised glass bottle and seal. Add 1 teaspoon of the rinse to a glass of water for a mouthwash.

ANISEED MOUTHWASH

Gargle with this refreshing mouthwash when you have eaten antisocial food, such as garlic or onions. Do not drink this mixture.

**2 tablespoons aniseed
100ml (3½fl oz) water
40ml (1½fl oz) vodka
50ml (2fl oz) rosewater**

Place the aniseed in a heatproof bowl. Boil the water and pour it over, then cover and leave to cool. Strain the liquid through a filter paper. Mix with the vodka and rosewater, then pour it into a dark glass bottle with a stopper and shake vigorously.

  After brushing your teeth, pour a few drops of the mouthwash into a glass of water and rinse your mouth and throat.

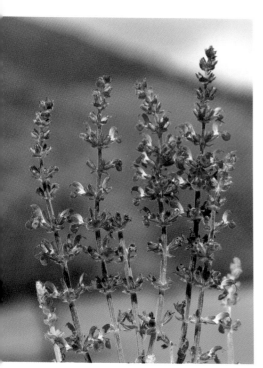

Healing plant The Romans regarded sage as a sacred plant because of its curative powers. As a mouthwash, it is a useful remedy for inflammation of the gums and throat.

HONEY LIP BALM

This natural balm prevents sensitive lips from drying out, keeping them soft and smooth.

2 teaspoons beeswax granules
30ml (1fl oz) jojoba oil
1 teaspoon honey

Heat the wax and oil in a bowl set over a pan of simmering water until they melt into a clear liquid. Heat the honey to 30°C (86°F). Add the honey to the wax mixture and leave to cool, stirring continuously. Pour the balm into a small glass screw-top jar.

LIP GLOSS

This rosewater lip gloss will give your lips a silky sheen, and protect them from the weather.

2 teaspoons beeswax
   granules
1 teaspoon rosewater
1 teaspoon grapeseed oil
2 teaspoons almond oil

Put the wax in a bowl and melt as for Honey lip balm (above). Remove from the heat and stir in the rosewater and oils. Allow the mixture to cool, then transfer it to a small glass jar with a lid.

Tried & Trusted
White teeth
- To ensure you have white teeth and firm gums, rub them with the inside of a piece of lemon peel.

- Remove nicotine stains from your teeth by brushing them once a week with salt. Even better, give up smoking.

Dental care
- Sugar, sweets and sugary drinks damage the teeth in many ways: they take vital calcium from the body and are the main cause of tooth decay. Try to see them as treats rather than eating them on a regular basis. And where possible, eat them as part of a meal, as our grandparents did.

- If you don't have the opportunity to brush your teeth after each meal, chew some sugar-free gum or eat a little fresh fruit, raw vegetables or cheese.

- To get rid of the smell of garlic on your breath, chew fresh parsley or aniseed.

- Use dental floss as part of your daily routine to help remove food remnants from between your teeth. Move the floss gently and carefully to and fro, at the same time gliding it under the edges of the gums.

Beautiful lips
- To keep the skin over your lips soft, gently massage it each morning with a soft toothbrush.

- Rough, chapped lips can be softened by rubbing them with softened cocoa butter or honey.

- Soothe cracked lips with a slice of fresh cucumber, cream or unsalted butter.

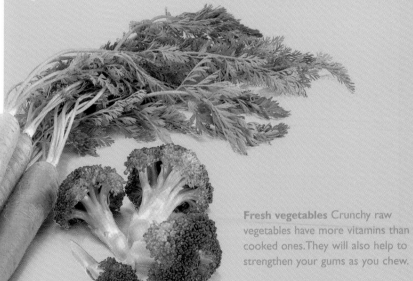

Fresh vegetables Crunchy raw vegetables have more vitamins than cooked ones. They will also help to strengthen your gums as you chew.

Hand and foot care

The condition of our hands and feet speaks volumes about the value we place on caring for ourselves. And a little cosmetic pampering can make a big difference to the way we feel.

Day in, day out our hands and feet are hard at work. Our hands are in constant use, often exposed without protection to extremes of weather or immersed in detergents and household chemicals. These strip out the hands' natural moisture.

Housework damages delicate skin and makes nails brittle, while stress also affects the way our hands look. They are the true mirror of a person's age because we can do little to repair the ravages of time if we haven't cared for our hands as the years go by. Regular care is essential to keep hands looking youthful and smooth, and nails healthy and strong.

The same applies to feet, which carry the bulk of our weight every day and are too often treated carelessly. Fortunately, there is no shortage of effective recipes to refresh tired feet and soothe chapped hands. Nature provides us with everything we need for their care and nourishment.

All-revealing hands

A person's touch, when you first shake hands with them, or when you hold hands, is very telling. Take care of your hands so they feel soft and look well groomed.

Soft to the touch

In addition to housework or gardening, frequent washing makes hands rough and dry. To minimise the risk of chapping, wear rubber gloves for household chores, and always use a mild soap and dry your hands well.

The delicate skin on the back of the hands, in particular, needs to be moisturised and nourished every time you wash. Cracked skin and chapped hands need extra care to protect them from daily damage.

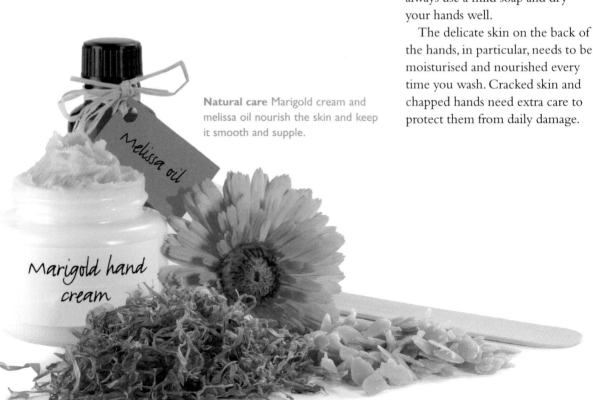

Natural care Marigold cream and melissa oil nourish the skin and keep it smooth and supple.

melissa oil

Marigold hand cream

NOURISHING LAVENDER HAND CREAM

Chapped, hard-working hands will benefit from the healing properties of this cream.

3 tablespoons beeswax granules
4 tablespoons almond oil
4 tablespoons coconut oil
6 tablespoons glycerine
6 drops lavender oil

Mix the beeswax granules with the almond and coconut oils in a bowl and place over a pan of simmering water until the wax melts. Stir thoroughly, then add the glycerine, drop by drop.

Remove the mixture from the heat and continue stirring until its texture becomes creamy. Stir in the lavender oil and transfer to a small pot with a lid. Seal and store in a cool place.

MOISTURISING NIGHT CREAM FOR HANDS

This cream is an ideal remedy for dry hands. Massage it into your skin before going to bed.

55g (2oz) honey
115g (4oz) lanolin
50ml (2fl oz) almond oil

Warm the honey in a bowl over a pan of boiling water, then stir in the lanolin. When the mixture is cool, stir in the almond oil and transfer it to a pot with a lid.

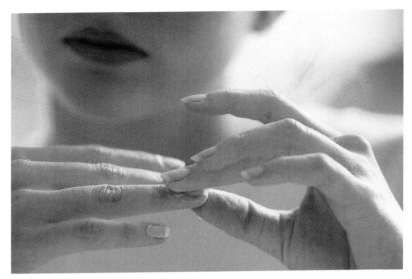

Extra care When applying hand cream, massage it carefully into the cuticles to keep them soft and supple.

MARIGOLD HAND CREAM

Marigold helps to make rough skin smooth and supple once more.

1 handful dried marigold flowers
100ml (3½fl oz) olive oil
15g (½oz) beeswax granules
4 drops melissa oil
or
4 drops lemon oil

Place the flowers and olive oil in a pan and simmer for 20 minutes. Strain the liquid through a fine sieve into a heatproof bowl.

Place the bowl over a pan of simmering water, then add the beeswax. When the wax has melted, take the pan off the heat and beat the mixture until it forms a creamy paste. Stir in the melissa or lemon oil. Transfer to a pot with a lid and store in a cool place.

MARSHMALLOW HAND GEL

Soften red and rough hands by gently massaging in some marshmallow gel after washing.

15g (½oz) dried marshmallow root
25g (1oz) dried marshmallow leaves
200ml (7fl oz) water
140ml (4½fl oz) witch hazel
15g (½oz) agar

Chop the root and place it with the leaves in a pan. Add the water and leave to soak for 4 hours. Bring to the boil and simmer gently for 10 minutes, stirring. You might have to add a little more water.

Strain through a sieve and press out the residue with the back of a wooden spoon. Heat the witch hazel in a bowl set over a pan of boiling water and slowly stir in the agar. Add the marshmallow lotion and stir. Transfer to a jar with a lid.

Well groomed – right to the fingertips

However naturally beautiful your hands may be, their appearance can be marred by torn cuticles and brittle nails. For healthy nails you need a diet that contains plenty of protein, vitamins and trace elements, such as zinc and iodine.

Problems, such as brittle nails, are sometimes due to a vitamin A deficiency; hangnails (torn dead skin at the side of the nail) can be a sign of too little folic acid.

There are plenty of tips and easy beauty treatments to keep nails healthy and looking good. These include natural treatments for strong nails and soft, untorn cuticles, which can also be used to pamper your toenails when you have a pedicure.

If you follow this beauty routine regularly and pay attention to your hands and nails, they will stay in tip top condition.

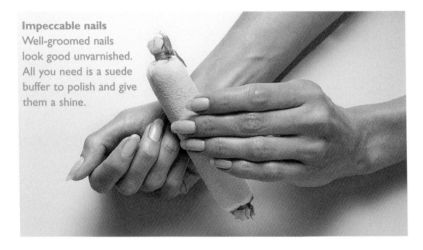

Impeccable nails
Well-groomed nails look good unvarnished. All you need is a suede buffer to polish and give them a shine.

CORNFLOUR PASTE FOR SWOLLEN HANDS

This traditional balm for swollen hands is sheer bliss.

55g (2oz) cornflour
85g (3oz) bran
few drops purified water

Blend the cornflour and bran with the purified water to make a thick paste. Smooth it onto your hands and leave on for 15 minutes. Place your hands alternately under warm and cold water until all of the paste has washed off. Pat dry.

PETROLEUM JELLY NAIL CREAM

Make split nails stronger and more resilient to wear and tear by treating them with this nail cream.

2 teaspoons petroleum jelly
2 teaspoons lanolin
½ teaspoon salicylic acid

Blend all the ingredients together in a bowl until they form a smooth paste. Store in a screw-top jar. Before going to bed, dip your nails into the cream, put on a pair of cotton gloves and leave the cream to work overnight. Continue this treatment for several days.

SMOOTH NAIL OIL

This protective oil treatment gives a boost to finger and toenails.

2 teaspoons soya bean oil
1 teaspoon avocado oil
1 teaspoon castor oil

Beat all three of the oils together for at least 2 minutes, then transfer the liquid to a small, clean, sealable glass jar. After cleaning your nails, paint on a thin coat of the nail oil with a cotton bud or small brush. Don't wash it off.

AVOCADO AND MILK PASTE

Treat your hands once a week to this nourishing paste, especially during the winter.

1 avocado
milk

Remove the skin and stone from the avocado, then mash the flesh and combine it with enough milk to form a smooth paste. Apply the mixture to both hands and leave for 15 minutes. Wash off, dry your hands and massage in hand cream.

Tried & Trusted

Beautiful hands

• Once a week bathe dry, chapped hands in lukewarm olive oil or sunflower oil for 5 minutes. Gently massage the oil into the cuticles.

• Rub petroleum jelly into cracked hands. A mixture of equal parts lemon juice, honey and glycerine is also very effective.

• Mix 1 teaspoon of isopropyl alcohol with 5 teaspoons of lemon juice. Pour the liquid into a cupped palm and massage it over damp hands. Repeat regularly.

• Remove nicotine stains from your fingers by rubbing the skin with lemon juice. Rinse off after a minute.

• If your hands smell of fish, onion or garlic, dip them in milk or rub them with coffee grounds or moist salt.

• Before chopping vegetables, rub olive oil into your hands to prevent them absorbing the smell.

• After washing your hands, apply massage oil or hand cream. Knead the fingers separately from the tip down, working over the palm and up over the knuckles. Put each hand on a flat surface and repeatedly stroke the back, from the fingertips to the wrist.

Perfect nail care

• Brittle nails and torn cuticles benefit from a soak in lukewarm almond oil.

• Oak bark tea is a reliable remedy for brittle nails that are prone to splitting. Simply bathe the nails in the tea. Alternatively, blend ground almonds with lukewarm water to make a finger bath.

• For a do-it-yourself manicure, file your nails into shape with an emery board. Soak them for a few minutes in a finger bath of warm vegetable oil. Carefully push back the cuticles with a wooden cuticle stick – never use a sharp object. Finally, smooth the surface using a nail buffer.

• Avocado oil is a rich base oil that can be used on its own as a vitamin-rich massage oil or blended with other oils or creams. Use regularly to coat the nails and massage into the nail beds.

Remedies for your feet

Did you know that during your lifetime your feet will cover a distance equivalent to walking around the world four times? During this mammoth trek, your feet are constantly carrying the burden of your body's weight.

For this service they deserve regular care, but in reality we often neglect our feet. However, it only takes a few days with a foot problem, such as a painful nail or cracked hard skin, to realise the importance of foot care.

ELDERFLOWER FOOT BATH

Elderflowers were once commonly used to relieve swollen, tired feet.

5 clusters fresh elderflowers
1 handful fresh
  peppermint leaves
1 litre (1¾ pints) water

Put the flowers and leaves in a pan, add the water and bring to the boil. Simmer for 30 seconds. Leave to cool, then pour into a bowl with 2 litres (3½ pints) of lukewarm water. Bathe your feet for at least 10 minutes, then pat dry.

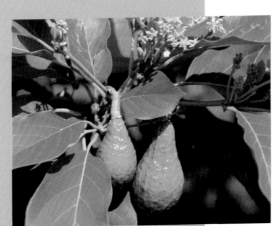

Tropical skin care
Avocados are rich in fat, nutritious plant oil and linoleic acid, which makes them ideal for soothing dry, sensitive skin.

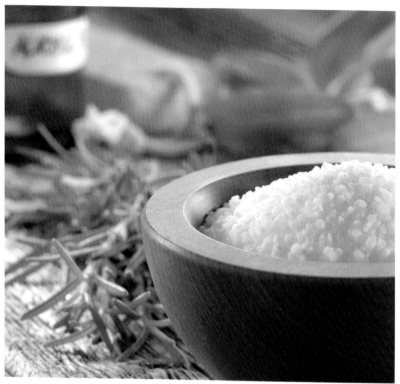

Instant relief When you've been on your feet all day, a footbath with your own homemade bath salts will be bliss.

BATH SALTS FOR THE FEET

A nightly footbath with these bath salts will cleanse your feet and stimulate circulation. This contains rosemary oil, so do not use if you are pregnant or suffer from high blood pressure or epilepsy.

1 teaspoon sage oil
1 teaspoon rosemary oil
4 teaspoons isopropyl alcohol
500g (1lb 2oz) sea salt

Dissolve both oils in the alcohol, then stir in the salt. Store in a container with a lid. To make up a footbath, dissolve 2 tablespoons of bath salts in 2-3 litres (3½-5¼ pints) of water in a basin and bathe your feet for 10 minutes.

TINCTURE FOR SWEATY FEET

Horsetail is rich in silicic acid, which is a proven remedy for sweaty feet.

100g (3½oz) fresh horsetail 'needles' and stems
100ml (3½fl oz) isopropyl alcohol

Mix the horsetail and alcohol in a bottle, seal and leave to infuse for three weeks. Strain the liquid through a fine sieve, then pour it back into the bottle and seal. Rub the tincture into your toes and the soles of your feet every day before getting dressed.

REVIVING FOOTBATH WITH ESSENTIAL OILS

If you want to refresh your feet for an evening out, but are short of time, try this footbath. It stimulates circulation and also acts as a disinfectant. After trying it, you're guaranteed to dance all night.

4 drops rosemary oil
3 drops lavender oil
3 drops cypress oil
5 litres (8¾ pints) water

Combine the essential oils with the water and heat in a pan until pleasantly warm. Pour into a basin and bathe your feet for 15 minutes.

FRUIT VINEGAR FOOTBATH

The acidity of fruit vinegar helps the skin to regain its protective anti-bacterial mantle. Sage and agrimony increase this effect because of their anti-inflammatory and astringent properties.

750ml (1 pint 7fl oz) fruit vinegar
pinch of dried sage leaves
pinch of dried agrimony

Put the vinegar and the herbs in a pan, bring to the boil and simmer for 30 seconds. Allow the mixture to cool to a temperature that is comfortable for your feet. Pour into a basin and soak your feet in this footbath for 30 minutes.

LIME FOOTBATH

Lime leaves and blossom have been used in herbal remedies since the 18th century. In earlier days, only the bark of the tree was used. The blossom and leaves have an anti-inflammatory, soothing effect. A regular evening footbath is both relaxing and refreshing.

25g (1oz) dried lime blossom
25g (1oz) dried lime leaves
500ml (18fl oz) water

Put the blossom, leaves and water in a pan. Bring to the boil and cool three times in succession. Cover and leave to go cold. Strain the liquid through a fine sieve. Pour it into a basin, add 2 litres (3½ pints) of hot water and soak your feet for 15 minutes.

Good practice For purposes of hygiene, it is always a good idea to use one set of manicure tools to look after your feet and a different set for your fingernails.

COLTSFOOT RUB FOR TIRED SWOLLEN FEET

This soothing rub is ideal for people whose work involves a lot of standing.

30ml (1fl oz) coltsfoot
    tincture
2 teaspoons lemon balm
    tincture
2 teaspoons marigold
    tincture
½ teaspoon melissa oil
    or
½ teaspoon lemon oil
30ml (1fl oz) witch hazel

Combine the tinctures in a glass bottle, then dissolve the oil in it. Add the witch hazel, seal and shake. Rub liberally over your feet in the morning and the evening.

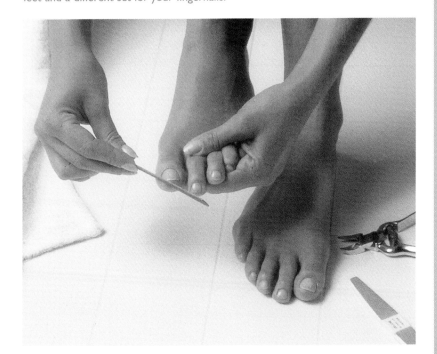

Tried & Trusted
Revive your feet

• **Fill two basins (each big enough for both feet) with water, one to a temperature of 38°C (100.4°F) and the other to 15°C (59°F). The water in each basin should come up to your ankles. Immerse your feet in the warm water for 5 minutes, then into the cold water for 10 seconds. Repeat.**

• **Shoe-free exercise is good for your feet: walk barefoot and wiggle your toes.**

Pamper your feet

• **Every now and then treat your feet to a massage. Using a massage brush or roller, massage the soles of your feet from the toes to the heels and then the instep. Massage cold feet every day.**

• **Give your feet a footbath, then rub off hard skin with a pumice stone and push back the cuticles with an orange stick. Finally, refresh your feet with a tincture, such as lavender, thyme or sage.**

• **Always cut your toenails straight across, to stop them from becoming painfully ingrown.**

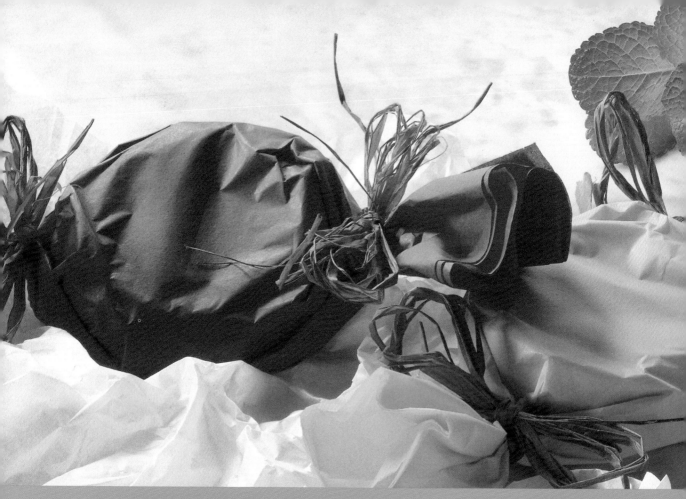

Herbal tea soap

Wrapped in decorative paper, this homemade soap will make a welcome gift. Choose different types of herbal tea to make soaps with unusual and fragrant scents.

Making your own soap is particularly satisfying, and continues a long tradition. As early as the 3rd millennium BC the Sumerians were making soap for washing cloth and to use as a medicinal ointment.

Today, all kinds of soaps are available but making your own allows you to control and experiment with the ingredients.

The key to this recipe is toilet soap, which suits all skin types. You can either buy it or make your own using this traditional recipe. Pour 50ml (2fl oz) water into a glass bowl and, wearing eye protection and rubber gloves, stir in 1 tablespoon caustic soda (sodium hydroxide) crystals. Melt 100g (3½oz) lard and add to the caustic soda liquid. Stir until it thickens.

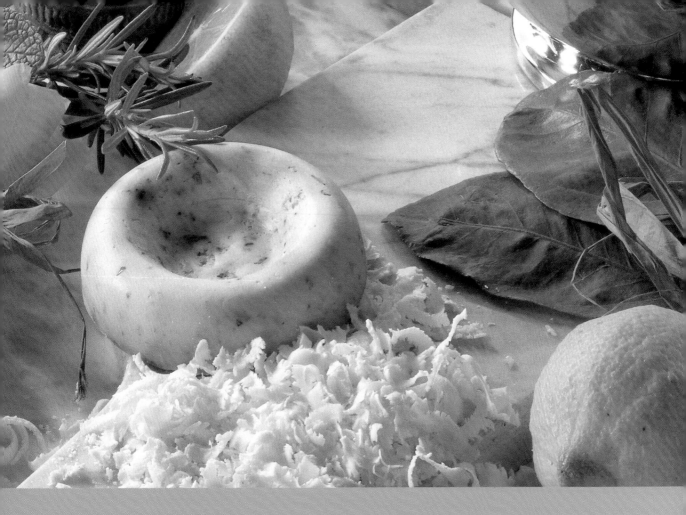

How to make your own herbal tea soap
Makes 4 bars, depending on the size of your moulds

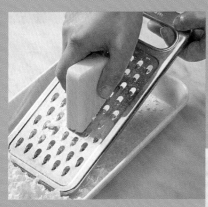

▲ Grate **150g (5½oz) fresh, soft toilet soap**, or **150g (5½oz) pure soap flakes**. Make **85ml (3fl oz) herbal tea** (camomile, peppermint or lime).

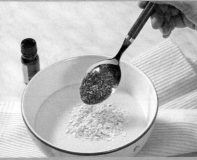

▼ Heat the tea with **40ml (1½fl oz) lemon juice** and the soap. Leave to cool. Add **1 or 1½ tablespoons** of freshly chopped **rosemary**, **1 tablespoon** of **oats** and **6 drops** of **essential oil** of your choice.

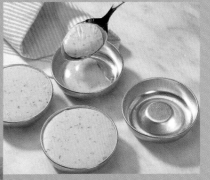

▲ Pour the setting soap mixture into individual moulds and leave to firm up in a dry, warm place for three weeks.

Total pampering for

Giving your entire body a treat needn't be a costly venture. Use simple, natural ingredients, such as flowers, herbs, milk and honey, in traditional recipes that pamper you from head to toe.

Like your face, your body needs regular care to keep the skin toned and supple as well as looking and feeling youthful.

The body has the same range of skin types as the face – oily, normal and dry – and each one needs a different treatment. The wealth of traditional body-care recipes means there's something for everyone.

You can make your own soap, relax in a fragrant bath, treat your whole body to a massage with essential oils, creams, lotions, powders and compresses. They are all made from natural ingredients to keep your skin healthy, and make you feel and look good.

Most of the ingredients can be obtained from a chemist or health shop, or from a mail-order herbalist. Where a herb or flower is not available, you can grow your own, but make sure you choose the right variety (see Garden herbs, pages 326-331).

All-over cleansing

Your body-care programme should start with gentle cleansing in the bath or shower. After this, your skin will benefit from a refreshing lotion, a soothing cream, a nourishing oil or talcum powder. You can even make your own mild deodorant.

Use only the best ingredients for these old recipes from times past and follow the instructions carefully. After all, it's no coincidence that elderly ladies often have smoother, softer skin than many 40-year-olds.

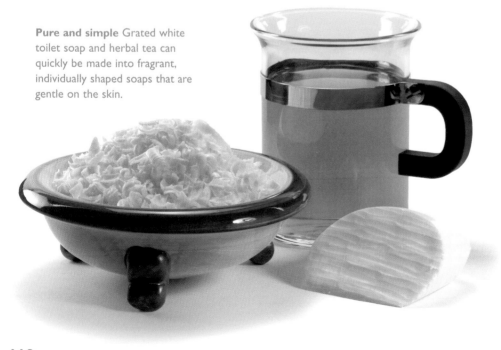

Pure and simple Grated white toilet soap and herbal tea can quickly be made into fragrant, individually shaped soaps that are gentle on the skin.

your body

Cleansing and caring for your body and mind

When you take time to care for your body, you are also taking time out for yourself – time to relax, unwind, to feel calm and tranquil. You'll find that by pampering your body, you will also be doing your mind a power of good.

LIME BLOSSOM SOAP

Pour this mixture into pretty moulds, such as heart shapes, to give as presents.

**350g (12oz) white
    toilet soap
300ml (10fl oz) strong lime
    blossom tea
4 tablespoons grapefruit juice
5 drops stock essence
4 tablespoons fine oats**

Finely grate the toilet soap and heat it in a pan with the lime blossom tea and grapefruit juice until the soap has dissolved. Remove the pan from the heat, then stir in the stock essence and oats with a wooden spoon. Continue stirring until the mixture cools and becomes creamy.

Pour the thickened mixture into individual moulds, cover them with a cloth and leave to harden in a dry, warm place for two to three weeks. Wrap the soap in tissue paper and store.

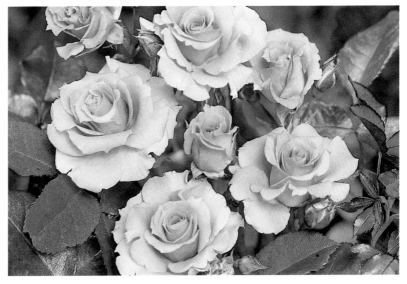

The queen of flowers The Crusaders introduced the rose to Europe and it has delighted gardeners ever since. Essential oil and water extracted from rose petals are used in a number of cosmetic products.

ENGLISH BEAUTY BATH

Three floral and fragrant scents are used to make this bath essence. You should feel elated and full of life after this bath.

**1 litre (1¾ pints) water
100g (3½oz) dried rosemary
    leaves
55g (2oz) dried rose petals
55g (2oz) dried lavender
    flowers**

Put the water in a pan. Add the rosemary and flowers and simmer for 15 minutes. Strain the liquid into bath water.

Hip bath

The advent of hot running water in Victorian and Edwardian times made baths popular among the wealthy. Styles ranged from basic wooden tubs lined with lead or copper to cast-iron and enamel baths such as the sophisticated 'Sitz' hip bath (below).

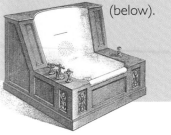

Steam baths

The benefits of a steam bath have been recognised for several thousand years; in Roman times a *calidarium* or 'steam room' formed part of the popular public baths.

More recently, steam baths, such as the 1940s example below, have been used to treat all kinds of conditions, from respiratory problems and rheumatism to nicotine addiction. The hot, humid air also cleanses the skin and aids relaxation.

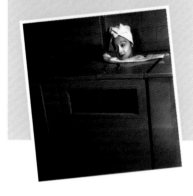

MILK AND HONEY BATH

Turn your bathroom into the land of milk and honey. This relaxing bath lotion, which Cleopatra is said to have bathed in, will leave your skin feeling smooth and soft.

2 litres (3½ pints) full-fat milk
350g (12oz) honey

Heat the milk in a pan, then dissolve the honey in it. Add the mixture to hot bath water, swirling it around with your hands.

BODY TONER WITH LAVENDER FLOWERS

Massage this lotion into your body after bathing to boost circulation.

1 handful dried
  lavender flowers
100ml (3½fl oz) isopropyl
  alcohol
300ml (10fl oz) water
1 tablespoon honey
4 drops lavender oil

Mix the lavender flowers and alcohol in a glass jar with a lid and store for four weeks in a dark place. Strain the liquid through a fine sieve. Heat the water in a pan then dissolve the honey in it. Stir in the lavender oil. Blend the water mixture with the infused alcohol and pour the toner into a dark glass bottle with a stopper.

PINE BATH SALTS

These relaxing and soothing bath salts are just the thing after a hard day. Pine oil is, however, not suitable for asthma sufferers.

400g (14oz) alum
200g (7oz) baking soda
few drops pine oil

Mix the alum and the baking soda together. Add a few drops of the pine oil and leave to allow the powders to soak up the liquid. Store the bath salts in a glass jar with a lid. Add a few tablespoons of the mixture to your bath water.

MILD DEODORANT

Apply this mild deodorant daily under your arms and feel pleasantly refreshed. It regulates the sweat glands in a natural way without suppressing perspiration.

¼ teaspoon menthol
30ml (1fl oz) isopropyl
  alcohol
50ml (2fl oz) rosewater
¼ teaspoon alum

Mix the menthol with the alcohol. Warm the rosewater in a pan and dissolve the alum in it. Combine both liquids and pour into a small glass bottle with a stopper. Shake thoroughly before applying a few drops under each arm.

RELAXING HERBAL BATH

Bath preparations made with scented flowers and herbs have stood the test of time.

150g (5½oz) dried
  camomile flowers
55g (2oz) dried
  peppermint leaves
55g (2oz) dried flag root
2 litres (3½ pints) water

Mix together the flowers, leaves and root in a heatproof bowl. Boil the water and pour it over them. Leave to infuse for 15 minutes, then strain the liquid through a fine sieve. Add the infusion to your bath water.

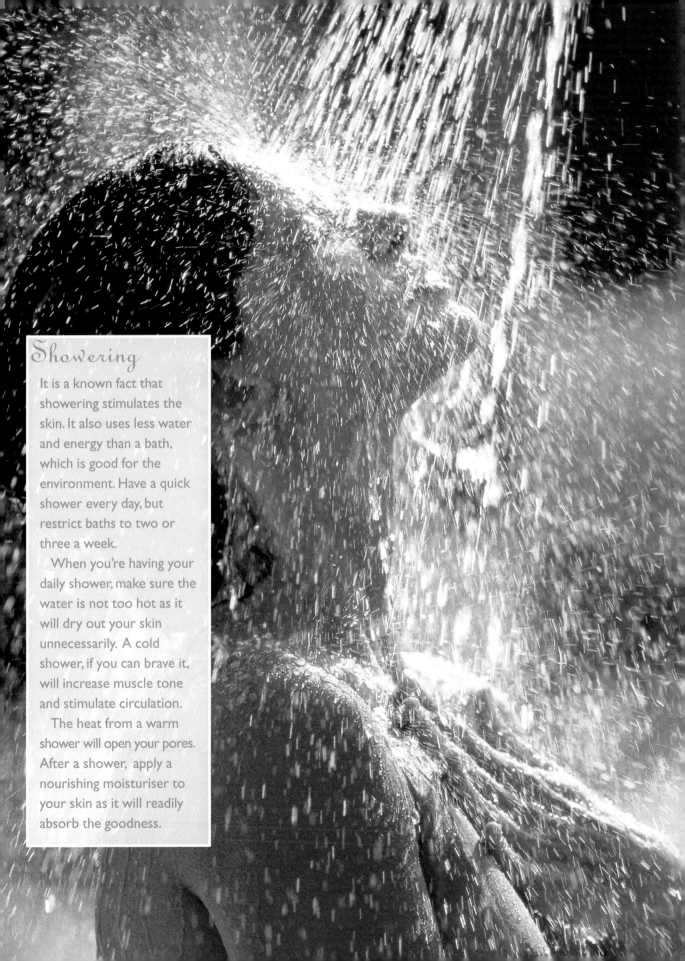

Showering

It is a known fact that showering stimulates the skin. It also uses less water and energy than a bath, which is good for the environment. Have a quick shower every day, but restrict baths to two or three a week.

When you're having your daily shower, make sure the water is not too hot as it will dry out your skin unnecessarily. A cold shower, if you can brave it, will increase muscle tone and stimulate circulation.

The heat from a warm shower will open your pores. After a shower, apply a nourishing moisturiser to your skin as it will readily absorb the goodness.

SOOTHING BODY LOTION

Apply this soothing body lotion after your bath or shower. For fragrance, choose from lavender, rose, apricot blossom or ylang ylang oil.

½ teaspoon lanolin
1 teaspoon cocoa butter
85ml (3fl oz) almond oil
3-5 drops essential oil of
    your choice

Melt the lanolin and cocoa butter in a bowl over a pan of boiling water. Add the almond oil. Heat until the mixture is clear, then remove from the heat and stir. Leave to cool, then stir in the essential oil.

BODY SCRUB

This scrub exfoliates the skin after showering or bathing, leaving it beautifully smooth and soft.

2 tablespoons double or
    whipping cream
1 tablespoon salt

Put the cream and salt in a bowl and beat to a smooth paste. In the shower or bath, gently rub the paste over your body using circular movements. Shower or sponge off the body scrub afterwards.

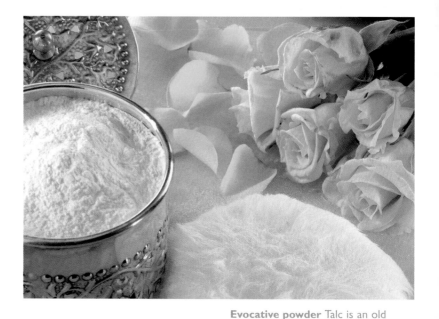

Evocative powder Talc is an old favourite which, depending on its scent, can be sporty or sensuous.

NOURISHING BODY OIL

Plant oils contain valuable nutrients that can revitalise your skin.

1 clove
25g (1oz) dried basil leaves
100ml (3½oz) almond oil
30ml (1fl oz) apricot
    kernel oil

Put all of the ingredients in a glass jar with a lid. Leave to infuse for two weeks, then strain the liquid. Pour the body oil into a dark glass bottle and store in a cool place.

PEPPERMINT TALCUM POWDER

After a morning shower, dust your body with this homemade talcum powder and you will feel fresh all day. For a more feminine scent use attar of roses or jasmine absolute instead of the peppermint oil.

1 tablespoon cornflour
2 drops peppermint oil
5 tablespoons talcum powder

Put all the ingredients into a tin with a tight-fitting lid and shake vigorously. Sieve the mixture through a fine mesh and return to the tin. Apply the powder with a wad of cotton wool, removing any excess powder with a paper tissue.

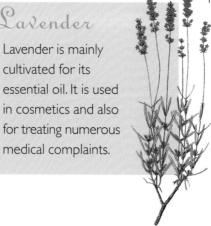

Lavender

Lavender is mainly cultivated for its essential oil. It is used in cosmetics and also for treating numerous medical complaints.

Tried & Trusted

The joys of bathing

- **Excessive perspiration can be reduced by adding an extract of oak bark to your bath water. It will make your pores contract, reducing the amount of sweat. Boil a handful of oak bark in 750ml (1 pint 7fl oz) of water for 10 minutes. Strain the liquid, then add the extract to your bath water.**

- **A lemon bath is relaxing and makes the skin feel soft. Cut three unwaxed lemons into slices, steep them in a bowl of water for a few hours, strain the liquid, then add it to your bath water.**

After-bath care

- **Follow up your bath with a natural deodorant. Add a few drops of lavender oil to 1 tablespoon of tap water and dab onto your skin.**

- **Enhance an ordinary body lotion or cream with fresh fruit. Mash half an apricot and blend it with the cream to make a mixture that can invigorate and smooth your skin. Two or three strawberries can be mixed in to add a cool and calming touch.**

BODY OIL FOR MEN

Male skin will benefit from good grooming. This mixture has a tangy, masculine scent.

50ml (2fl oz) jojoba oil
8 drops sandalwood oil
1 drop vetiver oil
4 drops geranium oil
4 drops bergamot oil

Pour the oils into a small dark glass bottle with a stopper. Seal and shake thoroughly before applying a few drops to your skin.

OLIVE OIL HERB SOAP

This soap is ideal for dry skin and rough hands.

15g (½oz) dried
  marigold flowers
15g (½oz) dried
  camomile flowers
50ml (2fl oz) olive oil
55g (2oz) toilet soap
100g (3½oz) white
  beeswax granules
50ml (2fl oz) purified water

Put the flowers and oil in a jar with a screw-top lid. Leave to infuse for two days. Filter the liquid through a fine sieve. Finely grate the soap and place it, with the wax, in a bowl set over a pan of simmering water. When melted, remove from the heat and leave to cool.

Add the oil to the soapy wax and heat over a pan of simmering water. Warm the purified water then add it to the mixture, beating until creamy. Pour into moulds while still warm and leave to set.

MOISTURISING OIL BATH

When you use this nourishing bath oil, there is no need to apply any lotion afterwards. Even very dry skin will benefit from this treatment.

6 tablespoons jojoba oil
8 drops jasmine absolute
1-2 tablespoons honey

Combine the oil and absolute in a small glass bottle with a stopper and shake thoroughly. Add 1 tablespoonful, together with the honey, to your bath water.

NOURISHING BODY PACK

A body pack should ideally be left to penetrate the skin for a few hours if it is to work effectively.

1 egg yolk
4 tablespoons almond oil
4 tablespoons avocado oil
2 tablespoons wheatgerm oil
juice of ½ lemon

Beat the egg yolk in a bowl and stir in the oils, drop by drop, until the mixture is firm. Add the freshly squeezed lemon juice and immediately smooth the paste over your body, from neck to toe. Cover rough patches, such as elbows, knees and heels, more thickly. Wrap your body in a linen sheet and relax while leaving the pack to work. Shower afterwards.

AVOCADO MASSAGE OIL

Avocado oil, when combined with lanolin, improves dry skin. Create your own massage oil with a scent of your choice: lavender, geranium, rose, petitgrain or ylang ylang.

2 teaspoons lanolin
85ml (3fl oz) avocado oil
few drops essential oil of
your choice

Melt the lanolin in a bowl over a pan of simmering water, then stir in the avocado oil. When the mixture turns clear, remove it from the heat. Leave to cool, then stir in the essential oil. Pour the oil into a dark glass bottle with a stopper.

Healing bath To make a soothing bath milk that removes skin impurities, mix 2 tablespoons of ground almonds and 1 tablespoon of almond oil with 125ml (4fl oz) milk. Add it to your bath water.

BRAN BATH FOR DRY SKIN

A bag filled with bran suspended in the water is a traditional remedy for dry skin. A wheat bran bath is also refreshing and reduces skin infections and irritations.

100g (3½oz) bran
1 muslin bag
175g (6oz) dried milk powder

Put the bran into a muslin bag or square of cheesecloth, tie the top securely and suspend it in a warm bath. Sprinkle the dried milk powder directly into the bath water and swirl it about with your hands. Squeeze the muslin bag occasionally like a sponge.

Mallow

A decoction of mallow flowers and leaves can be used externally to help soften patches of rough skin.

SPRING HERB BATH

This bath essence smooths, hydrates and invigorates dry skin.

1 litre (1¾ pints) water
100g (3½oz) dried
lavender flowers
100g (3½oz) dried
blackberry leaves
350g (12oz) honey

Boil the water in a pan, add the flowers and leaves, cover and leave to infuse over a low heat for 30 minutes. Strain the liquid, then add it to bath water with the honey.

SAVORY TEA

A cup of savory tea morning and night will help to relieve dry skin.

1-2 teaspoons dried
savory leaves
½ teaspoon dried thyme leaves
½ teaspoon dried mallow
flowers
250ml (9fl oz) water

Put the herbs in a heatproof bowl. Boil the water and pour it over them. Leave to infuse for 10 minutes. Strain the liquid and drink.

Tried & Trusted
Tackling dry skin

• **An instant beauty bath for dry, scaly skin: put 200g (7oz) of flour into a muslin bag, tie the top securely and place it in your bath water. Squeeze the bag frequently while you bathe.**

• **If the skin on your elbows or knees is rough, coat it with a mixture of 2 tablespoons of warmed honey and 1 tablespoon of lemon juice. Wash off after 30 minutes and massage in some skin cream.**

• **To exfoliate delicate skin, blend 3 tablespoons of olive oil with 2 teaspoons of sugar and rub over your body.**

• **Rough skin regains softness within weeks if it is regularly massaged first with buttermilk and then with suet.**

Tackling oily skin

• **Before showering, rub your body with fruit vinegar – it makes the pores contract and is refreshing.**

• **Pour 1 litre (1¾ pints) of boiling water onto 200g (7oz) of camomile flowers. Leave to infuse for 15 minutes, then strain the liquid. Add the infusion to your bath water.**

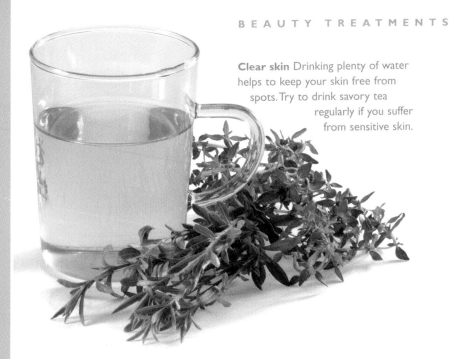

Clear skin Drinking plenty of water helps to keep your skin free from spots. Try to drink savory tea regularly if you suffer from sensitive skin.

Natural cleansing essences for oily skin

Since the production of sebum is controlled by hormones, oily skin often becomes a problem between the ages of 16 and 20. The most important treatment for oily skin is to cleanse it gently.

SAGE AND TEA TREE BATH ESSENCE

Sage and tea tree oil both have an antiseptic, healing effect.

200g (7oz) fresh sage flowers and leaves
1 litre (1¾ pints) water
4 drops tea tree oil
1-2 tablespoons runny honey

Place the sage in a heatproof bowl. Boil the water and pour it over the herb. Leave to infuse for 15 minutes, then strain the liquid. Pour it into warm bath water. Mix the tea tree oil with the honey, then add to the water.

REFRESHING LEMON VINEGAR BATH ESSENCE

This recipe for oily skin has been a favourite for generations and many women still swear by it. Lemon vinegar helps shrink enlarged pores, disinfects the skin and helps to regenerate the natural acid mantle that protects the skin against bacteria and infection.

3 unwaxed lemons
1 litre (1¾ pints) fruit vinegar

Wash the lemons and peel them thinly, making sure that there is no pith left on the peel. Place the peel in a wide-necked bottle and pour in the fruit vinegar. Seal with a stopper or cap and leave to infuse for two weeks in a warm place.

Strain the liquid and return it to the bottle and seal. Pour 250ml (9fl oz) of the lemon vinegar directly into your warm bath water.

SANDALWOOD AND JASMINE BATH ESSENCE

Both sandalwood oil and jasmine oil have antiseptic and anti-inflammatory properties. Because essential oils are not water soluble, they have to be mixed with a natural emulsifying agent, such as cream or a carrier oil, which also nourishes oily skin.

5 tablespoons cream
20 drops jasmine absolute
20 drops sandalwood oil

Mix the cream with the absolute and essential oil. Pour the bath essence into your warm bath water and relax for 15 minutes.

CYPRESS OIL

If you don't like the tangy, spicy smell of cypress oil, use geranium oil instead which has a milder sweet fragrance. Both essential oils are very good for oily skin.

75ml (2½fl oz) soya bean oil
2 teaspoons almond oil
1 teaspoon cypress oil

Fill a small glass bottle with the oils, seal with a stopper and shake the mixture vigorously. After your bath or shower, dry your body with a soft towel, then gently massage a few drops of the oil into the surface of the skin.

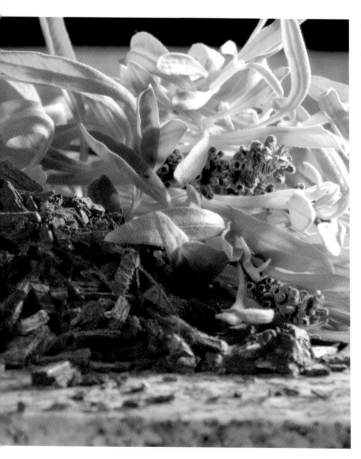

Ancient panacea
In India, dried and fresh sandalwood leaves and bark have been used in body care for more than 4000 years. The dried herb is also known as sanderswood.

'Orange-peel' skin

Cellulite, also called 'orange-peel' skin, affects many women. It is caused by a distortion of the skin's underlying tissue structure. Women are more prone to cellulite than men because the connective tissue which surrounds their body organs is softer.

Causes of cellulite can be metabolic disorders, hormonal changes or a weakened lymphatic system, which is why it often appears at puberty or at the menopause. The unsightly condition is most common on the buttocks, hips and thighs. Neither traditional recipes nor gels will get rid of the problem completely.

It can be improved, however, and the skin can be firmed by applying compresses to stimulate circulation and by cleansing the system with herbal teas.

HORSETAIL AND AGAR GEL

Agar, made from seaweed, melts in hot water to make a natural gel.

55g (2oz) dried horsetail
 'needles' and stems
250ml (9fl oz) water
½ teaspoon agar

Place the horsetail in a heatproof bowl. Boil the water and pour it over the herb. Leave to infuse for 10 minutes. Strain the liquid, stir in the agar and reheat until the mixture forms a gel. Pour it into a screw-top jar. Apply the gel daily, leaving it on your body for 15 minutes before rinsing with warm water.

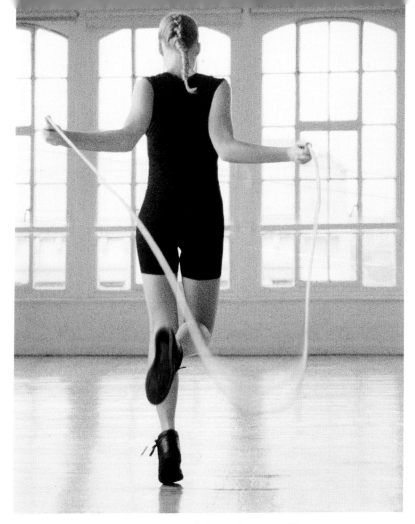

Essential body care Regular exercise helps to firm your skin and tone your muscles. This can also help to prevent cellulite or at least keep it in check.

ANTI-CELLULITE HERBAL TEA

Inner therapy is an important weapon in the battle against cellulite. As aromatic blackcurrant leaves and ash leaves both help to prevent water retention, this tea is considered a sound remedy for helping to reduce cellulite.

2 teaspoons dried blackcurrant leaves
2 teaspoons dried ash leaves
1 litre (1¾ pints) water

Place the leaves in a heatproof bowl. Boil the water and pour it over them. Leave to infuse for 15 minutes, then strain the liquid through a fine sieve. Drink three cups of this tea per day – one on an empty stomach and the others between meals.

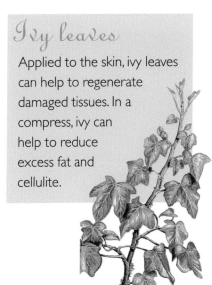

Ivy leaves

Applied to the skin, ivy leaves can help to regenerate damaged tissues. In a compress, ivy can help to reduce excess fat and cellulite.

IVY MASSAGE OIL

This oil can be used daily after a shower. Massage it into the cellulite using circular movements. Do not use when pregnant or if you have high blood pressure or epilepsy.

1 handful fresh ivy leaves
200ml (7fl oz) wheatgerm oil
2 drops rosemary oil

Put the ivy leaves in a jar and add the wheatgerm oil. Seal and leave for two weeks in a warm place. Strain through a fine sieve, add the rosemary oil, then pour the massage oil into a bottle and seal.

SEAWEED COMPRESS

Apply this compress three times a week to combat oily skin patches.

55g (2oz) dried seaweed
100g (3½oz) bran
115g (4oz) sea salt
water

Boil the ingredients in as much water as you need to make a pulp. Leave the mixture to cool a little then apply the compress to your skin. Cover with a linen cloth and leave for 5 minutes. Rinse off with warm water and dry thoroughly.

Creams and lotions for sunny days

Even 50 years ago, few people had heard of the ozone layer. And our grandparents didn't have to worry about whether too much sun was bad for them because they didn't sunbathe in the way we do today.

Most people now know that although sunshine is essential to help our bodies make vitamin D, it also has drawbacks. It is possible to use natural sun creams, but they offer little effective protection against harmful ultraviolet rays.

Traditional remedies are not suitable for serious sunbathing or for the delicate skin of babies and young children. In both cases it is best to use a commercial product with a high sun protection factor (SPF) of 20 or more.

Less is more

Prolonged sunbathing can be harmful. It is best to stay in the sun for short periods only and to spend most of your time in the shade.

These traditional lotions and oils should only be used if your skin is already used to the sun, and then only for moderate sunbathing.

Take care

Treat the sun with respect. Even sunbathing for a short time can accelerate your skin's ageing process. Suffering sunburn in adolescence can also double the chances of skin cancer in later life. Always protect young children's skin from the sun because it has less natural protection than adults'.

LEMON AND OLIVE OIL

Pure olive oil mixed with lemon juice and iodine will help to enhance your tan. This recipe comes from the Mediterranean and should only be used if you already have a suntan.

250ml (9fl oz) pure olive oil
10 drops iodine tincture
juice of 1 lemon

Mix all the ingredients together in a bowl, then pour into a dark glass bottle with a stopper. Shake before applying the oil to your skin.

SESAME SUN CREAM

Sesame oil contains an active agent that helps to absorb ultraviolet rays.

1 teaspoon beeswax granules
½ teaspoon cocoa butter
2 teaspoons lanolin
30ml (1fl oz) sesame oil
40ml (1½fl oz) purified water

Melt the wax, cocoa butter and lanolin in a bowl set over a pan of simmering water. When melted and clear, add the sesame oil and heat to 60°C (140°F).

Warm the purified water in a separate pan to the same temperature. Combine it with the wax mixture using an electric hand mixer on a low setting or beat with a fork until the cream is cold. Transfer it to a small screw-top jar. Store in a cool place.

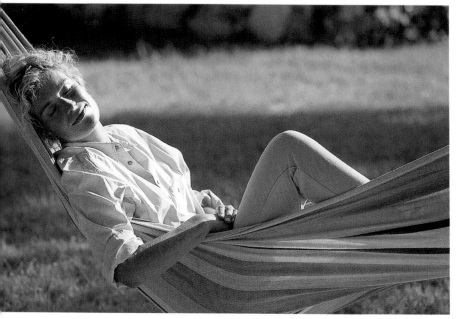

Safety first Enjoy the summer sun without putting your health at risk. Cover your skin or protect it with cream.

AVOCADO SUN OIL

This infused oil will give you warm, bronze-coloured skin. Use it to top-up your suntan.

1 teaspoon fresh
   lavender flowers
1 teaspoon fresh heather
   flowers
100ml (3½fl oz) avocado oil
50ml (2fl oz) carrot oil
8 drops cinnamon oil

Finely crush the flowers using a pestle and mortar. Put them in a glass jar. Add the oils. Seal the jar and leave to infuse in a warm place for 24 hours. Strain the liquid, then pour the sun oil into a dark glass bottle with a stopper.

Rich tones Avocado oil is rich in vitamin E, which will moisturise your skin as you sunbathe. Carrot oil and cinnamon essence are yellowish in colour and will help you tan more quickly, so protecting your skin.

REGENERATING AFTER-SUN LOTION

After exposure to the sun your skin will be in need of moisture and nutrients to relieve any possible damage. This old-fashioned wheatgerm lotion provides both. The lavender oil will also help to cool the skin.

2 tablespoons cocoa butter
2 tablespoons lanolin
5 tablespoons lavender oil
1 teaspoon wheatgerm oil
4 tablespoons black tea
1 tablespoon glycerine

Melt the cocoa butter and lanolin in a bowl set over a pan of simmering water, stirring continuously. Warm the two oils individually and stir into the mixture. Leave to cool, then add the tea and glycerine. Stir vigorously, then pour the lotion into a glass bottle, seal and store in a cool place.

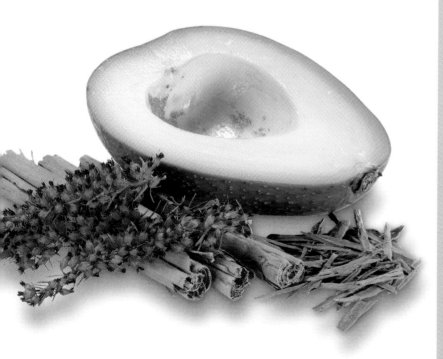

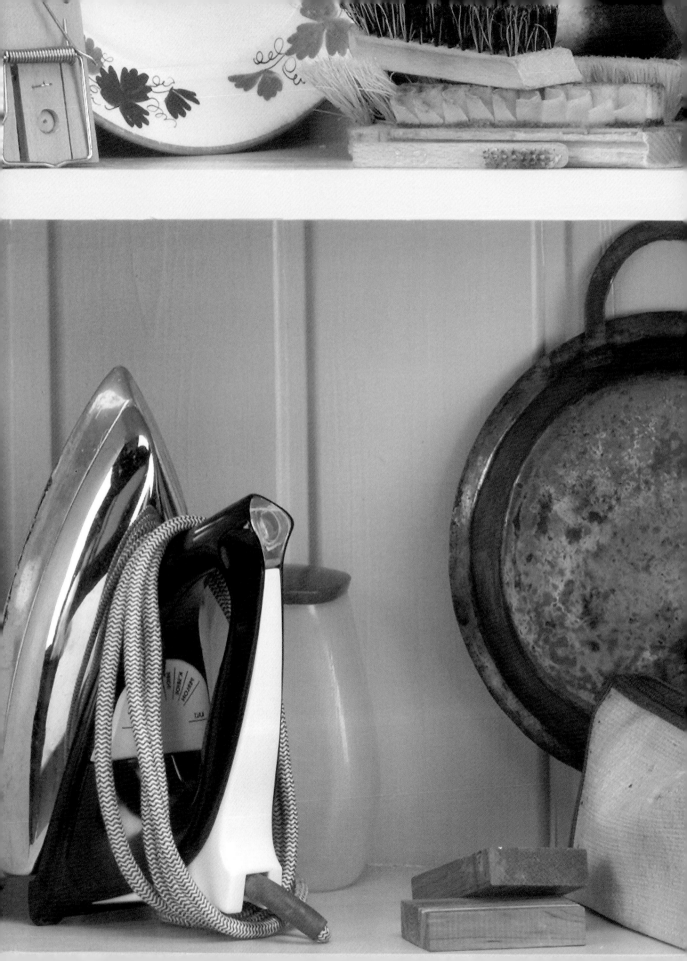

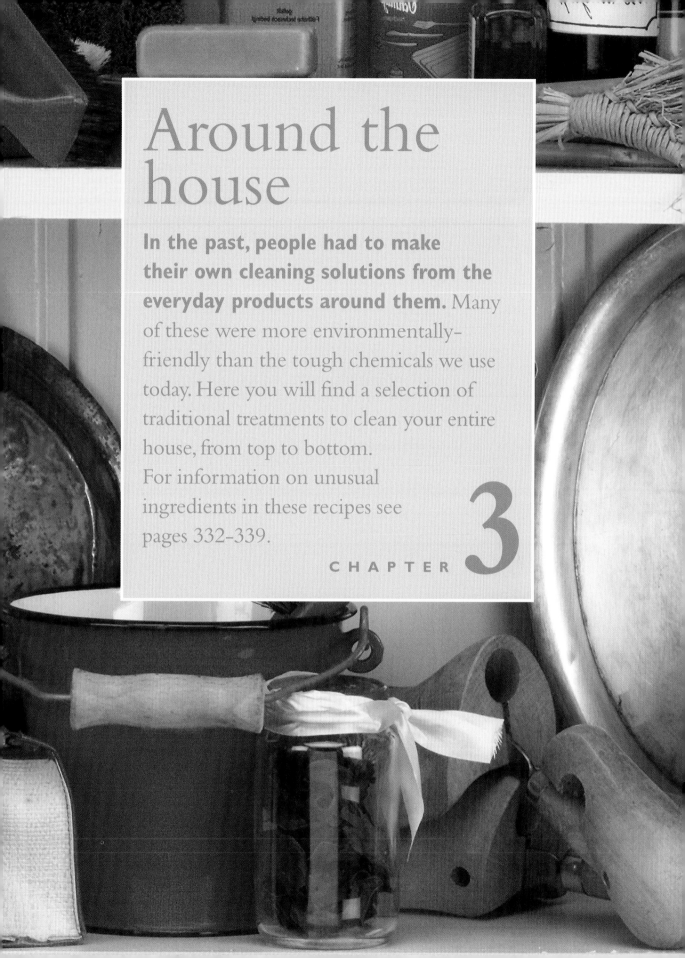

Around the house

In the past, people had to make their own cleaning solutions from the everyday products around them. Many of these were more environmentally-friendly than the tough chemicals we use today. Here you will find a selection of traditional treatments to clean your entire house, from top to bottom.
For information on unusual ingredients in these recipes see pages 332–339.

CHAPTER 3

Caring for furniture

Although our homes contain a wealth of different furnishing materials, old and new, the preparations our grandmothers used are still effective for many surfaces.

Whatever the style of your home, your furniture will need regular care to stay looking its best. You can buy a wide range of polishes, creams and other cleaning agents, but many contain mineral oils or solvents that pollute the atmosphere and can even cause allergies.

Natural alternatives, widely used in the past, care for your furniture just as well, but without side effects and without harming the environment. You can make up cleaning solutions and polishes for all kinds of materials and surfaces.

All the ingredients are available, though you won't necessarily find them on the supermarket shelf. A trip to the chemist, health shop or hardware store, or a phone call to a specialist mail-order company, may be required. See 'The main ingredients' listed on pages 332–339.

In some cases you'll need to be more resourceful. You can, for example, make paper ash and birchwood ash yourself, but do take sensible precautions. Light fires away from buildings and hedges and have access to a water supply in case of emergencies.

Many of the traditional recipes keep well, so you can make up a batch of them in advance. They will then be ready to use as and when you need them.

Softly, softly Be sure that you know what material you are treating before applying any cleaners or polishes.

the natural way

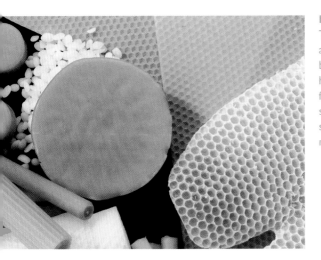

Natural beeswax
This can be bought as granules, discs, blocks and honeycomb sheets from hardware stores, craft suppliers and by mail order.

KEEPING DUST AT BAY

Keep dust from settling quickly on wooden furniture with this simple solution.

1 litre (1¾ pints) water
1 teaspoon vinegar
1 teaspoon glycerine

Mix the water, vinegar and glycerine in a container. Pour a little of the mixture onto a soft cloth and wipe it over your furniture.

First-class care for wooden furniture

It is generally easy to look after wooden furniture. Lift dust out of grooves and hollows with a fine paintbrush, then remove with a damp cloth. Never leave drops of water to dry on wooden surfaces, since these leave marks. The tried-and-trusted methods that follow will get rid of stains or scratches.

POLISH FOR OLD WOOD

This polish contains shellac, a natural resin made from the secretions of the Asian lac insect.

3 tablespoons shellac
3 tablespoons methylated spirits

Mix together the ingredients and apply the polish with a soft cloth. Buff with a lint-free cloth afterwards.

CARING FOR VENEERS

This polish can be used on all sorts of veneers, but it is only suitable for wooden surfaces.

200ml (7fl oz) olive oil
4 teaspoons fresh lemon juice, filtered

Use a funnel to pour the oil and the filtered lemon juice into a small glass bottle. Seal it with a cork stopper or cap and shake the bottle vigorously. Apply the polish to a wad of cotton wool then cover it with a linen cloth or tea towel. Polish the veneer using a circular motion, then dry it with a clean cloth. The polish will keep for a few weeks. Shake the bottle each time before use.

REVIVING DARK AND LIGHT WOOD

In the old days potash was a basic ingredient of soap. The ash in this polish helps to disguise scratches.

3 tablespoons beeswax granules
3 tablespoons turpentine
3 tablespoons raw linseed oil
3 tablespoons paper ash (for dark wood)
3 tablespoons birchwood ash (for light wood)

Place the beeswax in a heatproof bowl and stand it in a saucepan of water over a medium heat. Allow the water to simmer.
When the wax has melted, add the remaining ingredients and beat until smooth. Stir the mixture occasionally as it cools, then pour it into a glass jar and seal. The polish will keep for up to a year.

Domestic help

In the early 1900s most middle-class households had servants to help with the domestic chores. The average upper middle-class family usually employed a housemaid and a cook. Lower middle-class households were more likely to have one maid who did the cooking, cleaning and washing.

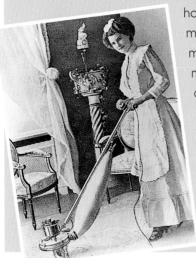

Even if a family could not really afford a maid, they employed hired 'help' as a status symbol. Maids were often badly treated and many girls preferred to work in factories with regular hours.

BEESWAX POLISH FOR LIGHT WOOD

Although dusting waxed wood with a soft cloth is usually sufficient, you can revive it with an occasional application of this polish.

2 teaspoons beeswax
  granules
100ml (3½fl oz) soya bean oil

Put the ingredients in a heatproof bowl and heat in a saucepan of water, as for 'Reviving dark and light wood' (see page 133). When the wax has melted, beat the polish with a whisk. Allow it to cool then pour it into a metal or glass container and seal. The polish can be kept for up to six months.

BEESWAX POLISH FOR DARK WOOD

In this recipe it is the turpentine that determines the consistency of your polish. If a thinner polish is needed, increase the amount of turpentine by one to two teaspoons. This polish can be used not only for wood, but also for bronze, iron, steel and leather.

½ teaspoon beeswax granules
1 teaspoon lanolin
4 teaspoons soya bean oil
1 teaspoon turpentine

Melt the beeswax in a bowl, then beat in the other ingredients as for 'Reviving dark and light wood' (see page 133).

REJUVENATING STAINED WOODEN SURFACES

This preparation can be used both to remove marks and to give a renewed shine to stained wood.

1 teaspoon salt
300ml (½ pint) boiled
  linseed oil

Add the salt to the linseed oil and mix well. Sprinkle drops of the mixture onto a cotton cloth and rub over the marks. Buff up the wood with a clean cloth.

CLEANING OAK FURNITURE

Dirty or stained oak can be cleaned with beer. If the surface has completely lost its shine, however, try the following.

1 tablespoon beeswax
  granules
300ml (½ pint) beer
2 teaspoons sugar

Melt the wax as for 'Reviving dark and light wood' (see page 133). Allow it to cool, but don't let it harden. Stir in the beer and sugar. Use a soft brush to coat the wood. Polish when dry.

Take care

Turpentine is a flammable liquid. Do not place it near a naked flame or heat it on its own directly on a cooker or hob. It combusts at only 40°C (104°F).

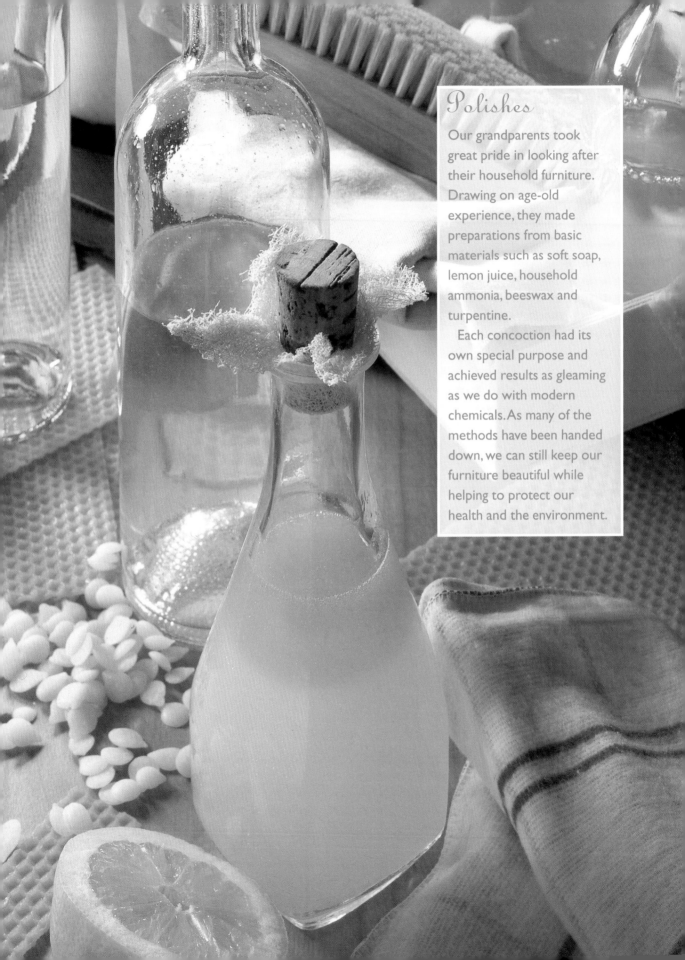

Polishes

Our grandparents took great pride in looking after their household furniture. Drawing on age-old experience, they made preparations from basic materials such as soft soap, lemon juice, household ammonia, beeswax and turpentine.

Each concoction had its own special purpose and achieved results as gleaming as we do with modern chemicals. As many of the methods have been handed down, we can still keep our furniture beautiful while helping to protect our health and the environment.

Tried & Trusted
Good for wood

- Treat light and dark unvarnished wood with teak oil. For reddish wood use boiled linseed oil.

- If a thick layer of dust has built up on wood, it can easily be rubbed off with cider vinegar.

- After dusting walnut furniture, polish it with a little milk on a soft cloth.

- To bring the shine back to wood painted white, such as window frames and doors, apply a mixture of whiting in warm water. Then polish with a soft cloth.

- Linseed oil is a useful ingredient of many recipes. It dries with a protective finish. Boiled linseed oil is a modern version that has had air passed through it so that it dries more quickly. Raw linseed oil is untreated.

Marks and scratches

- Treat scratches on light wood with petroleum jelly or 1 teaspoon each of vinegar and raw linseed oil mixed together. For darker wood use equal quantities of red wine and raw linseed oil.

- Scratches on light wood can be covered up with white or beige shoe polish. On darker wood use brown shoe polish; on ebony you can use black.

- Walnuts are not only good to eat, but can be useful too. Rub half of a kernel over scratches on walnut furniture to help fill them in.

- You can get rid of water marks on wood by rubbing them with toothpaste. For stubborn stains, add some baking soda, then polish with a soft cloth.

- Remove spilt wax by placing a piece of kitchen paper over it and pressing lightly with a warm iron. The wax should melt and be absorbed by the paper. Wipe over the area with a weak solution of water and vinegar and dry with a clean cloth.

- Marks caused by pressure can be treated by covering them with a damp cloth. Hold a warm, but not hot, iron over the cloth to absorb the moisture.

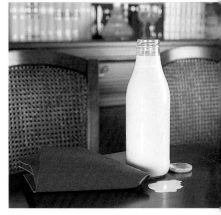

Milk for grained woods Use a little milk on a soft cloth to polish highly grained woods such as walnut and cherry.

MAKING THE BEST OF MAHOGANY

Use soapy water and a soft brush to remove surface dirt. Difficult stains can be treated as follows.

100ml (3½fl oz) methylated spirits
2 tablespoons raw linseed oil
2 tablespoons red wine

First rub the stains vigorously with the methylated spirits, then dry the wood. Stir the raw linseed oil and red wine together and use the mixture to polish the treated areas.

STUBBORN STAINS

Try this traditional method to remove heavy staining.

1 teaspoon petroleum jelly
2 teaspoons turpentine

Use a teaspoon to mix the ingredients together in a small container. Put a few drops of the mixture on a soft cloth and rub vigorously into the stains.

Varnished furniture

Because the finish is delicate, varnished wood needs special care. Never clean it with abrasive material, use soapy water and a soft cloth. However, do not allow the wood to become too wet.

Dull spots can be polished using a cloth dipped first in methylated spirits and then in raw linseed oil. Always test a new substance on the underside of your furniture – modern finishes react differently to those of yesteryear.

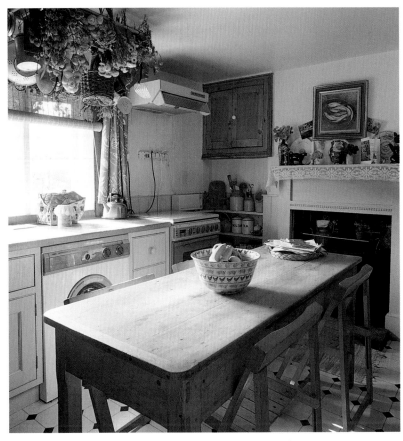

Scrubbed clean Kitchen tables and work surfaces made of pine need to be spotlessly clean and hygienic for food preparation. They can be cleaned with ammonia solution.

PROTECTIVE SHINE

This mixture will treat your wood.

55g (2oz) wheatgerm
I litre (1¾ pints) water

Put the wheatgerm and water into a heavy-bottomed saucepan and bring it to the boil. Allow to cool then push the mixture through a sieve with the back of a spoon. Apply with a soft cloth.

MILD CLEANER FOR WOOD

This mild solution is suitable for gentle wood maintenance.

I litre (1¾ pints) water
I tablespoon milk
I tablespoon washing-up liquid

Heat the water in a pan and stir in the remaining ingredients. Soak a soft cloth with the fluid and rub the dirty spots using a circular movement. Polish with a dry cloth.

STAIN REMOVER

This is a reliable method of removing stains from varnished wood. It appears in sections on furniture care in many old books on household management.

3 tablespoons raw linseed oil
3 tablespoons vinegar
3 tablespoons turpentine

Mix all the ingredients together in a bowl. Apply sparingly to a cloth and rub over the stains until they disappear. Finish by rubbing the area with a piece of kitchen paper.

STRONG CLEANING FLUID

Use this solution to clean very dirty wood, such as chopping boards and kitchen tables.

I litre (1¾ pints) soapy water
I tablespoon household ammonia
I tablespoon turpentine

Heat the water in a pan until it is lukewarm, then remove it from the heat. Mix in the ammonia and turpentine. Apply the mixture with a cloth or sponge to remove the dirty marks. Rinse well afterwards.

Cleaning fabric and leather upholstery

Dealing with the accumulation of dust is always the greatest problem when cleaning upholstered furniture. Dust inevitably collects deep in the fabric. The best solution is to vacuum upholstery once a week.

If possible, take smaller pieces of upholstered furniture outside from time to time and beat or brush them to remove the dust. You can beat leather upholstery, then wipe with a clean damp cloth to remove any lingering particles of dust.

Leather is a delicate material and if you are in any doubt about using any of the recipes, contact the manufacturer first.

Fabric care Dust will dull coloured fabrics, so vacuum them regularly. Use traditional preparations to clean stains and to restore faded colours.

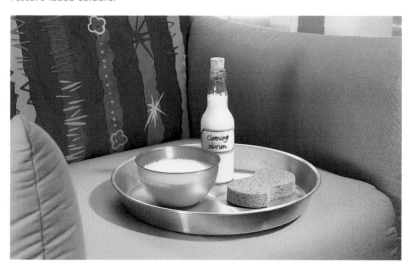

Take care

Household ammonia is an irritant. To avoid respiratory problems always use it in a well-ventilated room. Wear rubber gloves to protect your hands and wash off any splashes on your skin immediately.

BEAUTIFUL UPHOLSTERY

You can freshen up your fabrics with this gentle cleaning solution, which will keep for six months.

**1 litre (1¾ pints) water
25g (1oz) soap flakes
100ml (3½fl oz) glycerine
100ml (3½fl oz) methylated
  spirits**

Heat the water in a pan, stirring in the soap flakes until they have dissolved. Remove from the heat and allow it to cool, then mix in the glycerine and methylated spirits. Transfer the mixture to a glass container with a lid. Store the cleaner in a cool place.

To use, dissolve 1 tablespoon of the mixture in water and whisk vigorously. Apply the foam to the upholstery with a sponge, taking care that the fabric does not get too damp.

MULTI-PURPOSE SOAPSUDS

Heavily soiled fabrics can be cleaned with soap flakes.

**1 litre (1¾ pints) water
55g (2oz) soap flakes
1 teaspoon household
  ammonia**

Heat the water in a pan until it is hand-hot. Dissolve the soap flakes in the water and then add the ammonia. Apply the liquid with a brush, following the pile of the fabric. Brush with clear water and dry with a cloth.

INK STAINS ON LEATHER

Clean leather upholstery only when absolutely necessary, such as when stained with ink. Always treat marks immediately.

**milk
  or
white spirit**

Pour a little milk or white spirit on a cloth and wipe it over the stain. Dab lightly on the leather to avoid removing the colour. Do not allow any milk to spill into the seams as it will smell over time.

- Revive faded colours by rubbing the fabric gently with a weak water and vinegar solution (4:1).

- To remove fluff from upholstery, soak a chamois leather in white vinegar and rub it gently over the surface of the fabric.

- Fresh stains can sometimes be removed if you sprinkle them with salt or cornflour. Leave for 15 minutes to absorb the stain, then wash off.

- Stubborn stains disappear when they are rubbed with shaving cream. Let the cream soak in for a while, then rub down with a cloth and clean water.

- Clean synthetic upholstery with a cloth soaked in a solution made from 1 teaspoon of baking soda dissolved in 250ml (9fl oz) water. Rub down the upholstery and then, if necessary, sponge with a squirt of washing-up liquid diluted in 1 litre (1¾ pints) of water.

- Use a little glycerine soap on a damp cloth to give leather furniture a gentle clean. Rinse off.

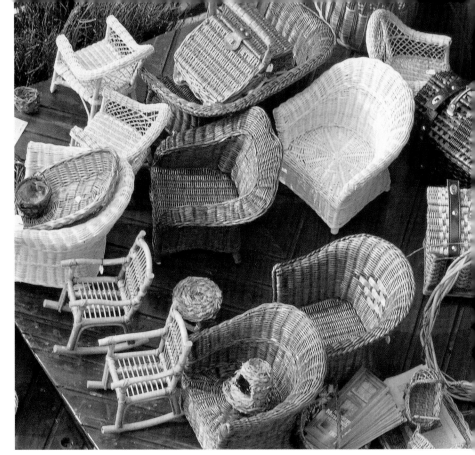

Woven wickerwork The flexible stems of plants such as willow can be woven or bent and tied to make all kinds of furniture.

Wickerwork and bamboo furniture

Wicker and bamboo are durable if well looked after. To clean small items of furniture, dip them in an ammonia solution then rinse and leave to dry.

WASHING WICKERWORK

Brush the wicker with a stiff brush to remove dust and surface dirt.

1 tablespoon household soap
hot water

Grate the soap into the water and swill it around to form a lather. Using a chamois leather, rub the soapy water over the wicker. Rinse it and leave to dry naturally.

BAMBOO CLEANER

Salt and lemon juice act like a gentle bleach and clean the bamboo without drying it out.

1 tablespoon salt
½ teaspoon lemon juice
300ml (½ pint) water
boiled linseed oil

Mix the salt and lemon juice with the water and apply it to the bamboo with a soft brush. Soak a soft, non-fluffy cloth with the boiled linseed oil and rub it over the bamboo.

After a few hours polish the bamboo with another lint-free cloth to a soft sheen.

Rustic furniture

Brightly coloured painted furniture has a traditional charm. Our forebears had just the recipe for keeping these colours looking fresh and at their best.

Painted surfaces should be wiped regularly with soapy water and polished with liquid beeswax.

**1 walnut-sized piece of
    beeswax
250ml (9fl oz) turpentine**

Melt the beeswax in a bowl over a pan of simmering water. Remove the bowl from the heat, then add the turpentine. Apply to the surface with a cloth. Polish with a fresh cloth to avoid a matt finish.

Painted folk art
Whether a valuable original or a modern piece, most painted furniture needs special care. If you have a precious item, always consult a specialist before using homemade cleaners or polishes.

Cleaning and polishing marble surfaces

Marble, a material prized for its veined texture, colouring and shine, has long been used both ornamentally and for surfaces such as floors and work surfaces.

Unfortunately, it is quite sensitive, especially compared with stone such as granite.

Take care

Use garden lime with caution. Although not as hazardous as slaked and unslaked lime, garden lime is still an irritant. Always wear gloves to protect your hands, and safety goggles to shield your eyes. Wash off any splashes immediately under running water. Use and store garden lime away from pets and young children.

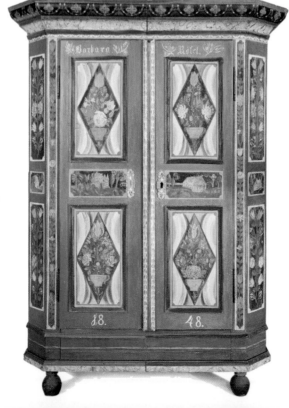

Marble surfaces therefore have to be well looked after, and spills should be dealt with immediately to prevent unsightly staining.

There is no need to buy expensive cleaners and polishes as you can make them yourself. However, if you have any antique marble, always consult a specialist.

MARBLE POLISH

Shine up dull marble with this basic polish.

**85g (3oz) turpentine
2 teaspoons liquid floor polish
½ teaspoon bone glue**

Mix the turpentine and floor polish. Make up the glue according to the manufacturer's instructions and then add it to the mixture. Apply the polish using a warmed lint-free cloth and rub in well.

REJUVENATING TREATMENT
FOR MARBLE

Never use a brush on marble as scrubbing takes away the shine. Try the following instead.

**4 tablespoons garden lime
1 tablespoon water
2-3 drops household ammonia**

Mix the lime with enough water to form a paste. Add the ammonia. Apply the polish evenly and leave it to work on the marble for two to three days. Wash it off with clean water and rub dry.

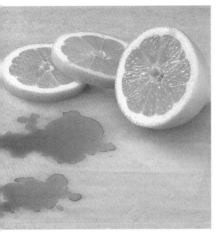

A natural cleaner Lemons contain citric acid, which removes stains from marble and enhances its fine grain.

STAIN REMOVAL

Most stains on marble come off with this handy remover, which is quick and easy to make.

½ lemon
1 tablespoon white vinegar

Squeeze the lemon and mix the juice with the vinegar. Wipe over the surface of the marble with the solution using a soft cloth.

SOFT SOAP TREATMENT

Soft soap has traditionally been used for cleaning marble.

½ teaspoon whiting
4 tablespoons soft soap
500ml (18fl oz) water
dash of household ammonia

Mix the whiting with the soft soap and apply evenly over the marble. Leave for a few hours. Heat the water, add the ammonia and wash the marble clean by removing the soap with the solution.

Tried & Trusted
Bamboo and wicker

- To clean bamboo, scrub it gently with a soft brush and lukewarm water. Leave the bamboo to dry, then apply a solution of 1 part raw linseed oil to 1 part turpentine.

- Wickerwork sometimes loses its tension with age and wear. It can be restored by wetting it liberally with hot water and leaving it to dry in a warm but shaded place. Small items can be left to soak in hot water, then dried in the same way.

Marble care

- White marble will not discolour if it is wiped with turpentine. Rinse and dry the surface with a cloth afterwards. Apply this treatment sparingly.

- Badly soiled marble tiles can be cleaned with fine pumice powder. Rub it into the tiles, then rinse and dry.

- To give your marble a beautiful bright shine, take 225g (8oz) of washing soda and 115g (4oz) each of pumice powder and chalk powder. Sift these through a fine sieve and mix to a paste with water. Rub this thoroughly over the marble, then leave for a few hours before washing it off with soap and water.

- Remove red wine stains from marble with a solution of a few drops of household ammonia and the juice of a lemon.

- Protect marble floor tiles by reviving their shine and making them waterproof with liquid floor polish.

- Marble can also be polished with furniture cream or with milk.

- Stains on matt marble can be removed by sprinkling them with fine pumice powder, then adding a few drops of vegetable oil. Leave the mixture to work for a few hours then rub off with a clean cloth.

Glass and chrome

- Clean greasy marks from glass surfaces with lemon juice. Then polish the glass with pieces of kitchen paper or crumpled newspaper.

- Clean chrome picture frames by rubbing them with a few drops of household ammonia.

- Very dirty chrome can be cleaned with turpentine or lighter fuel, then polished to a shine with a soft cloth.

Making soft soap

The art of soapmaking has existed since ancient Babylonian times, over four thousand years ago. Soft soap is a gentle, non–abrasive detergent.

For the Victorians, soap was a valuable commodity, as it was later during the World Wars. Pieces of soap were never wasted, and when a bar was too small for use, it was stored and then melted down with other leftovers to make 'soap jelly' or soft soap.

This type of soap is less acidic than ordinary household soap, and because it is basically solidified soapsuds it lathers up very quickly and efficiently.

Soft soap can be used for hand washing both clothes and fabrics, as well as for machine washing. It is also suitable for cleaning around the house and it can be added to cleaning recipes to boost the power of the detergent.

Today, soft soap is rarely available in high street shops, but it is very easy to make. You can also buy it from select craft suppliers for use in plaster casting.

How to make soft soap
Makes about 1 litre (1¾ pints)

▼ Add **1 litre (1¾ pints) cold water** and place the saucepan over a low heat. Bring just to the boil, stirring occasionally, then simmer gently for 15 minutes.

▼ Pour the hot soft soap into a tin or heatproof jar. Once the mixture has cooled, seal with a tight-fitting lid and leave for a day to form a gel.

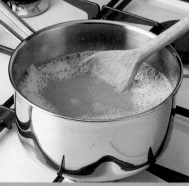

▲ Using a fine grater, grate **90g (3¼oz) good household soap** into an old saucepan. Unscented soap is best.

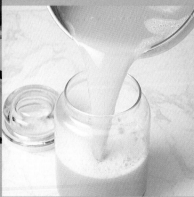

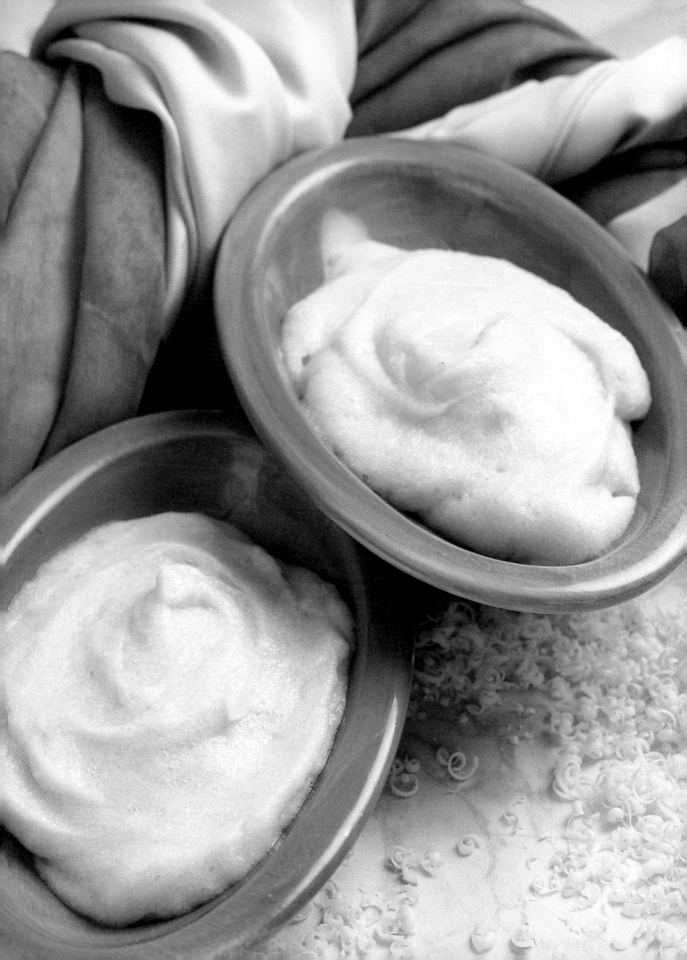

Easy ways to keep

Modern cleaning products are harsh but won't always shift food spills and stains. Try some of the tricks our grandmothers used to tackle stubborn grime and keep kitchens and bathrooms gleaming.

Because good hygiene is essential in kitchens and bathrooms and both get plenty of everyday use, these rooms require especially careful attention.

But you can save a great deal of time and energy by following a few basic principles and by organising your home sensibly. In the kitchen, crockery and utensils are best kept in cupboards or drawers, because anything left out will get covered in dust and grease.

Work surfaces should be smooth, so that they can be wiped easily and quickly. In the bathroom, too, it is best to store bottles of lotion and cleanser in cupboards, as the damp air condenses on bottles and jars trapping the dust, and can cause unsightly mildew.

For many surfaces you will find that the store-cupboard products our grandparents used, such as vinegar, salt and lemon juice, are just as effective today.

Taking extra care

For many people the kitchen is the centre of family life where everyone can relax around the kitchen table. However, this is an area that needs constant cleaning, as extra care has to be taken where food is involved.

For basic cleaning, soapy water or vinegar in water will do, but for more stubborn problems there are some useful tips in the repertoire of remedies from the past.

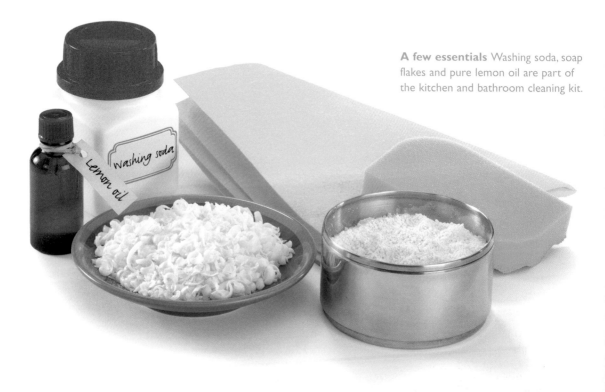

A few essentials Washing soda, soap flakes and pure lemon oil are part of the kitchen and bathroom cleaning kit.

your kitchen clean

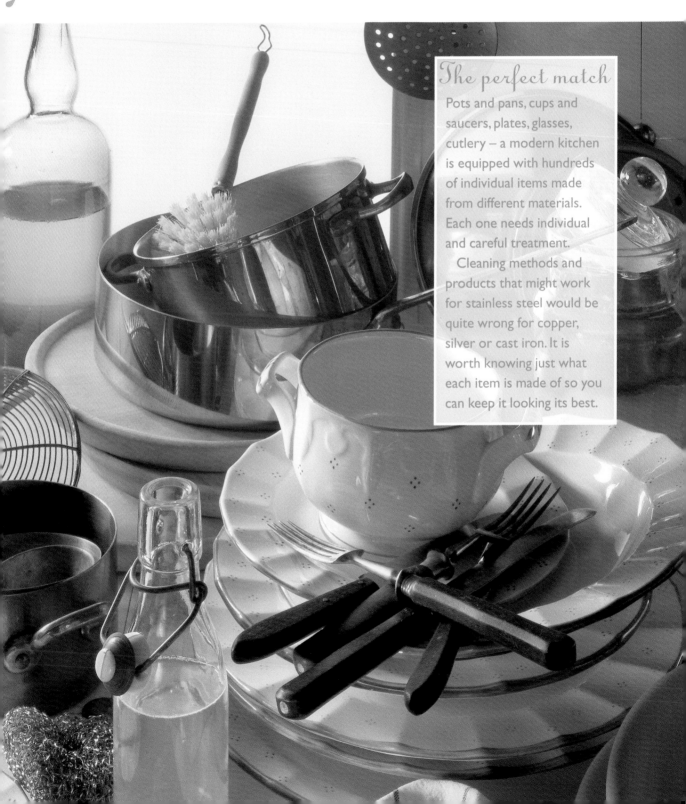

The perfect match

Pots and pans, cups and saucers, plates, glasses, cutlery – a modern kitchen is equipped with hundreds of individual items made from different materials. Each one needs individual and careful treatment.

Cleaning methods and products that might work for stainless steel would be quite wrong for copper, silver or cast iron. It is worth knowing just what each item is made of so you can keep it looking its best.

OVEN CLEANER

You can keep the oven clean by wiping it with soapy water after each use, while it is still warm. However, if you should have a spillage, this mixture will remove it without too much effort.

I tablespoon paraffin
2 tablespoons salt
I tablespoon washing soda
I litre (1¾ pints) warm water

Mix the paraffin with the salt. Wearing rubber gloves, rub the mixture onto stubborn stains with a sponge or a cleaning cloth until they have dissolved. Add the soda to the warm water and use the liquid to rinse the surfaces.

CLEANING PANS

If you have burnt some food in an aluminium or stainless-steel saucepan, fill with water and leave for an hour before trying this.

I onion
water
I tablespoon salt

Cut the onion into eight and drop the pieces into the saucepan with sufficient cold water to cover the burnt area. Add the salt and boil for 10 minutes. The burnt residue will dissolve and can be removed with a dishcloth. Boil for longer if the stain remains.

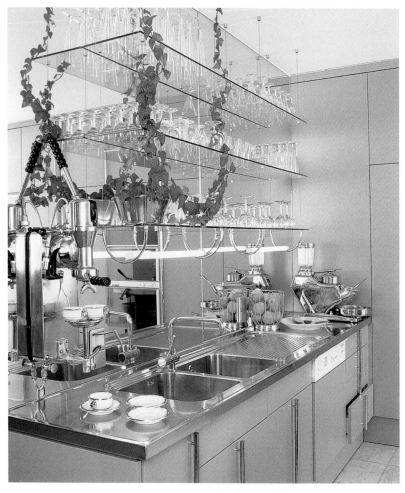

Old for new Traditional remedies work in the most modern of kitchens. Metallic surfaces, though considered modern, existed in Victorian times but only in the kitchens of the most wealthy households.

FINE SCOURING POWDER

This powder is suitable for cleaning delicate surfaces. It will keep for up to eight months.

55g (2oz) soap flakes
140g (5oz) whiting
85g (3oz) washing soda
5 drops pure lemon oil

Grate the soap flakes finely, and then mix with the whiting and soda. Finally, add the oil. Transfer to a bottle and shake well. Rub over the surface using a wet cloth.

Take care

Paraffin is a flammable liquid and care should be taken when using it. Always rinse ovens after using paraffin mixtures. Leave the door open and make sure the oven is thoroughly dry before using the appliance again.

A GLEAMING HOB

The cooker is the centrepiece of your kitchen. Ensure that it stays clean by using the following mixture. If required, this solution can be made up in larger quantities, as it keeps well for up to four months.

250ml (9fl oz) water
1 teaspoon soft soap
½ teaspoon glycerine
10 teaspoons vinegar
6 tablespoons whiting

Boil the water, then add the soft soap. Mix the glycerine and vinegar in a bowl and pour the boiling water into this mixture. Stir in the whiting then transfer to a bottle and seal tightly.

Hi tech – low maintenance In the old days, housewives rubbed the cooker with bacon rind to make it shine. The materials used for modern appliances make them easy to clean.

SPARKLING CROCKERY

Even if you have a dishwasher, there are always things that need to be washed by hand because they are very large, very dirty or very fragile. This traditional formula is environmentally friendly and will remove baked-on stains.

The lemon juice or rosemary oil will also make strong smells such as fish or onion disappear.

salt
85g (3oz) soft soap
85ml (3fl oz) water
juice of ½ lemon
   or
few drops rosemary oil

Using a damp cloth, apply a thin layer of salt over the stains. Leave for a few minutes. Dissolve the soft soap in the water. Add about 1 teaspoon of the soft soap mixture to washing-up water. Then add the lemon juice or rosemary oil.

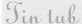

Tin tub

Many Victorian homes did not even have a stone sink in the kitchen. Plates and pots had to be washed up in a tin tub.

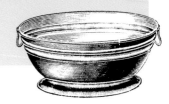

KEEP STAINLESS STEEL UNBLEMISHED

Stainless steel is hygienic, durable and easy to clean, but tends to get marked and scratched. With this special cleaning paste you can remove stains and even rub off little scratches.

1 tablespoon soft soap
1 tablespoon whiting

Blend the ingredients into a paste. Use a cloth to rub it onto the damp stainless steel, then polish.

EFFECTIVE RUST REMOVAL

Prevent cast-iron utensils from rusting by wiping them with cooking oil after washing. This mixture will remove any rust.

500ml (18fl oz) water
1 tablespoon citric acid

Mix the water and citric acid. Brush each spot with the liquid until all the rust has been removed from the surface, then rinse.

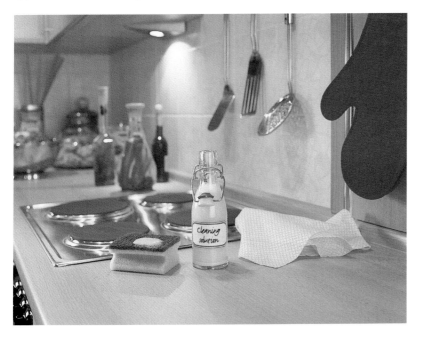

RESTORING FRESHNESS TO STORAGE JARS

Preserving jars and pots made of glass or earthenware can acquire a musty smell when they have not been used for some time. It is quite quick and easy to get rid of the smell by using this natural but effective method.

1 litre (1¾ pints) warm water
1 tablespoon baking soda
1 handful celeriac leaves

Dissolve the baking soda in the warm water and use to rinse the jars or pots. Dry them thoroughly with a clean tea towel.

Place the celeriac leaves into the bottom of the jars and stand them on a damp cloth.

Pour in boiling water and leave to stand. The damp cloth helps to prevent the jars from cracking when the boiling water is poured in.

Take care

Glass is a very good heat conductor and will become scorchingly hot when filled with boiling water.

REMOVING STAINS ON DRINKING GLASSES

If you rinse and dry glasses immediately, you shouldn't get any rings or water marks. But when you are entertaining and can't attend to the glasses straight away, marks soon form. This simple paste removes them effectively.

1 tablespoon vinegar
1 tablespoon salt

Mix the ingredients into a paste and apply with a damp cloth. Rinse with hot water and dry carefully.

GENTLE SOLUTIONS FOR NON-STICK SURFACES

Scouring powder and abrasive cleaning agents are not suitable for non-stick frying pans as they destroy the surface. This gentle but effective alternative makes use of baking soda.

125ml (4fl oz) water
2 tablespoons baking soda

Pour water into the pan, add the baking soda and bring to the boil. Pour the mixture away, rinse the pan thoroughly and then dry.

DESCALING PERCOLATORS AND ELECTRIC KETTLES

When tap water is heated, a residue of limescale remains. After a while a layer forms inside the kettle or percolator, which can reduce the efficiency of your appliance. Before using a commercial descaler, try this homemade mixture.

3 tablespoons citric acid
500ml (18fl oz) fruit vinegar

Dissolve the citric acid in the vinegar. Pour this mixture, undiluted, into the kettle or percolator and bring to the boil. Discard the liquid and rinse thoroughly or run clean water through the appliance again.

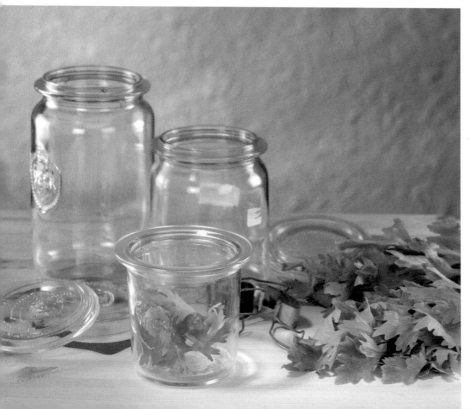

Multipurpose plant While the root of celeriac is excellent to eat, the leaves are a natural deodoriser.

NO MORE FURRY KETTLES

Prevent your kettle from furring up by placing a piece of marble, a pebble or a ball of wire mesh inside it. The following is a gentle solution to combat limescale.

300ml (½ pint) water
100ml (3½fl oz) vinegar

Pour both liquids into the kettle and bring to the boil. Let it cool, then pour away. If furring remains, repeat the process until all the limescale has disappeared.

CLEANING 'MILK'

This universal cleaning agent is based on a well-tried formula. It is gentle on both your kitchen and your hands and is particularly useful if you are sensitive to modern cleaning products.

1 tablespoon soft soap
200ml (7fl oz) water
1 teaspoon potash
15g (½oz) whiting
5 drops pure lemon oil

Put the soft soap, water and potash into a double saucepan over a low heat, stirring constantly until the soap and potash have dissolved. Whisk in the whiting. Add the lemon oil and pour this cleaning 'milk' into a bottle and seal. It will keep for up to three months.

Tried & Trusted

Cleaning cupboards

• Clean cupboard fronts with a mixture of 1 litre (1¾ pints) of water and 1 tablespoon each of vinegar and soft soap. This is suitable for Formica, wood, metal and glass.

• The interiors of units should be wiped once a year with a solution of equal parts of vinegar and water.

Sparkling hobs

• To clean dirty hotplates, switch them on at a low heat and sprinkle with baking soda. When cool, the surfaces can be cleaned with a wire pad.

• Marks on the hotplate disappear when they are sprinkled with salt and scoured with a damp brush. Rinse the surface afterwards with plenty of water and dry thoroughly with a cloth.

• Dirt on ceramic hobs can be wiped away with a damp cloth and a few drops of washing-up liquid.

Lemon wonder A freshly cut slice of lemon will remove fresh stains from worktops in an instant.

• To remove stubborn marks from ceramic hobs, use a special glass scraper, available from hob manufacturers and hardware stores. To retain the shine, polish the hob with vinegar.

Tips for other areas

• Wipe the inside of your fridge regularly with a water and vinegar solution (4:1).

• To prevent smells lingering in your fridge, place half an apple on the bottom shelf and replace it once a week. Used coffee grounds have the same deodorising effect.

• If kitchen pipes keep getting blocked, try pouring the hot water from boiled potatoes into the sink.

• Drainpipes can be kept clean by washing coffee grounds down the plughole.

• Stainless-steel sinks retain their shine if wiped with whiting and vinegar. Put some whiting in a bowl and pour on sufficient vinegar to form a paste. Apply the mixture to the sink. Wash off afterwards and polish.

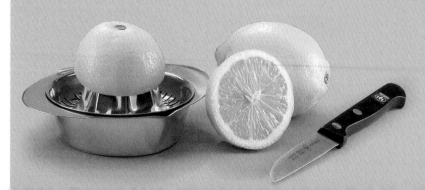

Bathrooms and showers that are clean as a whistle

The modern corrosive cleansers often recommended for bathrooms may give off vapours that can damage your respiratory system. Use these only as a last resort. Instead, try some of the following solutions to make your bathroom gleam. If you employ these regularly most marks and stains should disappear.

BRIGHTEN UP TILES AND BASINS

Dull tiles can be given a new lease of life if they are treated with this simple solution.

100ml (3½fl oz) raw linseed oil
30ml (1fl oz) turpentine

Mix together the oil and the turpentine. Apply the solution sparingly to a clean cloth and polish the tiles with it.

REMOVING YELLOW STAINS

Use this paste to lift any yellow stains under taps in basins and baths.

100ml (3½fl oz) vinegar
100g (3½oz) salt

Mix the ingredients to a paste, then apply to the stains. Leave on for up to half an hour depending on how stubborn the stains are. Rinse and re-apply if necessary.

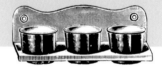

Storage jars

In days gone by, cleaning products such as scouring sand, soap and washing soda were bought in large quantities and enamel storage jars were topped up regularly for use.

GOODBYE TO LIMESCALE

Wipe off surface limescale with vinegar. Stubborn deposits can be shifted with this formula.

150ml (¼ pint) white vinegar
150ml (¼ pint) water
¼ teaspoon salt

Bring the vinegar and water to the boil. Add the salt and dissolve. Apply this liquid to the marks and directly to the fittings. Leave for at least an hour. Rinse with clean water and wipe dry.

PREVENTING BLOCKAGES

As a preventive measure, flush pipes regularly with soda water.

2 litres (3½ pints) water
3 tablespoons washing soda

Bring the water and soda to the boil and then pour it down the plughole. Repeat once a month for clear-running drains.

FREEING CLOGGED PIPES

Before calling the plumber, give this reliable method a try.

450g (1lb) salt
450g (1lb) washing soda

Mix the salt and washing soda in a bucket. Force the mixture down the offending pipe. After 30 minutes swill the pipe with boiling water, then flush through.

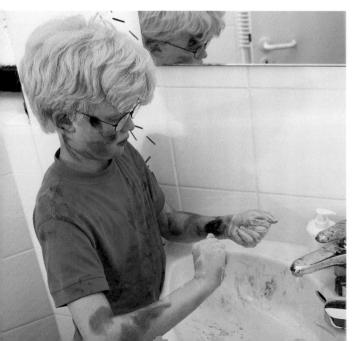

Grease and grime
An active family inevitably leaves dirty marks on baths, basins and fittings. These can be removed by wiping them with a few drops of paraffin.

If there is a blockage in the waste pipe under the basin and the water won't flow away, the usual remedy is to put a bucket under the trap, undo it and clean out the pipe. To avoid this rather laborious and unpleasant task, try clearing the blockage with the following solution.

140g (5oz) salt
140g (5oz) baking soda

Mix the salt and baking soda, then pour it down the plughole. Leave for a few minutes while the baking soda fizzes, then run the hot tap. If the water still won't run away, you can try the more aggressive method used in 'Freeing clogged pipes' (see left).

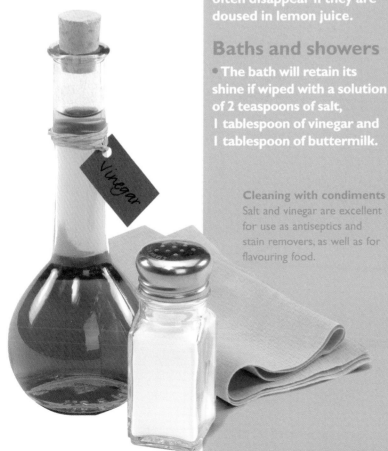

Tried & Trusted
Tiles and basins

- **Remove limescale deposits from tiles by wiping with white vinegar. Rinse with washing-up liquid or mild ammonia solution, then apply a little cooking oil to a soft cloth and polish the tiles to a shine.**

- **Restore the gleam by rubbing tiles with newspaper soaked in household ammonia. Take care to avoid the grouting.**

- **Make tiles and basins sparkle again with a cleaning paste of salt and turpentine (4:1).**

- **Yellow stains in the basin often disappear if they are doused in lemon juice.**

Baths and showers

- **The bath will retain its shine if wiped with a solution of 2 teaspoons of salt, 1 tablespoon of vinegar and 1 tablespoon of buttermilk.**

Cleaning with condiments
Salt and vinegar are excellent for use as antiseptics and stain removers, as well as for flavouring food.

- **Chrome fittings remain shiny if they are wiped with a mixture of ½ teaspoon household ammonia dissolved in 1 litre (1¾ pints) of water. They must then be rinsed and dried thoroughly. For everyday cleaning, just wipe with warm water. Always dry them afterwards.**

- **Limescale deposits will block up the spray holes of shower heads after a time. Fill a bowl with warm vinegar or salted water and immerse the shower head. Leave it in the solution until the limescale has dissolved.**

- **Wipe glass and plastic shower partitions with white vinegar to make them sparkle.**

- **Most shower curtains can be machine-washed at 30°C (86°F). Stubborn mildew and mould spots are best removed by brushing them with dry baking soda.**

Mirror, mirror

- **Hot water with a little white vinegar added is ideal for cleaning mirrors. Alternatively, rub the mirror with a potato, rinse it with clean water and polish it with newspaper.**

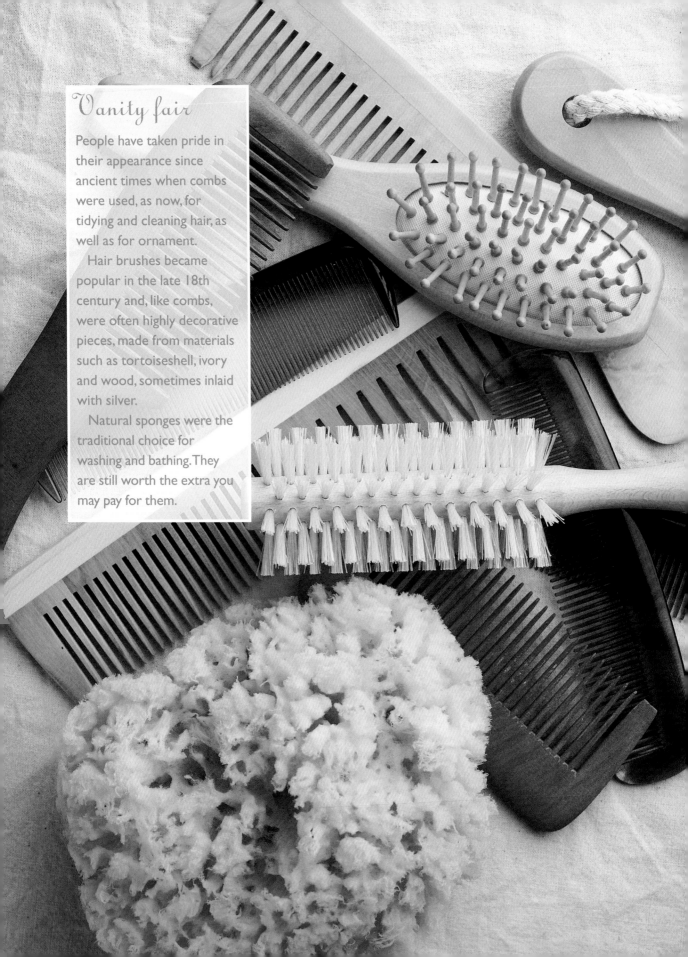

Vanity fair

People have taken pride in their appearance since ancient times when combs were used, as now, for tidying and cleaning hair, as well as for ornament.

Hair brushes became popular in the late 18th century and, like combs, were often highly decorative pieces, made from materials such as tortoiseshell, ivory and wood, sometimes inlaid with silver.

Natural sponges were the traditional choice for washing and bathing. They are still worth the extra you may pay for them.

CLEANING SPONGES

Natural sponges should be rinsed daily in clear, cold water. Once a week, clean them as follows.

125g (4½oz) salt
1 litre (1¾ pints) water

Dissolve the salt in the water and soak the sponge in the salt solution for 24 hours. Rinse thoroughly with cold water.

SPONGE CARE

After a while natural sponges will absorb a certain amount of grease from the skin and should be given an extra cleaning treatment.

1 tablespoon vinegar
500ml (18fl oz) water

Stir the vinegar into the water. Leave the sponge in this solution for a few hours, then rinse with clean water.

AMMONIA SOLUTION FOR BRUSHES AND COMBS

When washing wooden brushes, avoid getting the handles too wet. This solution will also clean glass, chrome and jewellery.

1 litre (1¾ pints) warm water
2 tablespoons household ammonia

Mix the ingredients in a shallow container. Wash the brushes and combs in this mixture. Rinse well.

The delights of bathing

A technical handbook from 1920 describes the two types of heating systems that were then generally in use for heating bath water – those that used coal and those that used gas.

In fact, the installation of a bath heater was very progressive at that time and confined to more affluent families. Most homes did not possess a bathroom at all. Instead people had to make do with a wash with water from a ewer (a large jug) in a basin in the corner of a bedroom.

Most ordinary households had a tin bath hanging in the kitchen which was used once a week. Water for the bath was boiled on the kitchen range and the heat from the fire provided welcome warmth during bathing.

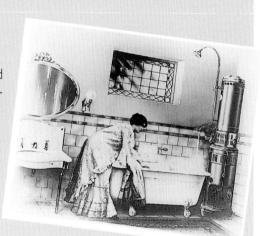

MAKING HARD BRISTLES SOFT AGAIN

If the bristles of your brush have become hard, use this special softener. It's worth conditioning all your brushes at the same time.

400ml (14fl oz) water
400ml (14fl oz) milk

Mix the milk and water and pour into a shallow container. Immerse the brushes for 30 minutes. Check the bristles and leave in for a little longer if they are not soft enough. Rinse in warm water and allow the brush to dry thoroughly.

CLEANING COMBS

Most antique combs are made of brittle tortoiseshell or horn. Unlike their modern equivalents, antique combs were never washed, as the water often split the teeth. Small, purpose-made brushes were sold for getting into the grooves.

However, modern combs can still benefit from an old-fashioned cleaning method. Wipe the comb with a cloth, then insert a piece of thin white cardboard and run it up and down between each tooth to remove any particles. Finally, wash the combs in the ammonia solution recommended (left).

Cleaning windows,

Create a sparkling first impression. A home with gleaming windows, doors and walls, both inside and out, will always be enticing to visitors and a joy to live in.

Of all household tasks, cleaning windows, doors and walls are among the least popular. Window cleaning can be particularly frustrating because, however much trouble you take, streaks always seem to appear when the sun comes out.

Doors and walls are no less problematic, so how can you tackle them successfully? The answer is don't leave it too long – catch the grime before it has settled.

Using the right cleaning materials also helps. Here you will find traditional tips and methods to make cleaning less of a grind. Most of the products used in the recipes are available in hardware stores or at supermarkets.

However, some ingredients that were common 50 years ago are now harder to find, but most can be bought by mail order or from specialist shops. Some of the suggested plants can be grown in your garden (see pages 326–331).

Sparkling clean windows

It helps to work in a methodical fashion when cleaning windows. First, clear the windowsills, then cover up furniture and floors. Start by wiping the window frames clean and then begin on the glass. Last of all, clean the sills.

Just as in the bathroom and kitchen, vinegar is the most effective ingredient for cleaning glass and is a completely natural product. For household use, white vinegar works best.

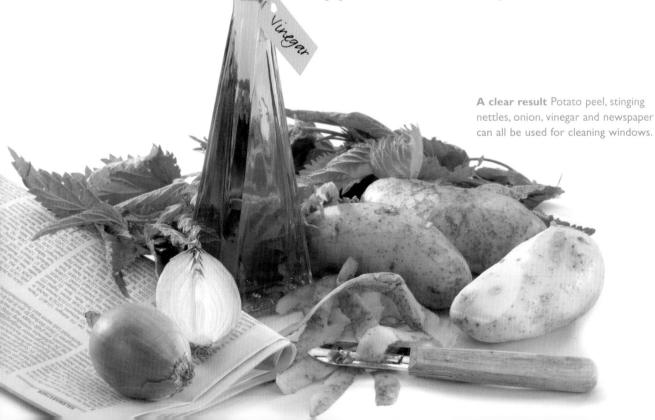

A clear result Potato peel, stinging nettles, onion, vinegar and newspaper can all be used for cleaning windows.

doors and walls

CRYSTAL-CLEAR PANES

This vinegar solution works well for general cleaning purposes, but if the windows are very dirty, use undiluted vinegar or rub them first with half an onion.

**1 litre (1¾ pints) water
250ml (9fl oz) vinegar**

Pour the water into a bucket, add the vinegar and clean the panes with a sponge. Dry with kitchen paper and buff with a handful of crumpled newspaper.

A QUICK SOLUTION

For a quick gleam in between thorough cleaning sessions, make up a supply of this window spray.

**1 litre (1¾ pints) water
squirt of washing-up liquid
1 tablespoon methylated
    spirits**

Pour the water into a spray bottle, then add the washing-up liquid and methylated spirits. Spray onto the window, wipe off with kitchen paper, then dry and buff with crumpled newspaper. Ammonia solution can be substituted for the methylated spirits.

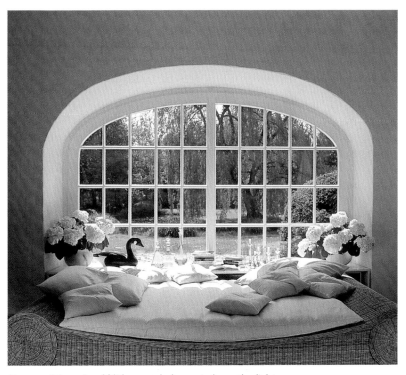

Room with a view With crystal-clear windows the light seems more intense and the room looks brighter and cleaner.

FOR AN EVEN CLEARER VIEW

A surprising way to clean windows is to use stinging nettles. Don't forget to wear protective gloves.

**1 litre (1¾ pints) water
dash of vinegar
1 bunch fresh stinging
    nettles**

Pour the water and vinegar into a bucket. Dip the leaves in the water, crunch them up, and quickly rub the windows with them. Dry with pieces of crumpled newspaper.

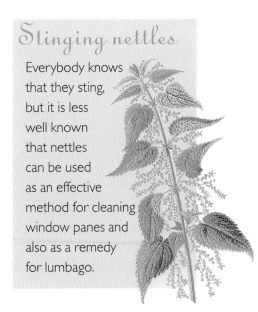

Stinging nettles

Everybody knows that they sting, but it is less well known that nettles can be used as an effective method for cleaning window panes and also as a remedy for lumbago.

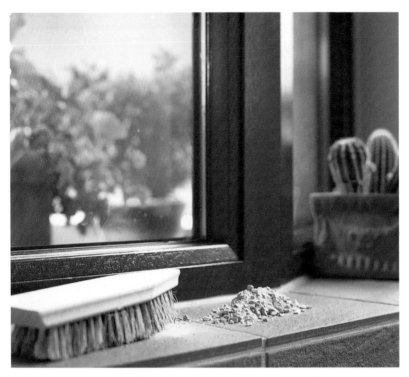

Spring clean Once winter is over, take plants off your windowsills and wash the sills down. Remove water marks from beneath pots of over-wintering plants by brushing with silver sand or rottenstone.

Cleaning doors and walls

How you clean your doors will depend on their finish. Today, doors are mostly veneered and varnished, or painted. Bare wood or stripped doors should be cleaned like wooden furniture.

Wallpapered walls should be vacuumed regularly and wiped with a dry sponge when necessary. For fabric wallpapers, consult the manufacturer or a specialist shop for care instructions.

Removing stains

Doors, paintwork and washable wallpaper only need to be cleaned with water. For more difficult stains use water with soft soap dissolved in it.

Soak encrusted dirt and grime in soft soap before washing down. Stains on woodchip wallpaper can sometimes be removed with a clean pencil eraser or by dabbing the stain with talcum powder.

LOOKING AFTER STONE WINDOWSILLS

Marks and scratches on stone sills and ledges can be removed with silver sand, the modern equivalent of scouring sand. Quantities will depend on the size of the surface to be treated.

silver sand
    or
rottenstone
water

Mix the ingredients to a thick paste and apply it to the marks and scratches. Using a bristle brush, work the paste in with even, circular movements.

A DEMISTING REMEDY

Condensation builds up on windows – especially in winter and in centrally heated homes.

1 tablespoon soft soap
½ teaspoon glycerine
1.5 litres (2¾ pints) water

Mix the soft soap and glycerine with the water. Wipe the window panes generously with the solution. Excess liquid can be soaked up with a sponge.

DIRTY WALLPAPER

Wallpaper that has become stained with smoke or dust can be cleaned in minutes.

medium-fine oatmeal

Rub the dry oatmeal gently into the stained wallpaper a little at a time, using a flannel and working in small, circular movements. Do not rub too hard or you may wear through the paper. Tie the flannel to the end of a mop or broom to reach high, inaccessible places.

This is ideal for heavily soiled areas.

2 tablespoons household
ammonia
2 tablespoons vinegar
2 tablespoons washing soda
4 litres (7 pints) warm water

Mix all the ingredients together
and wipe the wallpaper with this
solution. Dab dry with a sponge.

TILE CLEANER

This solution can also be used for
cleaning basins and floors. Do not
use on wood.

2 tablespoons washing soda
250g (9oz) whiting
2 tablespoons soap flakes
water

Grind the washing soda using a
pestle and mortar, then mix with
the whiting and soap. Add sufficient
water to make a thick liquid. Wash
the tiles, then wipe clean and dry.

Added protection Apply furniture
polish or boiled linseed oil to painted
doors to provide a weatherproof finish.

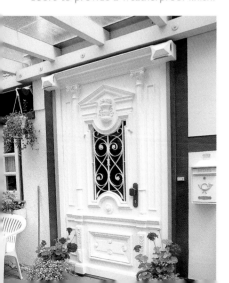

Tried & Trusted
Window cleaning

- **Add salt to your window-cleaning solution – it will give extra sparkle to your glass. Methylated spirits also does the trick, but tends to attract flies in summer.**

- **Try potato power: pour boiling water over clean potato peelings. Cool slightly, then use the warm water to wipe over your windows.**

- **Remove grease marks on glass with turpentine.**

- **Avoid cleaning windows when the sun is shining. Direct sunlight on drying panes can cause streaks.**

- **Glass can be cleaned by rubbing with damp crumpled newspaper.**

- **Wiping windows with a chamois leather wrung out in a mild solution of vinegar is another tried-and-tested method. Finish by buffing the glass with a cloth – an old towel is best.**

- **Always rinse your chamois leather in salted water after use. Soak in water, adding a few drops of ammonia to make the leather soft again.**

- **Dried-on paint can be scratched from windows with a razor blade. Remove oil-based paint by coating it with soft soap. Leave the soap to work for a few hours and then wipe it off.**

Frames and sills

- **Wipe untreated wooden window frames frequently with boiled linseed oil.**

- **Clean painted frames with a vinegar and water solution. Wipe them with neutral floor polish for anti-dust protection.**

- **Polish marble windowsills and ledges with neutral shoe polish, or use a paste made from cornflour and water.**

Tips for doors

- **Painted doors and window frames can be cleaned effectively with floor polish. This will restore the shine after frequent washes with soapy water, which quickly dulls gloss paint.**

- **Use an old toothbrush and a pea-sized blob of whitening toothpaste to take dirty marks off white paintwork.**

- **If a door squeaks, try greasing the hinges with petroleum jelly, or rubbing them with a pencil lead.**

Spotless floors

Many homes have a mixture of flooring materials. Most require a little regular maintenance but the traditional treatments will help to ensure lasting good looks.

Floors need extra attention because of the hard wear they take. The right treatment will depend on the material from which your floor is made. Many houses still have wooden floors, either floorboards or parquet flooring, which respond well to natural treatments such as homemade wax. But modern wood-effects such as strip flooring should only be wiped with a damp cloth. If badly stained, seek cleaning advice from the manufacturer.

Floors made of stone, tiles and marble, or covered with linoleum, are easily mopped and carpets must be regularly vaccuumed. But to keep them all looking their best and to give them a deep-down clean, try the recipes here.

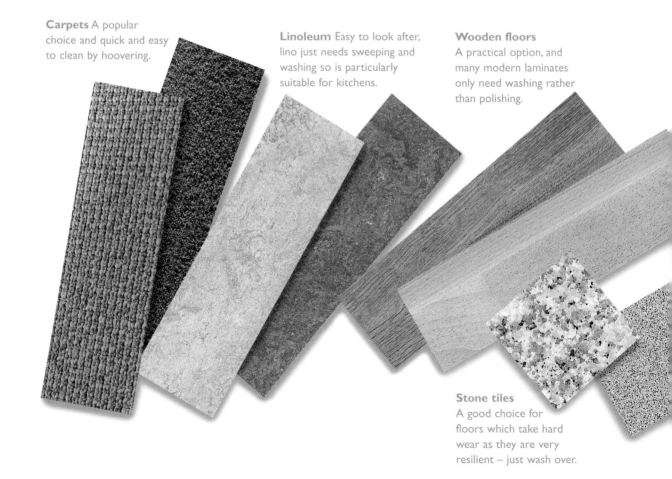

Carpets A popular choice and quick and easy to clean by hoovering.

Linoleum Easy to look after, lino just needs sweeping and washing so is particularly suitable for kitchens.

Wooden floors A practical option, and many modern laminates only need washing rather than polishing.

Stone tiles A good choice for floors which take hard wear as they are very resilient – just wash over.

Care for your flooring

To keep your floor looking good, ensure it is as dust-free as possible. Small sand particles will easily mark shiny floors if left to be ground in underfoot. Stone floors are easy to maintain: just sweep, wash and polish with a cloth.

To clean very dirty areas on ceramic floor tiles or marble and granite flooring, let the soapy cleaning water soak in for a few minutes. Rinse off with clean water and buff with a dry mop.

Sealed wooden floors and laminated flooring are also easy to clean. Just sweep up and then wipe the floor with water. But avoid cleaning polished wooden floors with water. Dry mopping and waxing should be sufficient. For this, use a homemade floor polish.

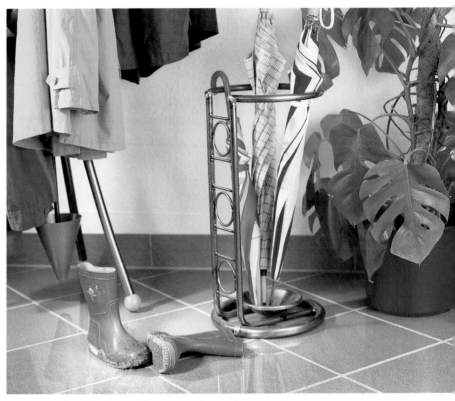

Easy-clean flooring Stone tiles just need sweeping, mopping with water and polishing with a dry cloth.

LOOKING AFTER MARBLE FLOORS

Rub soft soap into areas of flooring that are highly soiled. Wipe off with a damp cloth, then apply this cleaning paste. It will also restore the colour.

3 tablespoons non-abrasive cleaning powder
lemon juice

This amount is quite enough to clean 1m² (10 sq ft) of flooring. Add sufficient lemon juice to the powder to make a paste. Rub the floor with the paste and then rinse with clean water.

A NEW LEASE OF LIFE FOR STONE FLOORS

The time spent making this solution is rewarded by the results.

300g (10½oz) sieved wood ash
small sturdy fabric bag
10 litres (2¼ gallons) water

Carefully tip the wood ash into the bag and fasten it securely with a long piece of string. Place the bag in a bucket. Boil the water and pour it over the bag. Leave to soak for a few hours, then use the water to mop the floor. The bag can be used twice to make the washing solution.

HOMEMADE FLOOR POLISH

This excellent polish will really work wonders.

4 tablespoons furniture polish
6 tablespoons vinegar
10 litres (2¼ gallons) water

Mix all the ingredients together and wipe the floor with the polish. Use old tissue paper instead of a cloth – it won't soak up the liquid so quickly. Keep any surplus polish in a bottle for future use.

Tried & Trusted

Wood treatments

• Very dirty polished parquet flooring can be cleaned with a cloth dipped in turpentine. Rub along the grain. Re-apply wax and buff up with a clean cloth.

• If floorboards creak, try shaking talcum powder into the gaps.

• Light stains on wood floors can be removed with a paste made from a mixture of floor and shoe polish.

• Marks from shoes can be rubbed off with an eraser. For stubborn stains, use lighter fuel or turpentine on a cloth.

• Remove fresh grease stains by wiping with white blotting paper dipped in lighter fuel.

Stone floors

• Give dirty stone floors a good clean with ammonia solution. Soft soap dissolved in water also works well.

• Clean terrazzo flooring (marble chips set in cement) with soapy water.

• Stubborn stains on marble can be removed with a paste made from garden lime. Make sure that you wear protective gloves for this job.

• Remove dirt from grouting and gaps between tiles by rubbing with sandpaper.

Lino and cork floors

• Amazingly, the water from boiled potatoes can be used for cleaning linoleum.

• Remove scratches from lino by rubbing the marks gently with a fine grade sandpaper. Sweep up the dust and buff with boiled linseed oil.

• Black marks from rubber soles can be removed from lino with a cloth dipped in methylated spirits.

• Never allow linoleum, vinyl or cork tiles to become saturated. Water may cause the cork to swell and the tiles to lift.

• Sealed cork floors need only to be washed with a damp cloth from time to time.

• Polished cork flooring should be waxed twice a year at a minimum. Ideally, polish the floor every two months for maximum life.

Carpet and lino care

Vacuum your carpets at least once a week to prevent dust and grit from damaging the backing. Sponge off stains with warm water as quickly as possible to stop them penetrating the material. Wash linoleum when it gets dirty, then treat with floor polish.

CARPET CLEANER

You will find this carpet shampoo very effective.

3 tablespoons soap flakes
500g (1lb 2oz) potato starch

Grind up the soap flakes finely using a pestle and mortar and mix with the potato starch. Sprinkle the mixture over the carpet and work it in with a scrubbing brush. Leave for 30 minutes, then vacuum.

Polished or varnished? Make sure you know the finish on a wooden floor before applying a cleaner.

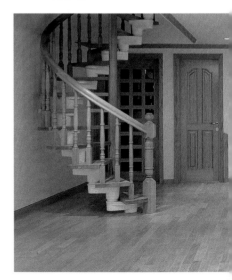

PEPPING UP YOUR CARPET

This is ideal for cleaning a carpet and restoring its colour.

1 litre (1¾ pints) water
1 tablespoon household
   ammonia
fine wood shavings

Mix the water with the ammonia. Add the wood shavings and leave them to absorb the liquid. Sprinkle on the carpet, scrub in with a brush, then vacuum up.

GETTING RID OF STAINS

Remove any stains before cleaning a carpet.

115g (4oz) household soap
2 tablespoons vinegar
1.2 litres (2 pints) boiling
   water

Grate the soap into a bucket, add the vinegar and then pour on the water. Apply the suds to the stains using a brush. Blot off excess water after cleaning. Finish by wiping over with a damp cloth.

KEEPING LINO SUPPLE

To keep linoleum from cracking, rub it with this oil mixture.

1 litre (1¾ pints) raw linseed
   oil
1 litre (1¾ pints) vinegar

Combine the oil and the vinegar and rub the solution into the surface of the floor.

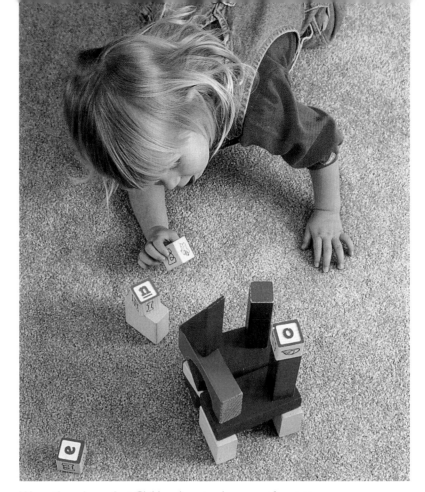

Warmth and comfort Children love to play on a soft carpet, so keep carpeted areas clean by vacuuming regularly and dealing with spills at once.

SOAPSUDS FOR LINOLEUM

Linoleum gets less dirty if it is given a regular treatment with floor polish.

2 tablespoons soap flakes
15 litres (3¼ gallons) water
2 tablespoons liquid floor
   polish

Mix the soap with three-quarters of the water and scrub the floor with a scrubbing brush. Pour and stir the polish into the remaining water and rinse the lino.

SHINY LINO

Ground-in stains on linoleum floors can be removed with fine wire wool dipped in turpentine. After rubbing off the stains, restore the shine with this polish.

1 litre (1¾ pints) milk
1 litre (1¾ pints) water

Combine the milk and water and stir well. Apply the mixture with a soft cloth and polish.

Scented candles

Candles were once the only source of light
when darkness fell. Now they are enjoyed
for their warm romantic glow.

Although gas had provided lighting
in most towns since the 1850s, in many
rural areas candles and paraffin oil lamps
continued to be the only means of lighting
until the 1920s and 1930s, when electricity
became more widespread.

Today wax candles come in all shapes,
sizes and colours. To make your own unique
candles, all the materials are readily available
from craft and specialist shops.

For these candles you will need old
saucepans for melting the wax and
watertight, heatproof containers for the
candle moulds. You will also need wire or
paper-cored wicks suitable for the candle
diameter, and wick sustainers to weight
down the wicks in the molten wax.

Prime the wicks first by dropping them
into a little melted wax for 5 minutes and
then leaving them to dry on foil.

How to make scented candles
Makes three candles

▼ Pour **40g (1½oz) stearin
powder** into an old saucepan.
Place this pan in a larger pan of
water. Bring the water to the boil
and allow the stearin to melt.
Add ¼ **disc wax dye**.

▼ Thread a wick sustainer onto
a wick and tighten it with pliers.
Cut the wick to a length slightly
longer than the height of the
container and tie it onto a
skewer. Drop the wick into the
container, pour wax in nearly to
the rim, then suspend the skewer
across the rim. Leave the wax to
set, then cut the skewer free.

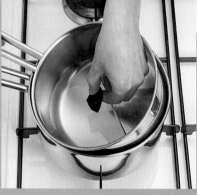

▲ Add **400g (14oz) paraffin
wax granules** and heat to
80°C (176°F), stirring
continuously. When the wax
has melted, add a few drops of
candle scent or an **essential
oil** of your choice.

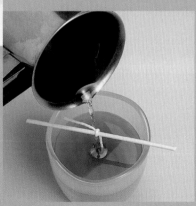

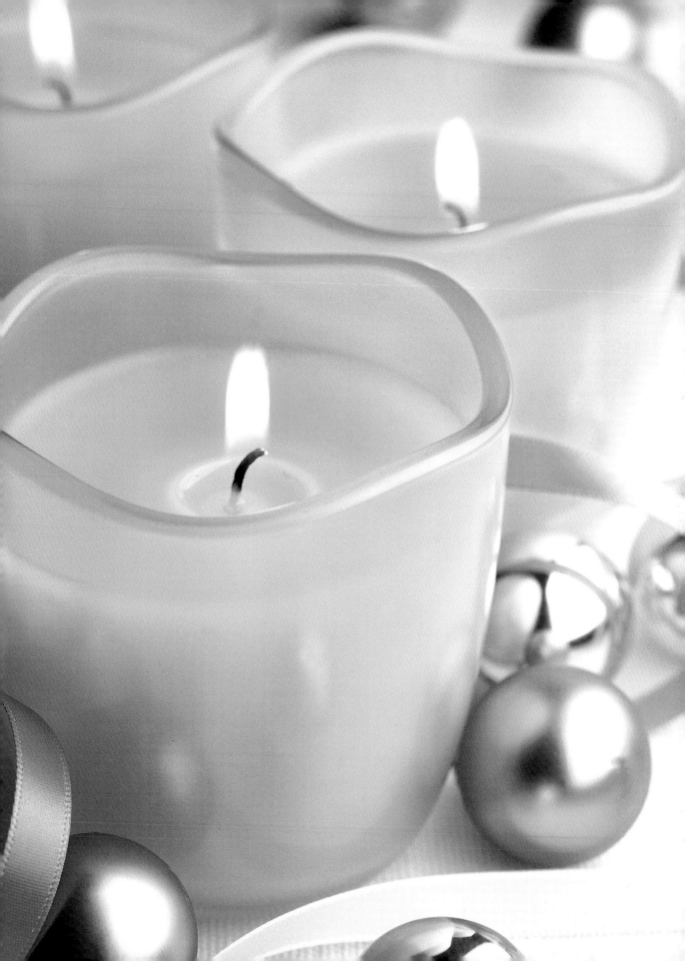

Washday wonders

Many of today's vast array of harsh washing powders, liquids, conditioners and stain removers can be replaced by a few milder preparations, made from natural ingredients.

For the majority of our grandmothers, 'washday' meant a hard day's work at the washtub. Clothes were scrubbed on a washboard, boiled in big coppers and then put through a mangle that was hand operated. Washing machines, detergents and dryers have made life considerably easier, but at a price. Countless gallons of soapsuds and harmful chemicals clog up our drains and pollute the environment which means that it is worth making the effort to achieve clean laundry in a more environmentally friendly way.

Past and present

A number of tips from times past will help to reduce the pollution. Some of the old methods not only make washing easier, but also make chemical detergents superfluous.

However, you'll need to seek out a few of the more unusual ingredients at the chemist's and remember to think ahead if pre-soaking is required.

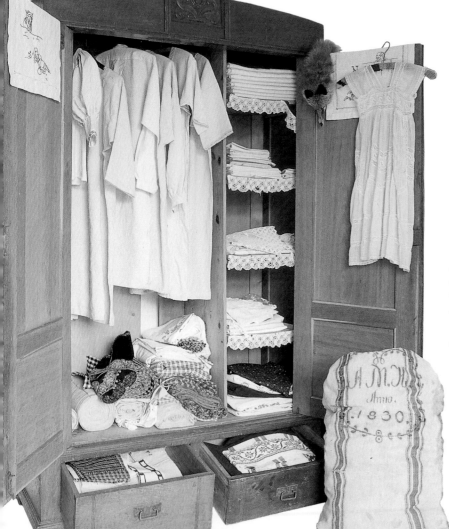

A labour of love In the 1920s it took considerable time and effort to keep the family linen laundered. Even with the advent of the washing machine, removing stubborn stains still involves special treatment.

Gentle washing

Nobody would want a return to the days of the washtub, but you can still show some environmental awareness when using your washing machine.

Choose only biodegradable washing products and use a little less than recommended. Try to do more hand-washing and next time you wash something by hand, use your own homemade soap.

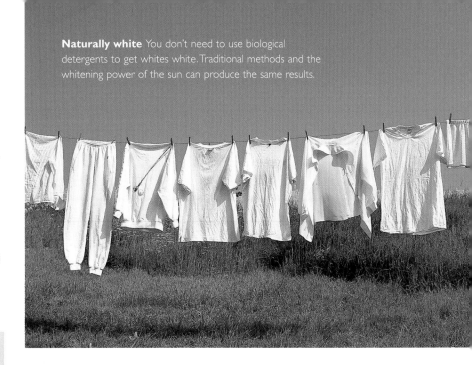

Naturally white You don't need to use biological detergents to get whites white. Traditional methods and the whitening power of the sun can produce the same results.

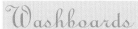

In the early 20th century, clothes and linen were rubbed 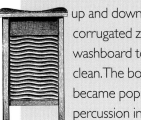 up and down against a corrugated zinc washboard to get them clean. The boards also became popular as percussion instruments.

PRE-SOAKING SOLUTION

Soaking greasy and heavily soiled clothes overnight in this solution will enable you to wash them with normally soiled items.

7 litres (12¼ pints) water
225g (8oz) garden lime

Fill a large saucepan with the water. Add the lime and heat. When the lime has dissolved, boil the solution for 2 hours. Take off the heat, cool slightly and add your washing. Wear protective gloves when using the limed water and wash any splashed solution off your skin.

SOFT SOAP FOR CLOTHES

Many coloured fabrics should only be washed in soapsuds.

1kg (2¼lb) household soap
7.5 litres (13 pints) water
500g (1lb 2oz) washing soda

Grate the soap and combine with the water and washing soda in a large pan. Bring it to the boil, stirring constantly, until the soapsuds become smooth. When slightly cooled, add the washing.

CLEAN NET CURTAINS

For best results, net curtains should always be pre-soaked.

500g (1lb 2oz) washing soda
10 litres (17½ pints) water

Dissolve the washing soda in the water and leave the curtains to soak in the liquid for a few hours. Rinse in plenty of warm water.

NO MORE GRUBBY WHITES

This excellent bleach combats yellowing and restores whiteness. Bleaching your washing in this way takes quite a long time but is worth the wait.

4 onions
25g (1oz) household soap
1 litre (1¾ pints) white vinegar
100g (3½oz) sieved wood ash

Peel and chop the onions. Grate the soap. Mix the onions, soap and vinegar with the ash, and bring everything to the boil in a saucepan. Pour the mixture into a tub and soak all the items for 12 hours, then rinse and wash. Individual stains and dirt marks can be rubbed off with the suds.

Tried & Trusted

... for softness

- Adding salt or white vinegar to the final spin will soften your washing.

- Towelling becomes beautifully soft if it is left overnight in hot water with a little vinegar added.

...for whiteness

- Pre-soak heavily soiled items in washing soda (see manufacturer's instructions for specific quantities).

- Add a tablespoon of baking soda to your washing powder for an extra white, fresh wash.

- Tennis socks regain their former whiteness if you add some lemon peel in a small linen bag to the wash.

- A gentle method of starching curtains and delicate fabrics is to place them in a bowl of water strained from boiled rice.

... for lasting colour

- Always check the colour fastness of new fabrics. To do this, wet the fabric and then rub it with white paper. If any dye comes off on the paper, hand wash the item with soft soap.

- When articles are new, the dye often runs. To avoid this, add a dash of vinegar to the water in the first wash.

- Prevent colours from running by adding salt to the final rinse.

- Add vinegar to the final rinse to restore dull colours.

- Pre-soak coloured curtains in salted water to prevent them fading in the wash.

- Restore the colours of cotton fabrics by soaking the garments for a few hours in skimmed milk.

... for delicates

- Woollens stay soft if you add a few drops of vinegar to the last but one rinse and a similar quantity of glycerine to the final rinse.

- To ensure that they don't shrink it is best to wash woollens in warm water without soap, adding a little borax or diluted ammonia.

Whiter than white
Fill a small linen bag with eggshells, tie it securely and boil it with your white wash for dazzling results.

KEEPING COTTONS WHITE

You can stop white items, such as shirt collars, turning yellow by adding this cleaner to the wash.

1 tablespoon methylated spirits
1 tablespoon turpentine

Mix the methylated spirits with the turpentine, then add it to the final rinse, or to the water used for starching. This quantity is sufficient for one bucket of water. For larger loads adjust accordingly.

BLEACHING LINEN FABRICS

It is best to do this on a sunny day when you can hang out the washing, as the sun helps the bleaching process.

10 litres (17½ pints) water
100g (3½oz) washing soda

Put the water, soda and linen into a pan and leave to simmer on the lowest heat for a few hours. Rinse well, wash and rinse again. If more bleaching is required, boil again in the same water.

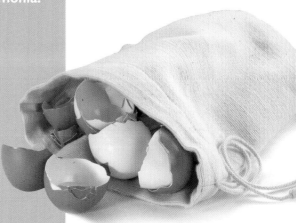

STARCH FOR USE IN THE WASHING MACHINE

Starching makes linen fresh and crisp. It also helps to stop dirt from soaking into the fibres of the fabric.

1 litre (1¾ pints) water
2 teaspoons potato flour

Pour the water into a large jug then add the potato flour. Gently whisk the liquid until the flour has dissolved. Add this starching liquid to your washing machine just before the final rinse.

WASHING LACE

Slip dirty lace into a pillowcase to protect it from damage when you wash it in the machine. As an added precaution, spray on this starch solution.

300ml (½ pint) water
1 tablespoon cornflour
salt

Combine the water, cornflour and a little salt in a container. Fill a spray bottle with the solution and douse the lace thoroughly before placing it in your washing machine.

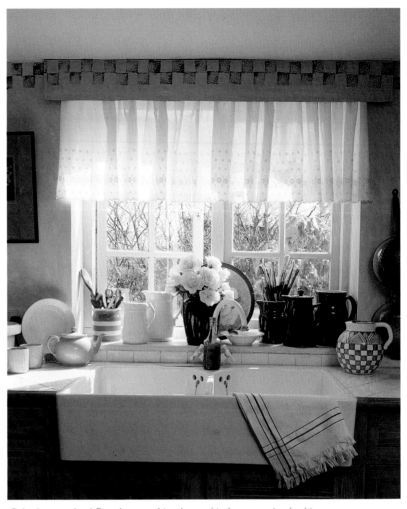

Crisply starched Regular starching keeps kitchen curtains looking good and helps to stop them from absorbing dirt and cooking smells.

Take care

Special care should be taken with antique lace and lace-embroidered table linen. Even if you are using appropriate traditional methods, seek expert advice before attempting to remove stains and clean them, as you may risk reducing their value.

WATER-REPELLENT CLOTHES

Alum is known for its water-repellent qualities. It is also used to treat leather.

1 teaspoon alum
2 litres (3½ pints) water

First wash the article. Dissolve the alum in the water, then dip the garment once or twice in the solution and leave it to dry.

WASHING LIQUID FOR KNITS

Knitwear should be washed in warm water to prevent the fibres clinging together and becoming felted. This liquid will remove light felting.

1 teaspoon borax
1 teaspoon glycerine
cold water

Dissolve the borax and glycerine in a basin of water. Wash the knitwear in it, then rinse thoroughly.

The laundry room

By the 1920s mechanical advances meant that the ideal laundry room had to accommodate a wash-boiler, a table, a washing machine and a mangle.

The first electric washing machines had an engine under the drum. The machine could only heat water and move the washing about. After washing, the dirty water was poured away and the machine refilled with clean water for rinsing.

KEEPING WOOLLENS FRESH

Before you start this treatment, hang out your clothes on a washing line to air for a few hours.

200ml (7fl oz) water
100ml (3½fl oz) household ammonia

Blend the ingredients. Moisten a cloth and gently rub the clothes with the ammonia water. Adjust the quantities depending on how many clothes you are treating and their size.

UNWANTED SHINE

To prevent woollen fabrics from becoming shiny, they should be ironed on the wrong side, or with a damp cloth placed over them. If you forget, and disaster strikes, this solution will get rid of the shine.

25g (1oz) salt
25ml (1fl oz) household ammonia
250ml (9fl oz) water

Mix all the ingredients. Sponge the garment with the solution then rinse thoroughly but gently with warm water and dry flat.

Take care

Always check the care label on woollen and silk garments to make sure they can be hand or machine-washed. Never use washing powder or liquids on items that need to be dry-cleaned.

SILK TREATMENT

Dark-coloured silk should be carefully sponged with black coffee and ironed while damp. Silk can also be cleaned with this solution.

1 part household ammonia
3 parts water

Prepare the solution. Dip a cloth into it and rub it over the silk using straight strokes along the grain of the fabric. Turn the garment inside out and iron it on the wrong side with a medium-hot iron until dry.

SILK CONDITIONER

After washing a silk garment in mild soapy water, use this conditioner to soften it.

dash of methylated spirits
water

Add the methylated spirits to a basin of water and rinse the silk. Iron the item while it is still damp.

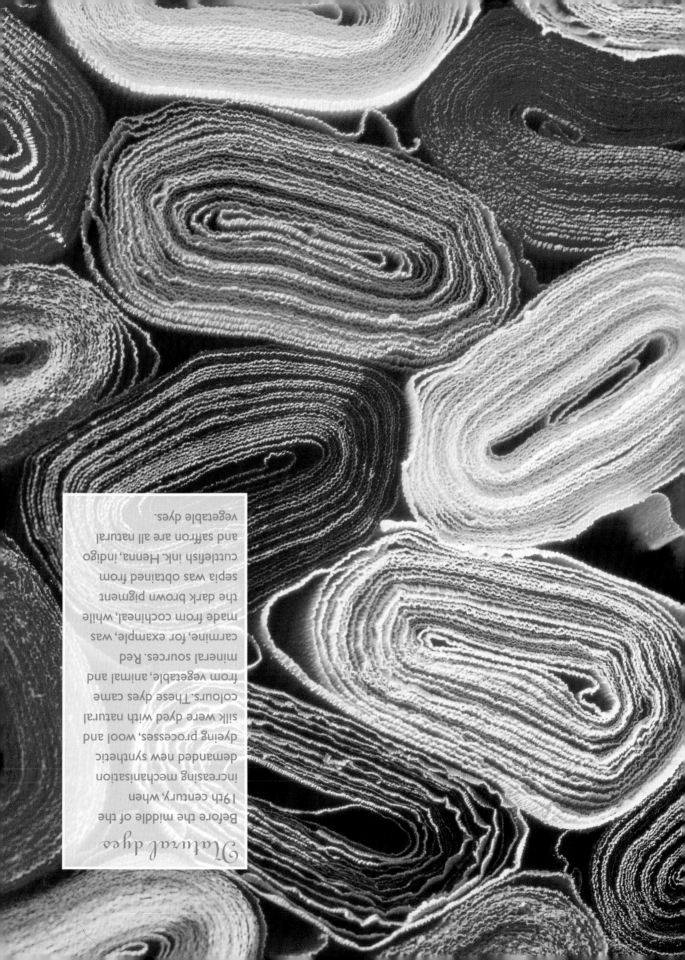

Natural dyes

Before the middle of the 19th century, when increasing mechanisation demanded new synthetic dyeing processes, wool and silk were dyed with natural colours. These dyes came from vegetable, animal and mineral sources. Red carmine, for example, was made from cochineal, while the dark brown pigment sepia was obtained from cuttlefish ink. Henna, indigo and saffron are all natural vegetable dyes.

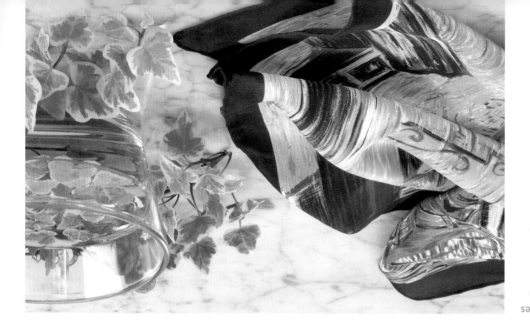

Leaf shine Ivy leaves help to restore the finish to silk. If salt and vinegar are added, silk fabrics become colourfast.

RESTORING SILK

Silk that has lost its shine will benefit from this treatment, although it is not suitable for white and very pale colours.

1 handful ivy leaves
3 litres (5¼ pints) water
1 tablespoon vinegar
salt

Wash the ivy then boil in the water for 5 minutes. Leave to cool, then add the vinegar and wash the silk in it. Rinse the silk in salted water.

PREVENT DENIM CLOTHES FROM FADING

Faded denim can be washed with new jeans to restore its colour. Salt water helps to prevent fading.

5 tablespoons salt
5 litres (8¾ pints) cold water

Dissolve the salt in the water and leave the jeans to soak for an hour. Wash in cold water.

VELVET COLLARS

Velvet collars tend to get grease marks around the edge and inside. These can easily be removed.

chalk
sheets of blotting paper

Grate the chalk finely. Place a piece of blotting paper on the collar and sprinkle over the chalk. Cover with another piece of paper and press with a hot iron until grease marks appear. Renew the blotting paper until all the grease is absorbed.

PRE-SOAKING FOR COLLARS

If collars on shirts are very dirty, loosen the grime before washing.

coarse salt
1 tablespoon isopropyl alcohol

Dissolve the salt in the alcohol and apply it to the collar with a sponge. Leave to soak in, then rinse with water and wash as usual.

WASHING GLOVES

Clean pale-coloured woollen gloves in this soapy water.

soft soap
lukewarm water

Dissolve a small quantity of soft soap in a basin of water. Gently swirl the gloves around and then rinse well. Leave to dry on a flat surface away from direct heat.

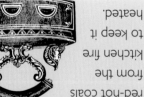

Irons
The weight of the iron used to make ironing particularly hard work as it was filled with red-hot coals from the kitchen fire to keep it heated.

Tried & Trusted
Clothes care

- **Whiten discoloured collars** with a paste made from 1 tablespoon of vinegar and 1 teaspoon of baking soda. Apply it to the collar and then wash out.

- **Coloured knitwear** can be given a new lease of life if soaked in buttermilk and then washed.

- **To stop a sweater irritating**, place it in the deep-freeze overnight. Alternatively, wash it with a mild shampoo, immerse for 10 minutes in water that has hair conditioner added and then rinse.

- **An out-of-shape felt hat** can be restored if you hold it over a steaming kettle and press it back into shape.

- **Restore the sheen of velvet garments** by brushing them with salt.

Ironing tips

- **Sprinkle your ironing** with warm water before you start. It makes ironing much quicker and easier.

- **When you iron delicate fabrics**, such as crêpe, silk or net, cover them with a thin piece of tissue paper.

Take care

To prevent unpleasant smells from building up, run your washing machine on a hot, clean water-only cycle every few months and leave the door open after each wash to let it dry.

CLEANER FOR SILK TIES

You don't necessarily have to have silk ties dry-cleaned. Try out this potato cleaner instead.

4 raw potatoes
water

Grate the potatoes into a linen cloth and squeeze out the juice over a medium-sized bowl. Add warm water to the potato liquid and wash the ties. Rinse the ties with clean water.

LIMESCALE-FREE WASHING MACHINES

Washing machines should be descaled regularly. The build-up of limescale results in higher energy consumption and reduced washing efficiency.

2.5 litres (4¼ pints) vinegar
2.5 litres (4¼ pints) water

Pour the vinegar and water together into the washing machine and run it on the hot cycle at 95°C (203°F). If you use vinegar regularly in your machine as a fabric softener, you will not need to descale so often.

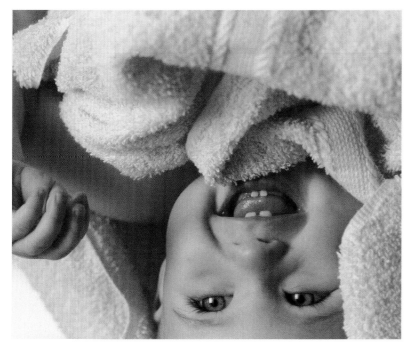

Baby-soft towels Before you hang your towels on the line, shake them out to fluff up the fibres. With the help of a gentle breeze, the towels will feel soft again.

Herb sachets

For centuries, herbs have had a wide variety of household uses. Homemade herb sachets will keep drawers and cupboards smelling fresh.

Valued for their perfume, flavour and medicinal qualities, herbs are highly versatile plants. In the garden they encourage the growth of other plants by keeping pests at bay – and they are just as effective in the house. Place small sachets filled with herbs in the linen cupboard to discourage insects.

Lavender smells lovely and keeps moths away, and its use goes back centuries. 'Your breath is lovelier than balsam, your scent as sweet as lavender flowers in a linen trunk,' reads the description of a beautiful woman written in the 14th century. Rosemary, southernwood, orris root and tansy are equally fragrant.

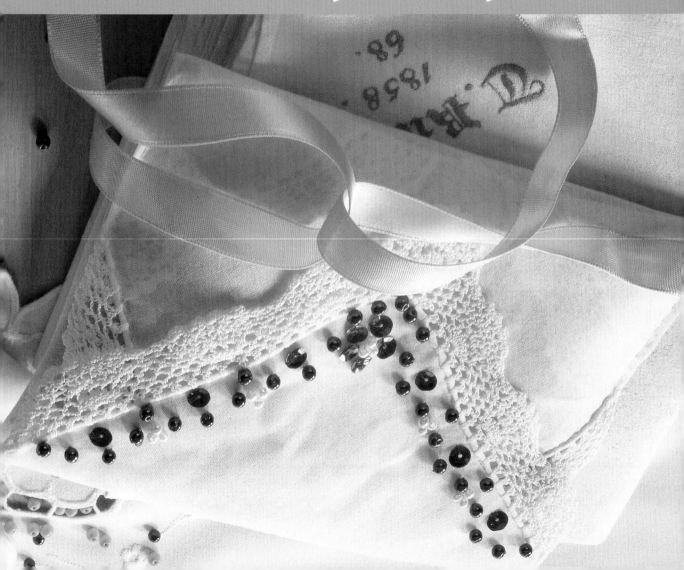

How to make herb sachets
Makes one sachet

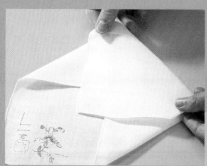

▲ Fold opposite corners of a **white handkerchief** into the middle, overlapping slightly; press with an iron. Fold up the bottom corner to form an envelope.

▼ Sew along the overlapping edges with matching **cotton thread** and invisible stitching. Decorate the flap by sewing on small **beading pearls**.

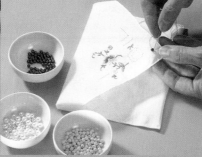

▲ Fill with 4 parts each of **tansy** and **southernwood**; 2 parts of **lavender flowers**; 1 part of **rosemary** and ½ part of **orris root powder**. Fold over the flap to close the envelope. Stitch on a small press-stud to secure.

Tried & Trusted
Rules for fabrics

• **If possible, always treat stains immediately. To protect fabric and absorb the stain, place a soft, absorbent cloth or piece of kitchen paper underneath the stained area.**

• **Stain removers should be tested first on a 'hidden' part of the fabric, at the hem or an inside seam for example. This way you can ensure that the fabric will not be damaged or bleached by the cleaning agent you use.**

• **To avoid making rings, apply cleaning liquid in a circular motion working from the outside of the stain towards the centre.**

• **If you are using diluted ammonia or turpentine, rinse the garment in water after treating the stain.**

Gentle remedies

• **Fruit stains can often be removed with buttermilk.**

• **Fizzy mineral water can be a handy and effective stain remover. Pour it over the stain, leave it to soak in for a few minutes and then blot dry with a cloth.**

Successful stain removal remedies

In the past, tradesmen who specialised in stain removal went from village to village offering their services. Now we turn to professional dry-cleaners and the many different stain-removing products on the market. To save money and to clean more gently use the old-fashioned methods, many of which work very well.

ATTACK STAINS

This is very effective for removing stains from everyday cottons. As when using any solvent, rinse the fabric afterwards and wash as usual.

4 tablespoons household ammonia
4 tablespoons isopropyl alcohol
1 tablespoon salt

Mix the ingredients thoroughly and lightly dab the solution on the stain.

FOR INSTANT ACTION

If you keep methylated spirits to hand, you can try this speedy stain removal remedy.

2 tablespoons water
1 tablespoon methylated spirits

Mix the water and methylated spirits in a small cup and use to remove the stain.

Take care

A number of chemicals, such as household ammonia, methylated spirits and isopropyl alcohol are potentially dangerous and should be stored safely. Keep them out of reach of children.

Universal solvent Mix 15g (½oz) salt and 500ml (18fl oz) isopropyl alcohol to remove stains on coloured fabrics. Check for colour fastness on an inconspicuous area before use.

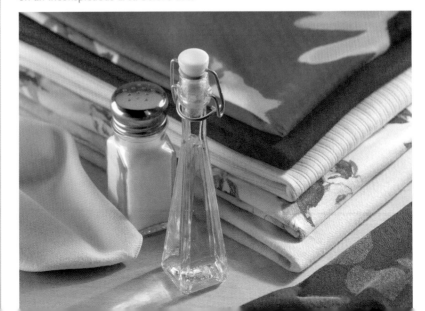

TACKLING SCORCH MARKS

Rubbing a white onion on fabrics singed by an over-hot iron will sometimes remove the scorch marks. If that fails, try this solution.

¼ teaspoon borax
100ml (3½fl oz) water

Dissolve the borax in the water. Soak a clean cloth in the solution and rub it over the burn mark. Rinse with clean water.

TREATING OLDER STAINS

If you cannot deal with a stain immediately, try this remedy.

2 tablespoons liquid detergent
3 tablespoons vinegar
1 litre (1¾ pints) warm water

Mix everything together in a bowl. Apply the solvent to the stain and leave to dry. Repeat the process until the stain disappears.

MOULD STAINS

If necessary, re-apply this solution to remove the stain completely.

1 tablespoon household ammonia
1 tablespoon salt
200ml (7fl oz) water

Stir the ammonia and salt into the water. Work this solution into the stain with a cloth. Leave the article to dry, then wash as usual.

Messy eater Most food stains come out easily if dealt with promptly. Tomato, like many other stains, should be rinsed in cold water and then soaked in a soap-flake solution before being washed as normal.

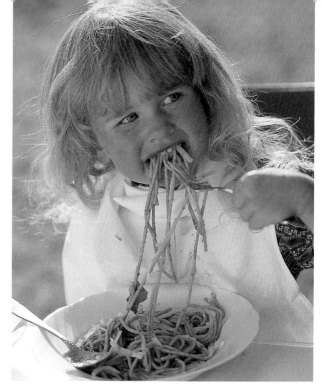

GRASS STAINS

Do not use water to wash off grass stains as it fixes them and makes them harder to remove.

methylated spirits
or
isopropyl alcohol
soapy water

Dab the stain with methylated spirits or isopropyl alcohol. Finally, wash out with soapy water.

BALL-POINT PEN

Most ink stains can be removed with warm lemon juice. If not, try this basic stain remover.

1 teaspoon white vinegar
1 teaspoon methylated spirits

Soak a cloth in this solution and rub off the stain. Then rinse thoroughly with clean water.

INK SPOTS ON THICK FABRIC

Materials with a heavier pile, such as upholstery fabric, are difficult to clean at any time. Try this remedy for ink spots.

salt
skimmed milk

Pour salt over the ink stain, then moisten it with milk. Leave for several hours before brushing it off and sponging with water.

MEDICINE STAINS

Apply this cleaner to the medicine stain before washing.

4 teaspoons fuller's earth
1 teaspoon household ammonia

Mix the ingredients to a paste and brush over the stain. Leave to dry then wash in cold water.

Tried & Trusted
Stain removal

- **Beer stains on a tablecloth: remove with very hot water.**

- **Beer stains on clothes: remove with a cleaning solution of equal parts of household ammonia and methylated spirits.**

- **Bloodstains: rinse and soak immediately in cold water. For stubborn stains add a handful of salt to the water. Wash the item as normal.**

- **Carrot juice on baby clothes: pour a few drops of baby oil on the stain and then wash as usual.**

- **Chewing gum: harden the gum by placing the article of clothing in the freezer for an hour. Scrape off.**

- **Egg: for egg white use cold water; soak egg yolk in a glycerine solution and then wash in warm water.**

- **Fruit juice: rinse in cold water and treat with a glycerine solution.**

- **Craft glue: soften the adhesive in warm water, wipe the stain with vinegar and then rinse. Some permanent glues may be more stubborn.**

- **Grease and oil: sprinkle stains with cornflour or talcum powder. Brush it off when the grease is absorbed and rinse in cold water. Finally, wash at as high a temperature as possible.**

- **Milk: sponge with cold water. Old milk stains can be removed with a solution of diluted ammonia.**

PERSPIRATION MARKS

Try soaking stains in a lukewarm solution of diluted white vinegar. Alternatively, use this method.

water
household ammonia
vinegar

Mix equal parts of water and ammonia. Soak the stains in the solution and then rinse. Add 1 tablespoon vinegar to 600ml (1 pint) water and apply to the stains. Wash as normal.

FRUIT STAINS

First try washing the stained articles with methylated spirits. If that doesn't work, try this alternative method.

2 tablespoons household ammonia
2 tablespoons buttermilk
1 teaspoon lemon juice

First warm the ammonia with a little water and apply it to the stain. Then mix the buttermilk with a little lemon juice and leave the item to soak overnight. Wash out the next day and rinse well.

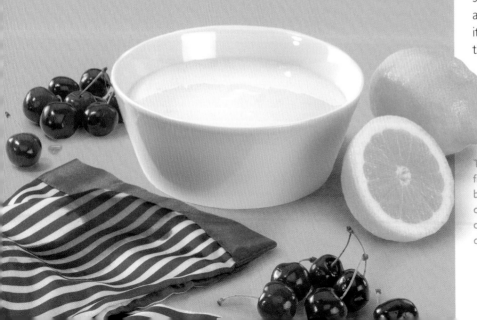

Troublesome marks Stains from cherries, mangoes and bananas are particularly difficult to shift. This is because of the fruit acid and natural dyes they contain.

OIL-BASED PAINTS

Paint hardens quickly, so act immediately for the best results.

turpentine
household ammonia

Scrape off as much paint as you can. Mix together equal amounts of turpentine and ammonia and dab onto the stain with a cloth. Keep re-applying the mixture with clean areas of the cloth to prevent smudging. Rinse well.

CANDLE WAX

Before treating wax stains with a solvent, flake off as much wax as possible with your fingernail or a palette knife. Then try the following method.

methylated spirits

Apply the methylated spirits to the stain using a linen cloth. Dab gently at the wax as it dissolves, removing it slowly.

MUD STAINS

Allow mud to dry before brushing it off, otherwise the dirt will become ground into the fabric.

potato water

Remove the surface mud, then rub the stain with strained water in which potatoes have been boiled. If the stain still remains, try a weak ammonia solution with ¼ teaspoon of borax added.

Caring for leather and suede shoes

Leather is a natural, hard-wearing material that has been used for thousands of years. Suede is slightly softer leather, produced by rubbing the flesh side of the hide. Many of the old methods for keeping these materials supple are still effective.

Regular cleaning and polishing keeps leather looking good and protects it from the elements and everyday wear, prolonging its life. Don't buy expensive proprietary polishes – with a few ingredients you can make your own.

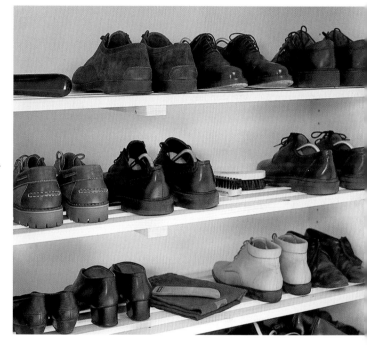

Keep shoes in shape Use shoe-trees to keep your shoes at their best. Store them in an airy shoe cupboard or on a large shoe rack where they won't get dusty or crushed.

EVERYDAY SHOE POLISH

If this polish hardens when stored, soften it in a warm oven.

150g (5½oz) petroleum jelly
2 teaspoons beeswax granules
2 teaspoons water
1 teaspoon soap powder

Melt the petroleum jelly and beeswax in a bowl over a pan of simmering water. Blend the water with the soap powder, then add to the wax. Stir and leave to cool.

NEUTRAL SHOE POLISH

This polish is particularly good for pale-coloured shoes.

1 teaspoon beeswax granules
5 heaped teaspoons lanolin
2 tablespoons soya bean oil

Gently heat all the ingredients in a bowl placed in a pan of simmering water until the wax melts. Cream the mixture with a hand blender set at a low speed, then transfer to a tin. It will keep for eight months.

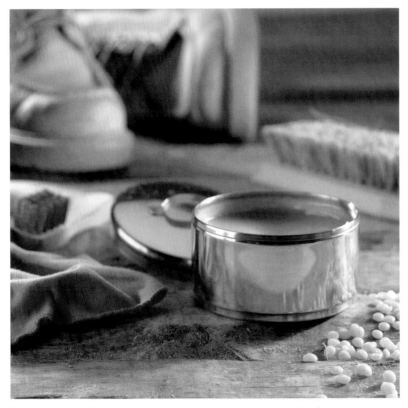

Natural protection Beeswax granules, lanolin and soya bean oil make a wonderfully effective and protective cream for leather shoes.

GENTLE CARE FOR WHITE LEATHER

You'll find the two ingredients for this protector in your kitchen.

1 tablespoon milk
egg white

Mix the milk and the egg white. Moisten a light-coloured cloth with the mixture and apply evenly to the leather.

RESTORER FOR PATENT LEATHER SHOES

Cream can be a treat for shoes. Use single or double cream to make this mixture.

30ml (1 fl oz) raw linseed oil
50ml (2fl oz) cream

Mix the linseed oil with the cream. Dip a soft cloth into the liquid and rub onto the leather until it shines.

PATENT-LEATHER SOFTENER

Patent leather needs to be maintained to prevent it from drying out and becoming hard.

juice of 1 lemon

Rub the freshly squeezed lemon juice over the patent leather using a lint-free cloth. When the surface is dry, rub the leather with a soft rag, then polish as usual.

BLACK SHOE POLISH

Soot is needed for this polish. If you happen to have an open fire and chimney, you might want to give it a try.

1 egg
1 teaspoon vinegar
2 teaspoons beer
1 teaspoon soot
few drops paraffin

Whisk the egg and stir in the remaining ingredients. Apply the cleaning fluid with a soft cloth.

CLEANING BROWN SHOES

This mixture for cleaning brown leather shoes takes only minutes to make. Prepare only as much as you need, as it does not keep.

3 teaspoons skimmed milk
1 teaspoon turpentine

Mix the skimmed milk with the turpentine. Soak a cotton cloth in the cleaning solution and rub it over the shoes. Buff with a duster.

SPRAY FOR SUEDE

Stains on suede shoes can be removed with fine sandpaper. For protection and care use this spray.

1 tablespoon fruit vinegar
175ml (6fl oz) water

Pour the vinegar and water into a spray bottle and douse the shoes. Leave to dry before brushing them with a wire suede brush to raise the nap.

SUEDE PROTECTOR

This variation on the suede spray above gives added protection against the rain.

1 tablespoon glycerine
1 tablespoon fruit vinegar
5 tablespoons water

Mix all the ingredients together and pour into a spray bottle. Apply it to suede shoes, then allow them to dry naturally.

Well travelled Keep luggage in tip-top condition by removing dust and dirt from leather suitcases with a solution of milk and turpentine.

LEATHER PROTECTION AGAINST MOISTURE

Protect your boots and shoes against rain, snow and slush in the winter months.

2 tablespoons beeswax granules
1 tablespoon lard or dripping

Melt the beeswax and lard in a double saucepan. When the mixture is cool, apply to the leather with a cloth. Leave overnight, then polish with a soft cloth.

Take care

Leather and suede becomes damaged and marked when soaked through. Wet shoes should be sponged clean, stuffed with crumpled newspaper and left to dry naturally, away from direct heat to prevent white marks forming.

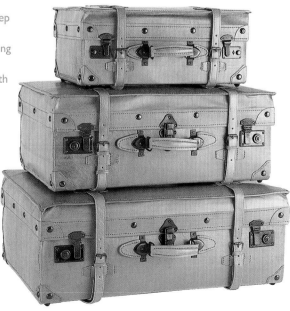

Tried & Trusted

Removing stains

● Restore stained leather shoes by rubbing them with half an onion. Polish them with a soft cloth.

● If your shoes become scuffed, rub the leather with the inside of a banana skin and dry it with a soft tissue.

Rain protection

● Rub leather uppers with castor oil to waterproof shoes and boots.

● In autumn you can quickly dry out damp shoes by putting chopped conkers in them.

● Apply a thin coat of matt varnish to leather soles to make them waterproof and to help them to last longer.

Other items

● Grease on suede collars and cuffs can be rubbed off with a pencil eraser.

● Clean fur-lined shoes with talcum powder. Sprinkle the powder over the fur lining and then shake it out again after a few hours.

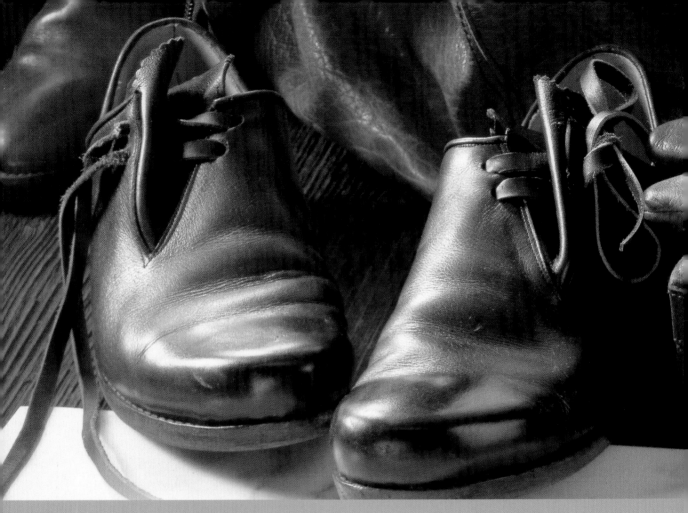

Waterproofing shoes

Rain, snow and slush can ruin leather shoes, but by using this special solution made with natural ingredients you can protect your shoes and keep them looking good in all weathers.

Even at the end of the 19th century, when leather shoes were being industrially manufactured, they remained a precious commodity. Most working folk wore simple wooden clogs. People learned how to look after their leather shoes to make them last as long as possible.

Every day, people would give the soles and heels of their shoes a thorough brushing, then clean and polish the leather uppers. In winter, shoes were often waterproofed with a homemade solution made from beeswax to prevent hardened leather from cracking. This can still be used today.

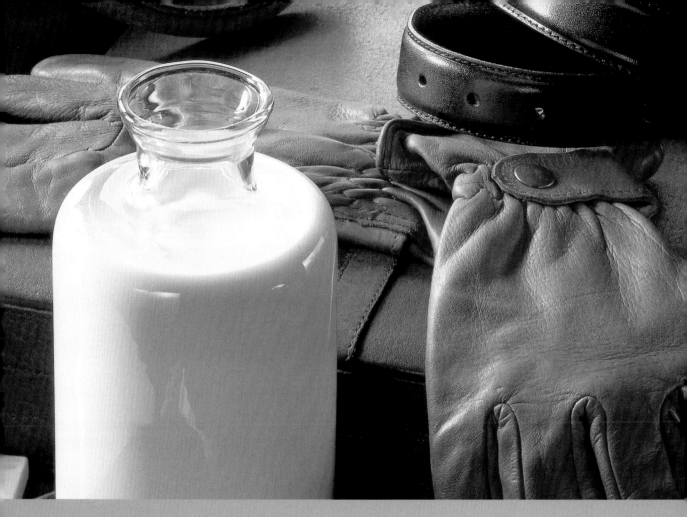

How to waterproof leather shoes
Makes approximately 1.2 litres (2 pints)

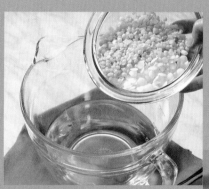

▼ Add **25g (1oz) soap flakes** to **600ml (1 pint) water** and heat gently until the soap flakes have dissolved.

▲ Measure **85g (3oz) beeswax** and **25g (1oz) white beeswax granules**. Put in a bowl and stand in a pan of simmering water. Heat gently, stirring, until all the wax has melted. Add **600ml (1 pint) turpentine** and stir.

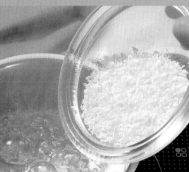

▲ Blend the soapsuds with the wax and turpentine solution. Whisk vigorously until it has a smooth and thick consistency. Pour it into a bottle, seal and label. Wipe over shoes with a cloth and buff with a dry duster.

Caring for precious

We all have treasured ornaments, pictures, jewellery
and glassware. To keep them looking their best,
use natural polishes and cleaning solutions.

During Victorian times, it was customary for a new bride to be given a book such as Mrs Beeton's *Book of Household Management* which was a popular gift from its publication in 1861.

In other cases a beautifully bound booklet might be given, handwritten by the bride's mother, who used it to pass on all her own knowledge and experience of housekeeping. The introduction to this booklet would usually expound the housewifely virtues, and was followed by important aspects of household management, including cooking, needlework, entertaining and child care, as well as tips on the purchase and maintenance of machines.

Pages were also devoted to subjects such as washing and cleaning. Looking after gold, silver, copper, brass and pewter objects was particularly important, as every housewife took pride in keeping valuable items sparkling.

Beautiful frames

When hanging heavy paintings, attach two small blocks of wood or cork to the back of the picture frame. These will protect the wall and allow air to circulate, thus stopping moisture getting into the picture and the frame. Rub polished wood frames with a damp cloth. Gold frames require careful treatment, as the fine layer of gold rubs off easily.

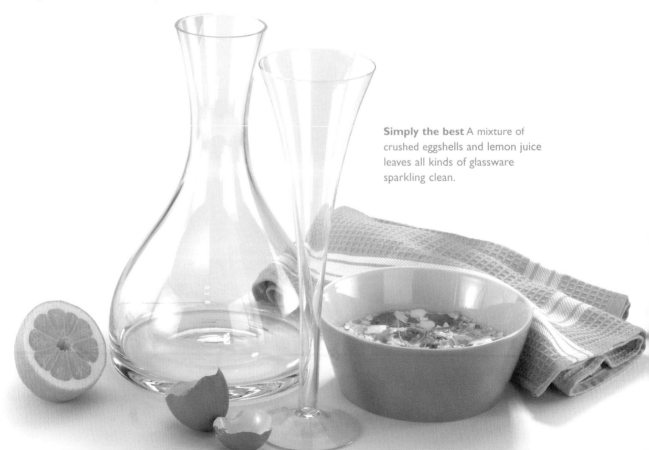

Simply the best A mixture of crushed eggshells and lemon juice leaves all kinds of glassware sparkling clean.

household objects

GENTLE CARE

This cleaner is suitable for silver and gold frames.

**2 tablespoons household
 ammonia
250ml (9fl oz) lukewarm
 water**

Add the ammonia to the water, mix well and apply it with a sponge to the metal frame.

CLEANING BRASS FRAMES

If a brass frame becomes tarnished, make it look like new without removing the lacquer.

**300ml (½ pint) turpentine
300ml (½ pint) methylated
 spirits
200ml (7fl oz) sunflower oil
150ml (5fl oz) vinegar**

Pour the ingredients into a glass bottle, seal with a cork stopper or cap and shake vigorously. Rub the cleaner over the brass with a cotton cloth. Polish off with a soft duster. Store in a cool cupboard and shake before use.

Special treatment
Ornate gilt mouldings need a delicate touch. Dust them regularly with a soft dry watercolour or make-up brush to stop dirt from building up. If the frame needs cleaning, use a cloth or cotton bud dipped in turpentine. For valuable frames, seek expert advice.

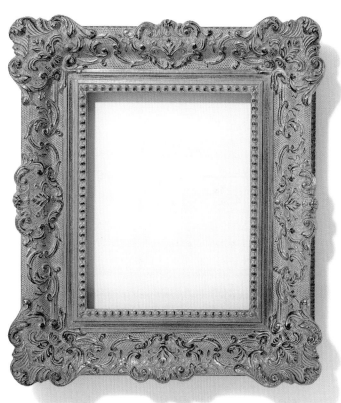

Keeping your glassware glittering

Everyday glass can be put in the dishwasher, but valuable crystal should be washed by hand. Use warm soapy water, rinse each item, then dry and polish it.

Bottle brush

The handy bottle brush is still a most useful kitchen item. It comes in a range of sizes to suit different purposes.

CLEANING AWKWARDLY SHAPED GLASS

Intricate glass vessels are often difficult to clean. Try this method.

**eggshells
lemon juice**

Adjust the quantities to the size of the vessel. Scrunch up several eggshells, then cover with lemon juice. Leave to infuse for two days. Fill the vessel with the liquid and swirl it gently around until the glass is clean.

183

FOR BEAUTIFUL GLASS

Remove occasional stains by rubbing them with the cut surface of a raw potato. For badly stained glass use this cleaner.

1 litre (1¾ pints) water
¼ teaspoon potash
few drops household
ammonia

Mix the ingredients and pour them into the glass vessel. Leave the solution to stand for several hours, then rinse thoroughly.

TO REMOVE GREEN ALGAE

Use this tea solution to remove the green algae that cling to a vase when flower stems begin to rot.

1 handful black tea leaves
vinegar

Drop the tea leaves in the glass vase and pour over sufficient vinegar to quarter-fill the vessel. Swirl the liquid around until all the algae have been removed. Then pour it away and rinse well with warm soapy water.

Take care

Avoid putting cut glass or fine crystal in the dishwasher. There is always a danger that the dishwasher detergent will cause 'etching' – white marks on the surface of the glass which are impossible to remove.

SCRATCHED MIRROR GLASS

Achieve a high gloss finish on your mirror glass by polishing it with an old pair of tights dipped in methylated spirits. To hide scratch marks use the following remedy.

silver polish
or
brass polish
toothpaste

Blend together equal quantities of silver or brass polish and toothpaste on an old saucer. Apply the paste to the scratches using a lint-free cloth. Leave for 5 minutes, then polish off the excess.

Keep your gold and gold plate glittering

In time, both silver and gold get tarnished and turn black. One old method of removing this layer is to wipe it with fine whiting moistened with ammonia or alcohol.

CLEANING GOLD JEWELLERY

You will need softened water – ideally cooled, boiled water – for this jewellery cleaner.

2 tablespoons household
ammonia
500ml (18fl oz) softened
water

Combine the ingredients in a pan, then place the jewellery in the solution. Simmer for about 10 minutes. Drain, then rinse with cold water and polish with a chamois leather.

The best silver

In Victorian and Edwardian times, a silver tea service, silver cutlery and fine china would be on display in the best households. However, they would only be used on very special occasions.

Gold-plated objects can be placed in a solution of water and soft soap. Clean all jewellery worn next to the skin regularly to keep it sparkling.

UNTARNISHED GOLD

Before you start cleaning gilded items, make sure that they are made with real carat gold.

1 tablespoon grated
household soap
water
household ammonia

Dissolve the soap in the water, then add a few drops of ammonia. Dip an old toothbrush into the solution and gently scrub the gold. If the tarnish is obstinate, increase the strength of the ammonia.

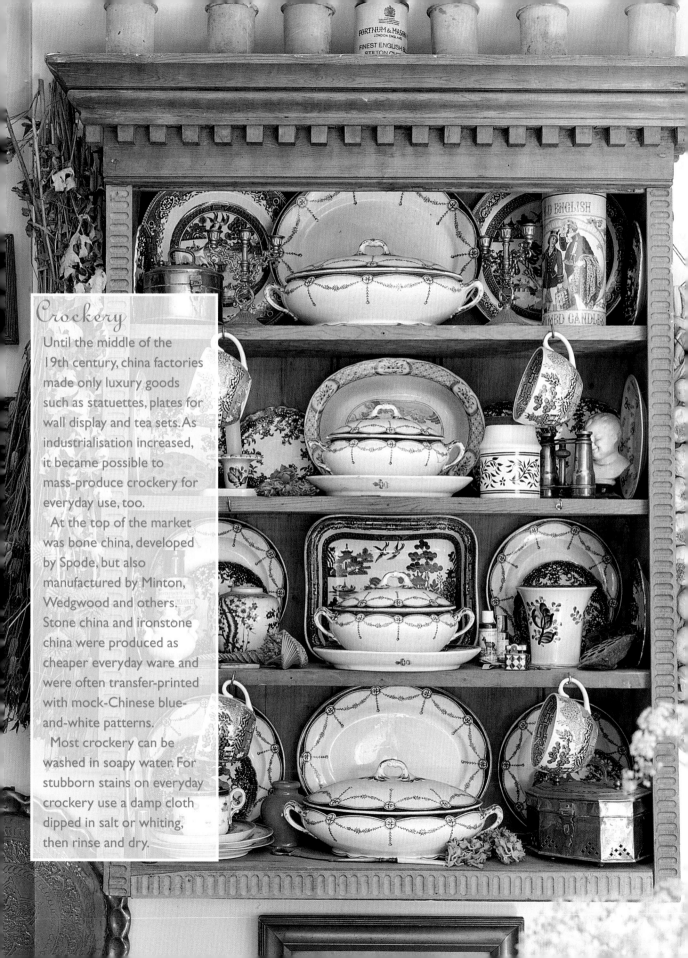

Crockery

Until the middle of the 19th century, china factories made only luxury goods such as statuettes, plates for wall display and tea sets. As industrialisation increased, it became possible to mass-produce crockery for everyday use, too.

At the top of the market was bone china, developed by Spode, but also manufactured by Minton, Wedgwood and others. Stone china and ironstone china were produced as cheaper everyday ware and were often transfer-printed with mock-Chinese blue-and-white patterns.

Most crockery can be washed in soapy water. For stubborn stains on everyday crockery use a damp cloth dipped in salt or whiting, then rinse and dry.

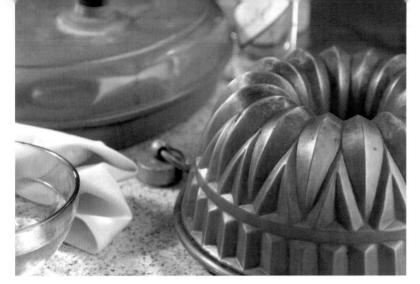

Decorative copper In the past copper moulds were practical utensils used for jellies and blancmanges. Now these moulds are also put to decorative use and are often lacquered to keep them looking good.

Polishing copper

Traditionally, every self-respecting household boasted a kitchen filled with shiny copper utensils. The disadvantage of copper is that a layer of verdigris, which is poisonous, forms on the metal when it comes into contact with acids and fats in food. This is one reason why nowadays copper is lined with stainless steel.

Old copper pots and pans were unlined. If verdigris formed on the surface it was removed immediately using this effective cleaning solution.

250ml (9fl oz) water
½ teaspoon salt
dash of household ammonia
chalk powder

Mix the water, salt and ammonia. Dip a cloth into the liquid and wipe off the verdigris. Polish the copper with the chalk and a cloth.

Silver, brass and pewter

To prevent tarnishing, it is best to wash and polish silver cutlery as soon as possible after use. Keep it in a drawer lined with velvet, or in a cutlery box or canteen. Brass mounts and door handles should regularly be rubbed with a chamois leather. Pewter is now mainly used decoratively and needs only occasional cleaning.

Take care

Always proceed with caution if you have any items that you believe to be valuable. Oil paintings, jewellery and antique silverware can be irretrievably damaged by cleaning and polishing.

FOR GLEAMING SILVER

This is an effective method of cleaning and polishing silver.

4 teaspoons salt
4 teaspoons baking soda
1 litre (1¾ pints) water

Add the salt and baking soda to the water. Soak the silver for 10 minutes in the solution. Rinse each item carefully. Dry thoroughly with a clean tea towel and polish the silver with a chamois leather.

STOCKING UP ON SILVER POLISH

With this recipe, you won't run out of silver polish for a while.

70g (2½oz) chalk powder
85ml (3fl oz) household ammonia
125ml (4fl oz) methylated spirits
500ml (18fl oz) water

Mix all the ingredients together and pour into a glass bottle. Seal and shake before use.

SHINING UP BRASS

Copper cleaning agents are also suitable for cleaning brass.

few drops paraffin
few drops methylated spirits

Mix together the ingredients in equal amounts. Dip a cloth into the solution and wipe it over the brass.

TAKING CARE OF PEWTERWARE

Common horsetail, which is also called scouring-rush, is found in fields, on dunes and on roadsides.

1 handful fresh horsetail 'needles' and stems
1 teaspoon vinegar

Mix the crumbled horsetail with the vinegar. Rub on the pewter and leave overnight. Rinse, then polish with a soft cloth.

CABBAGE AND LEEKS FOR CLEANING PEWTER

For this recipe use the outer leaves of a cabbage.

few cabbage leaves
green leaves of a leek

Chop the cabbage leaves finely and use to rub down the pewter. Rinse with clean water and then rub with the leek. Rinse again with clear water and dry with a soft cloth.

Tried & Trusted

Paintings and glass

• To clean an oil painting, wipe it very gently with a raw potato cut in half. Alternatively, dab the surface with fresh white breadcrumbs, then brush off.

• Another method is to carefully wipe the oil painting with a soft cloth dipped in warm milk, then dry the picture with a piece of silk.

• When washing crystal by hand, add a little household ammonia to the washing-up water to make the glass sparkle like new.

• To give sparkle to your glassware, rub a paste of vinegar and salt (1:1) over the surface; rinse and dry.

• Clean glass and plastic bottles with rice. Drop a few grains into the bottle, add a little water and then shake well. Rinse thoroughly.

• Small limescale deposits in glasses can be removed by rubbing with vinegar.

Copper and brass

• Shine copper with a cloth dipped in vinegar and sprinkled with a little salt.

• If you wipe brass taps, door handles and curtain rods with wax polish, they keep their shine for longer.

Gold and silver

• Polish gold and silver jewellery with toothpaste and it will gleam again.

• Keep a piece of chalk in your jewellery box to stop metal items from tarnishing so quickly.

• Wipe tarnished silver with household ammonia and then polish it.

• Keep silver cutlery looking bright by wiping it with petroleum jelly after it has been cleaned.

• Very dirty pewter can be cleaned with warm beer. Scrub it with a soft brush and then rub.

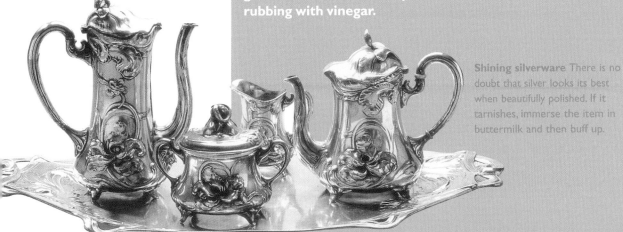

Shining silverware There is no doubt that silver looks its best when beautifully polished. If it tarnishes, immerse the item in buttermilk and then buff up.

Fragrance all round

Whether you want to get rid of an unpleasant smell or create a fragrant one, there are many old recipes that can help. Both dried and fresh plants can be used to make an intoxicating scent.

A room that smells of flowers or spices is welcoming and relaxing. In the past, a variety of flowers and herbs were used to make sweet-smelling posies, or perfumes and potpourris for elegant salons and bedrooms.

Wealthy people had special rooms for growing the plants and a maid responsible for their care who provided a constant supply of dried flowers and herbs.

With scented sachets, dried flowers and herbs, you can still create a fragrant home without using artificial sprays.

Many recipes make use of essential oils that have a perfume characteristic of the plant or tree from which they come. They are commonly used in aromatherapy and are easy to buy (see The main ingredients, pages 332-339).

Fresh air for every room

Get rid of the smell of tobacco smoke and other unpleasant odours with a special air freshener.

HELP FROM DOWN UNDER

Eucalyptus leaves, from plants native to Australia, are available in florist shops or gardens.

200g (7oz) fresh eucalyptus leaves
1 litre (1¾ pints) vinegar

Place the leaves and vinegar into a jar with a screw top. When needed, heat a few tablespoons of the mixture in an oil burner and leave it to vaporise in the room.

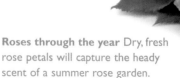

Roses through the year Dry, fresh rose petals will capture the heady scent of a summer rose garden.

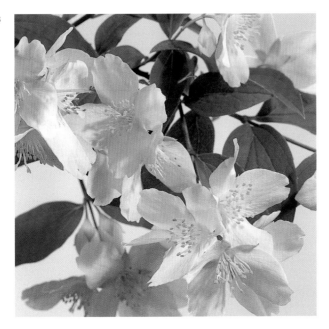

Scented petals
The white flowers of the 'mock orange', *Philadelphus coronarius*, have an intense fragrance.

CLEARING THE AIR

The most common use for essential oils is as room fragrances. Pine oil can also be used as an inhalant to relieve colds.

cotton cloths
pine oil

Sprinkle the oil onto the cloths and hang them up in the room.

UNPLEASANT ODOURS

Even when a room has been aired, tobacco smells often linger. This essence will get rid of them.

I tablespoon ammonia solution (see page 153)
I tablespoon lavender oil

Mix the ammonia solution and lavender in a bowl and leave in the room until the smell has gone.

COMING UP ROSES

For this, fragrant old roses, such as Bourbon and Damask, are ideal.

I handful dried rose petals
I teaspoon salt
few drops isopropyl alcohol

Place the rose petals in a plastic container and sprinkle the salt over them. Add the alcohol and mix well. Put the mixture into a jar with a lid and leave in a cool place for a few weeks. Stand the open jar in your room to release the scent.

REMOVE MUSTY SMELLS

The oils in lemon or orange peel are released by heat.

fresh citrus peel

Place the orange or lemon peel on top of a radiator.

Tried & Trusted
Air fresheners

• **Essential oils are distributed quickly and more effectively if bowls of water with a few drops of oil are placed on windowsills beside warm radiators.**

• **Unpleasant paint smells will disappear overnight if you leave out bowls filled with salt or halved onions.**

• **Place empty perfume bottles in the cupboard. The small amount of remaining scent will give your clothes a delicious fragrance.**

• **If there is a musty smell in your cupboard, put in a few coffee beans or a whole orange stuck with cloves.**

• **Shoes won't make the cupboard smelly if you use wooden shoetrees treated with cedarwood oil.**

Fragrances

• **Lavender bags impart a delightful smell. Place one in the linen cupboard and enjoy its fragrance. An alternative is to fill several bags with a fragrant potpourri mixture.**

Herbal and floral potpourri for the home

A potpourri usually consists of three elements: fragrance, fixative and filling. The fragrance is created by oils and spices; the fixative, such as orris root powder, stops the scent from fading and the filling adds eye-catching appeal.

Adapt the following recipes according to your taste, using flowers and herbs from your own garden or from a florist's.

Refer to pages 326–331 for a chart on growing herbs and flowers traditionally used for potpourris, or rely on old favourites such as rose petals and lavender. To dry your own filling, spread fresh flowers and foliage on newspaper and leave in a warm place for a week or so. Keep them out of the sun and any draughts.

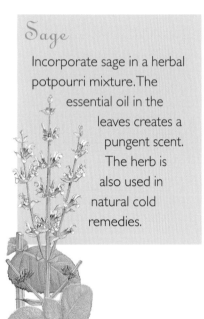

Sage

Incorporate sage in a herbal potpourri mixture. The essential oil in the leaves creates a pungent scent. The herb is also used in natural cold remedies.

SUMMER POTPOURRI

You can buy these flowers and petals dried, or dry them yourself.

200g (7oz) lavender flowers
125g (4½oz) lemon verbena leaves
55g (2oz) jasmine flowers
1 tablespoon orris root powder
1 tablespoon ground cinnamon
3 drops lavender oil

Mix the dry ingredients in a bowl, then add the essential oil. Leave it in a cool place for a few days.

HERB AND FLOWER POTPOURRI

The ingredients in this recipe are all fragrant. Myrrh has a distinctive scent while the dried herbs release a strong perfume.

1 tablespoon myrrh gum
1 tablespoon thyme leaves
25g (1oz) woodruff leaves
25g (1oz) scented geranium petals
25g (1oz) peppermint leaves
25g (1oz) orris root powder
25g (1oz) vervain leaves
55g (2oz) angelica root
100g (3½oz) rosebuds
115g (4oz) lavender flowers
essential oil of your choice

Place the leaves and flowers in a bowl or basket. Add a few drops of essential oil. Freshen up every now and then with additional drops of the essential oil.

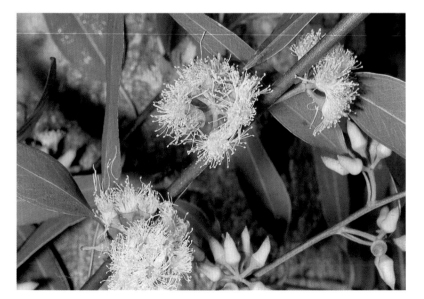

Natural aromas Many plants have aromatic leaves as well as flowers. The attractive foliage of the eucalyptus is often used in flower arranging and has a distinctive, clarifying perfume.

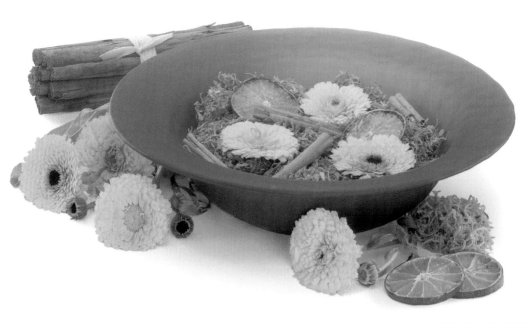

ENGLISH ROSE POTPOURRI

Roses are particularly good for a potpourri. They look and smell good for months. If you keep your dried potpourri inside a paper bag in the dark for two weeks, it will develop an even stronger and more lasting perfume.

1 stick cinnamon
1 tablespoon allspice
1 tablespoon cloves
400g (14oz) rose petals and rosebuds
200g (7oz) lavender flowers
100g (3½oz) rosemary flowers
25g (1oz) orris root powder
3 drops attar of roses
1 drop rosemary oil
1 drop geranium oil

Crush the cinnamon, allspice and cloves coarsely using a pestle and mortar. Put aside a few rosebuds. Mix the remaining dry ingredients. Add the attar of roses and essential oils. Position the rosebuds decoratively on top.

GARDEN POTPOURRI

Create your own individual mixture with flowers and herbs from your garden or window box.

Lasting fragrant mixtures to try are aster, carnation, jasmine, geranium, lily of the valley, hollyhock and violet. Good leaf mixtures include lavender, mint, rosemary, liquorice, hyssop and lemon balm.

300g (10½oz) flowers of your choice
100g (3½oz) rose petals
100g (3½oz) fragrant leaves
½ vanilla pod
25g (1oz) orris root powder
1 teaspoon ground cinnamon
½ teaspoon ground allspice
5 anise flowers
2 drops lavender oil
2 drops clove oil
2 drops camomile oil

Dry the flowers, petals and leaves. Cut the vanilla pod into small pieces. Arrange the mixture in a bowl. Add the oil, drop by drop. Leave the mixture to mellow in a cool place for six weeks.

Take care

Use essential oils with extreme caution; they are highly concentrated and only a few drops are needed.

POTPOURRI OF SPICES

You can buy these spices in most supermarkets. All these ingredients are dried and also available from specialist herbalists.

100g (3½oz) cinnamon sticks
25g (1oz) tarragon leaves
25g (1oz) cloves
25g (1oz) bay leaves
100g (3½oz) peppermint leaves
25g (1oz) sage leaves
55g (2oz) camomile flowers
55g (2oz) nutmeg flowers
55g (2oz) hops

Crush the cinnamon coarsely using a pestle and mortar. Mix the dried leaves, petals and flowers with the spices in a bowl.

Spicy pomanders

In times past pomanders were given as presents and used to ward off infections. Now they are a popular way to perfume rooms and cupboards.

For our grandparents, the period leading up to Christmas holds some of the fondest childhood memories. The whole family would sit down together to make things for the festive season.

Women would knit and embroider presents for family and friends, while men carved and sawed. Children cut, stuck and folded together amazing decorations. Even the youngest members joined in to paint nuts and make pomanders. Fruits such as oranges, lemons and apples were stuck with spices to create a Christmas atmosphere. Pomanders can easily be made from an orange stuck with cloves. It is best to use fruit with thick skin.

In this recipe the orange is rolled in a mixture of powdered spices, then placed in a paper bag and kept in a drawer for four weeks. This way the spices penetrate the skin of the fruit, enhancing the fragrance and ensuring its long-lasting effect.

How to make spicy pomanders
Makes three pomanders

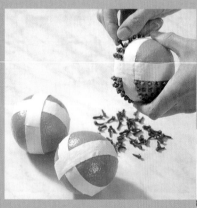

▼ Blend a mixture of **nutmeg**, **cinnamon** and **orris root powder**. Roll the oranges in the spices. Wrap them in a paper napkin and leave in a warm place for four weeks.

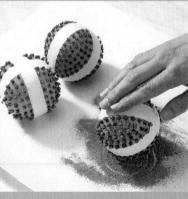

▲ Wind two strips of **sticky tape** all round each **orange**. Stick **cloves** into the uncovered orange skin. It is best to pierce a hole for each clove first, using a knitting needle or cocktail stick.

▲ Carefully pull off the strips of sticky tape and tie **silk ribbons** round the fruit in its place. Make a loop for hanging.

192

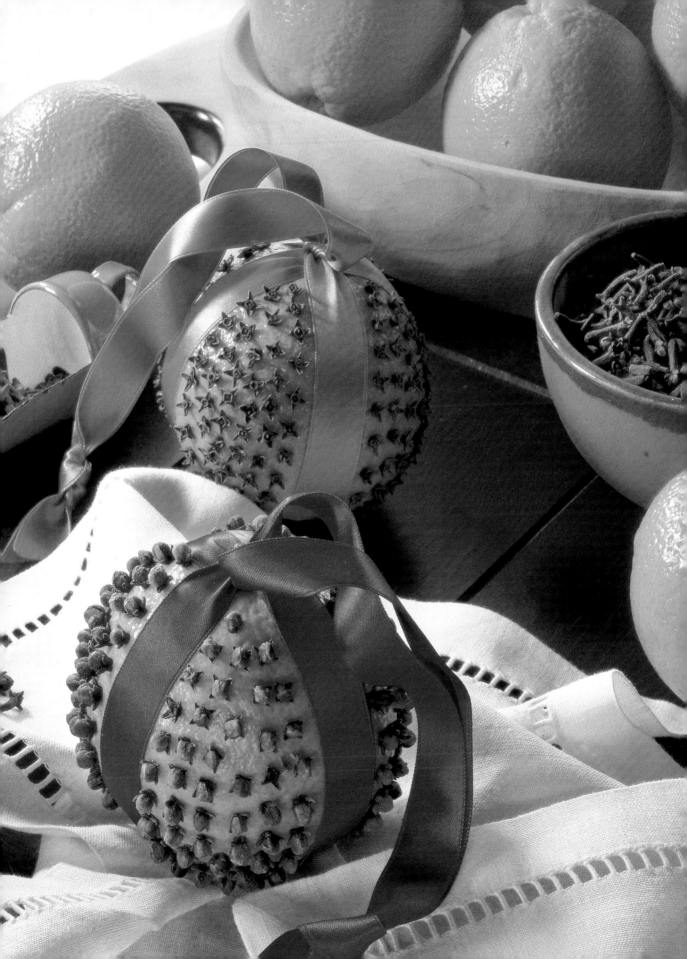

How to take care of

Even the most beautiful summer's day is seldom completely problem-free as flies, wasps and midges accompany the good weather. Pests are a fact of life no matter how you try to avoid them.

Not all uninvited guests are harmful or dangerous to your home. Spiders make themselves useful as flycatchers and daddy longlegs (crane flies) are simply attracted by bright lights. If you don't like these creatures in the house, it is best to catch them and simply take them outside. It would be inappropriate to use chemical poisons in this case and might well damage your own health.

However, there are many pests that must be dealt with decisively and immediately because they are a health risk. The simple household fly spreads dirt and disease, while a mouse or cockroach can quickly multiply into an infestation. So action should be taken sooner rather than later.

Rather than buying ready-prepared chemical mixtures there are several homemade pest control methods you can try. You may need to order some of the ingredients, and take great care in using them as many are highly toxic. If they do not prove to be successful, or if the exact nature of the pest is unclear, then it is best to turn to a pest control expert.

Controlling pests

Establish exactly what kind of pest you are dealing with before deciding upon a remedy and use your common sense. Simply vacuum up the odd ant, for example, if you want to keep your distance.

To prevent pests returning, ensure that all food is stored away in the kitchen and that any cracks are filled to reduce the number of hiding places.

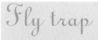

Fly trap

This glass container is cleverly shaped so that flies can get in through the narrow opening, but then cannot find their way out.

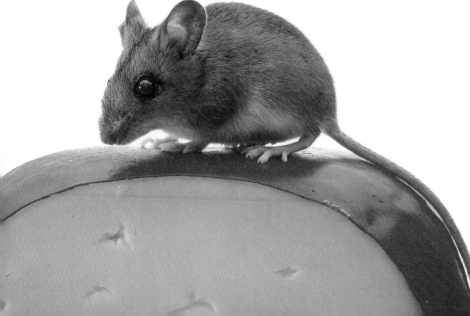

Trick or treat Cheese or bacon were traditionally used to lure mice and rats into a trap. If you use these, put the food out without the trap for a day or two to entice the vermin before using it as bait.

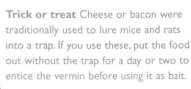

unwelcome guests

ARRESTING ANTS

As a preventive measure, scatter cloves near all entrances to the house. If the ants are already in the house, make up this trap.

1 tablespoon sugar
2 tablespoons dried yeast
500ml (18fl oz) water

Dissolve the sugar and yeast in the water. Pour into shallow containers and distribute them throughout the house or flat.

SERIOUS ANT INFESTATIONS

Borax was traditionally used to kill all kinds of insects and pests. Store it out of the reach of children and keep them, and pets, well away when it is applied.

1 tablespoon borax
1 tablespoon icing sugar

Mix the ingredients and place it near the entrance to the ants' nest. Remove and discard the mixture as the ants die. Repeat with more mixture as necessary.

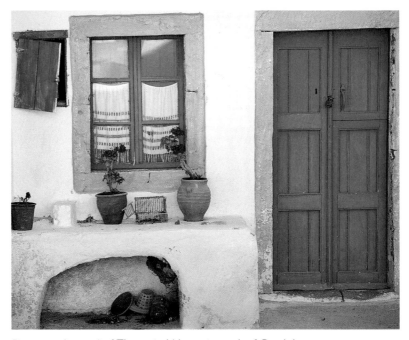

Pretty and practical The typical blue paintwork of Greek houses looks good and serves a purpose – flies avoid the colour blue and so are kept away.

GETTING RID OF ANT HILLS

It is best to tolerate ant hills in the garden as ants destroy a number of plant pests. Ants' nests in or near the house, however, should be dealt with as soon as possible.

1 part camphor oil
9 parts methylated spirits

Mix the camphor oil and methylated spirits. Pour the liquid over the ant hill. If the nest is in a hollow space, pour in pure camphor oil.

CATCHING FLIES ON A ROPE

Mastic is a gum exuded from the bark of a Mediterranean tree. It is now available as an essential oil.

50cm (20in) long rope
1 piece of resin
sunflower oil
few drops mastic oil

Melt the resin in a bowl placed inside a saucepan of boiling water. Mix it with about half as much sunflower oil and stir in the mastic oil. Soak the rope in this solution and hang it up in the kitchen.

Tried & Trusted

Keeping pests away

- Ants make themselves scarce if they smell tomato leaves or fresh chervil.

- A clean sponge sprinkled with sugar makes a sweet trap for ants. They will soon make their way to the sponge, which can then be dropped into boiling water.

- Sprinkle ant runs with salt, baking soda or garden lime.

- To keep flies away, stand castor-oil, tomato or basil plants on a windowsill. Alternatively, a few drops of peppermint oil in a jug of water will do the trick.

- Wood lice can be lured with hollowed-out potatoes, which you can then dispose of on the compost heap.

- Use camphor oil to drive cockroaches from their holes and crevices. Then fill in all their hiding places.

- Kill cockroaches by washing kitchen and bathroom floors with a solution in the ratio of 225g (8 oz) borax and 4 litres (7 pints) water. The cockroaches die when they come into contact with the borax residue on the surface of the floor. Do not use this remedy if young children or pets are about.

- Keep a room free of mosquitoes with an open bottle of clove oil.

- If you have mice, you don't necessarily need a mousetrap. Instead, put down bunches of fresh peppermint or camomile, or saucers containing a little peppermint oil.

- Protect yourself from mosquito, midge or gnat bites when gardening by rubbing a sprig of parsley over your exposed skin.

Pest-free pets

- If a bird has ticks, hang a thick white cloth on one side of its cage. The ticks will collect on the cloth, which can then be thrown away.

- If a dog has fleas, scatter fresh walnut leaves on its bed or in its kennel. Rid your dog and cat of fleas with this solution. Pour 2 tablespoons of vermouth into 1 litre (1¾ pints) of water and bring it to the boil. Cover the container and leave for a few hours. Rub the mixture into your pet's coat. Rinse off thoroughly and finally comb it through. If the fleas prevail take the pet to the vet for further treatment.

Wood lice cause little damage but they can be a nuisance if you have a lot of them in the house.

pieces of rotting wood
moss
boiled potatoes
flowerpots

Moisten the rotting wood and moss. Place both in flowerpots, along with pieces of boiled potato. Lie the flowerpots on the floor with their open tops about 4cm (1½in) from the wall. When wood lice have crawled into the pots, throw the contents onto the compost heap.

Moths avoid cupboards that are regularly aired. They also dislike the strong smell of certain herbs, such as southernwood, camphor, tansy and woodruff.

piece of fine cotton
   material
herbs

Cut the material and use it to make small sachets. Fill these with any mixture of herbs, tie with string and lie them in your linen cupboard and drawers. Mothballs were traditionally made using camphor oil.

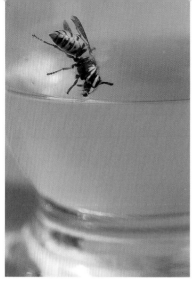

Sugar solution In summer, wasps are drawn to sweet drinks. To keep them from yours, prepare a trap of honey and water.

ANTI-MOTH FRAGRANCES

Aromatic herb sachets will help to keep cupboards moth-free.

**silk material
dried lavender flowers
 or
dried elder flowers**

Use the material to sew together a 20 x 20cm (8 x 8in) bag. Fill the bag with the flowers, sew it up, then hang it among your clothes.

GETTING MOTHS OUT OF UPHOLSTERY

If moths have got into your upholstery, try laying a trap to catch them.

**small cardboard box
pieces of soft fabric**

Cut several holes in the box, each about 2cm (¾in) in diameter. Push in the fabric pieces. After a week, empty the trap and repeat.

NO MORE COCKROACHES

Cockroaches are attracted by damp but will keep away if you use this mixture.

**2 parts borax
1 part flour
1 part sugar**

Mix the ingredients together and sprinkle on the appropriate areas. Repeat as necessary, keeping children and pets well away.

GETTING RID OF SILVERFISH

Silverfish are nocturnal insects, so use this remedy at night.

**white cotton cloths
powdered plaster**

Dampen the cloths with water, sprinkle on the plaster, then place them in the affected rooms. Next morning shake the cloths outside.

REMOVING WASPS' NESTS

Wasps will sting if you come too close to their nest so it is best to remove a nest that is in or near the house. If in any doubt call out a pest control expert to do the job.

turpentine

After dark, when the wasps are in their nest, soak a cloth in turpentine and wrap it around the end of a long pole. Push the cloth firmly into the entrance of the nest. Leave in place and do not approach for 24 hours.

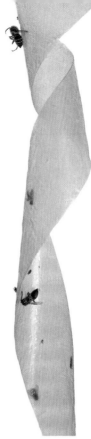

Homemade fly papers Combine 100ml (3½ fl oz) of golden syrup with 1 tablespoon each of brown and granulated sugar. Cut six strips of brown paper. Soak the paper in the mixture overnight. Scrape off excess syrup, make a hole in the top of each strip and hang up near windows and doors.

MAKING A WASP TRAP

If there is an invasion of wasps, or if a member of your family is allergic to stings, make your own trap.

**250ml (9fl oz) water
4 teaspoons honey
dash of vinegar
dark-coloured bottle with a
 narrow neck**

Heat the water and dissolve the honey. Allow it to cool, then add the vinegar and pour the solution into the bottle using a funnel. Stand the trap in the room where the wasps are gathering.

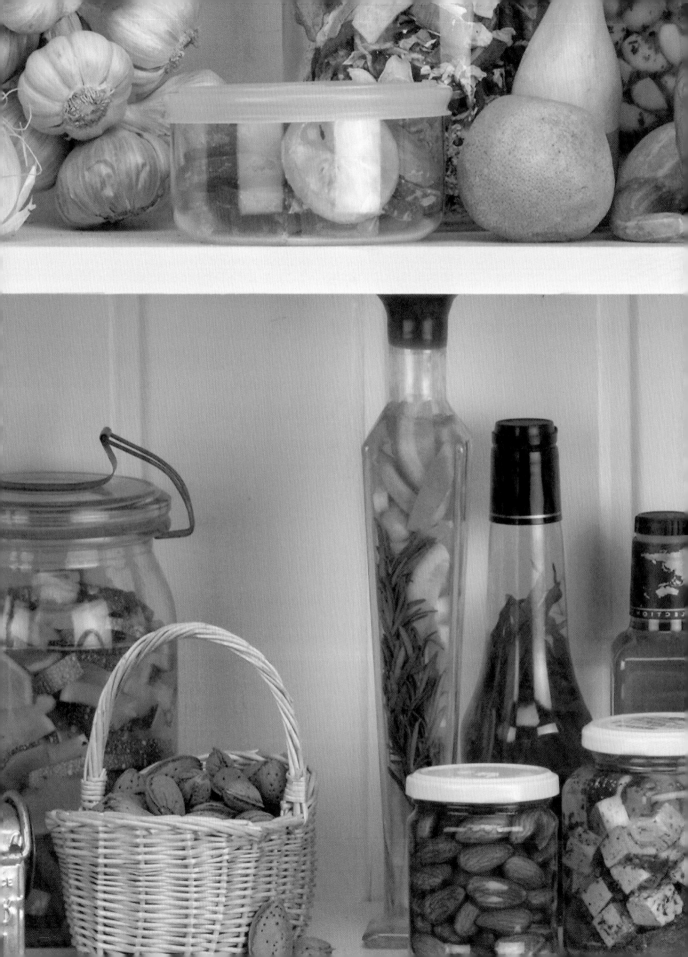

Kitchen secrets

In days gone by, many of the cook's ingredients were home-grown. Garden produce was dried or bottled, bread was home-baked and seasonal fruit, vegetables and fresh herbs were added to oils, vinegars and syrups.

In this chapter you will find a variety of recipes handed down through the generations, as well as a number of handy tips for guaranteed success.

Taste the difference!

CHAPTER 4

Drying fruit, herbs

Take a leaf out of grandmother's recipe book
and dry your own fruit and vegetables. Drying
concentrates the flavour, making them ideal as snacks
or as ingredients in other recipes.

Long before other methods of preservation were known, our ancestors would dry food in times of plenty and store it for later use.

Early civilisations were familiar with simple drying techniques. Ancient history records how fresh figs were crushed, then shaped into loaves and dried in the hot sun. Our grandmothers, too, dried their own harvest of fruit and vegetables.

Unfortunately, this skill has largely been forgotten. But with the ever-growing interest in a healthy, vitamin-rich diet, supermarkets are once again stocking dried fruit such as bananas and pineapples as well as familiar figs and apricots.

However, shop produce is often treated with preservatives, which you can avoid if you use classic recipes to dry home-grown fruit, vegetables, mushrooms and herbs. The methods are simple, although

they require a little time and patience. And the results are well worth the effort.

Store your dried produce in airtight containers in a cool, dry place. If using clear jars, these are best kept in the dark.

To rehydrate fruit and vegetables for use in other recipes, soak them in cold water. Plump fruits and vegetables are best soaked overnight, or at least for a few hours; sliced mushrooms and onion rings need just 30 minutes or so.

Golden harvest Dried fruits are a nutritious treat. Apple rings can be oven dried on bamboo canes then taken off and left to cool.

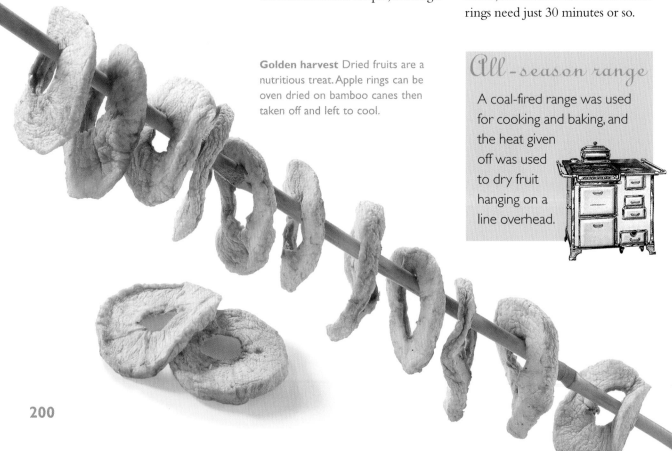

All-season range

A coal-fired range was used for cooking and baking, and the heat given off was used to dry fruit hanging on a line overhead.

and vegetables

Summer fruit – winter joy

Apples, apricots, peaches, grapes, pears and quinces are all ideal fruit for drying. For the best results, you need clean, good quality fruit.

Slice or cut it into pieces, then thread it onto clean bamboo canes or spread it out on cloths and racks to dry in the oven.

If it is stored in a dry, cool place, dried fruit will keep for several months. It should feel springy and velvet soft, with no moisture exuding when pressed and no signs of mould.

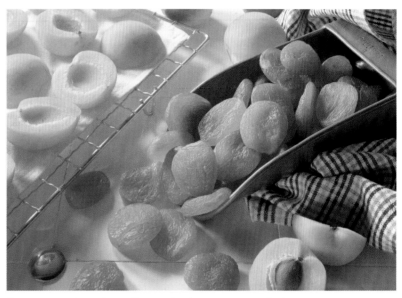

Concentrated goodness During the drying process, which can take up to two days for stone fruit such as apricots, all the juice will evaporate and the fruit will lose half their volume.

APPLE RINGS

Set the oven to a low temperature: 120°C (250°F, gas mark ½).

juicy dessert apples
1 teaspoon salt
1 litre (1¾ pints) water
bamboo canes

Peel and core the apples. Cut them into rings and put immediately into a bowl of salted water to prevent the flesh from turning brown.

Cut bamboo canes to fit the width of your oven. Remove the apple rings from the water, pat dry and thread them onto the canes. Remove the oven shelves and slide the canes into the oven, balancing them on the shelf rests. Leave to dry for 4-6 hours, keeping the oven door slightly open to prevent a build-up of condensation.

APRICOTS, PEACHES AND PLUMS

Stone fruits shrink considerably during the drying process.

apricots, peaches and plums

Wash the fruit. Leave plums whole, but halve and stone apricots and peaches. Stretch a square of muslin or cheesecloth over a wire cake rack and spread the fruit over it in a single layer with the cut surfaces uppermost. Place the rack on a shelf in the oven and dry as for Apple rings (see left). Cool the fruit at room temperature and, depending on its size, leave to continue drying for up to 48 hours.

PEARS

Williams pears are the best choice of pear for drying.

1 litre (1¾ pints) water
1 tablespoon vinegar
pears

Pour the water and vinegar into a bowl. Peel, quarter and core the pears. As you work, drop the pear quarters into the vinegar water to stop the flesh discolouring. Pat dry, then place on a muslin-covered wire cake rack and dry as for Apple rings (see left).

Drying vegetables and mushrooms

Mushrooms, onions, peas and beans are all suitable for drying. Root vegetables, such as carrots and celeriac, are better stored in boxes of sand, and most other vegetables can be preserved either by freezing or bottling.

Vegetables should be dried as soon as possible after harvesting to ensure maximum vitamin retention.

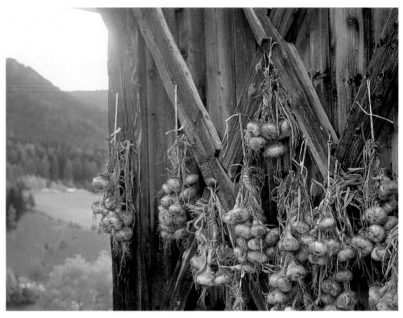

Time-honoured tradition Onions and garlic can be stored by hanging them on strings. Onions can also be cut into slices and dried.

MUSHROOMS

You can dry any edible variety of mushroom – ceps and horn of plenty are particularly good wild varieties to choose. Store dried mushrooms in small portions ready to add to casseroles, risottos and sauces. Chillies can be dried in the same way.

fresh mushrooms
long, thick needle
thin string

Wipe the mushrooms with a damp piece of kitchen paper and remove the stalks. Very large mushrooms can be cut in half. Thread them onto the string by pushing the needle through the middle of each mushroom, pushing the mushroom along the string and making a knot after each one.

Hang up the strings of mushrooms in a well-ventilated, warm place until they are dry and shrivelled. Store them in a jar or plastic tub in a cool place (see Tools for drying, page 203).

ONION RINGS

Dried onion rings are handy for adding to sauces and soups.

1 kg (2lb 4oz) medium-sized
onions
2-3 litres (3½-5¼ pints) water

Peel the onions, cut into 5mm (¼in) thick slices and separate into rings. Pour the water into a pan and bring to the boil. Blanch the onions for 30 seconds in the boiling water. Drain and pat dry with kitchen paper. Spread out the onion rings on muslin-covered wire cake racks and dry in the oven on the lowest possible setting for 3 hours.

PEAS AND BEANS

Dried peas and beans are a good traditional store-cupboard stand-by. They are especially good if you use home-grown produce.

peas
or
beans (broad, haricot and fava)
water

Shell the peas and beans. Put 5cm (2in) water in a pan and bring to the boil. Place the vegetables in a sieve, cover with a cloth and steam over the pan for 2-3 minutes. Alternatively, blanch in boiling water. Immerse the beans in very cold water, then dry on a muslin-covered wire cake rack as for Apple rings (see page 201).

Drying aromatic herbs

Pick herbs intended for drying in the morning, as soon as the dew has evaporated. See page 278 for alternative ways of drying herbs.

To microwave-dry herbs, spread out 15g (½oz) rinsed fresh leaves between two sheets of kitchen paper. Microwave on FULL for 4–6 minutes until brittle with a small bowl of water alongside.

MIXED HERBS

Before drying herbs, examine each sprig for dead flowers and leaves. These need to be removed.

fresh small-leaved herbs
2–3 litres (3½–5¼ pints) water
paper bags

Tie the herbs in small bunches. Bring the water to the boil and dip the bunches into the water for a few seconds. Shake off the water and pat dry on kitchen paper. Put in paper bags to stop the herbs getting dusty and hang up to dry.

A handy jar Keep a jar of dried mixed herbs ready for use when fresh herbs are not available.

Tried & Trusted

Tools for drying

- Cover food laid out to dry in the sun with a thin piece of cloth such as muslin or cheesecloth to protect it from birds and insects.

- Aluminium and other metal containers are unsuitable for storing dried fruit or vegetables because the metal reacts with the oxygen they give off. Use screw-top jars, plastic boxes, glazed pottery containers, paper or muslin bags.

- Don't forget to label your containers; always note the contents and the date they were dried.

Fruit and vegetables

- After drying, fruit and vegetables must be left for at least five days before being packed into containers. This should help to prevent them from sticking together.

- Fruit and vegetables can be dried in the airing cupboard. It takes longer than in the oven, but uses less energy and leaves the oven free for everyday cooking.

- Fan-assisted ovens are ideal for drying, because fruit and vegetables can be spread out on a number of shelves and dried at the same time.

- Peeled, dried fruit keeps better if sugar is sprinkled between each layer of fruit when it is packed.

Culinary herbs

- The length of time herbs take to dry depends on how thick the stalks and leaves are, as well as on the humidity and temperature at the time.

- Before storing dried herbs, remove hard stalks and ribs of leaves by rubbing the herbs between the palms of your hands. Discard the woody pieces.

Bottling fresh fruit

Picking home-grown produce in season and bottling it makes sound sense. You know its origins and quality and can feel immensely proud to offer it to family and friends.

Today, supermarkets offer a year-round supply of fruit and vegetables of every kind. But because their stock is bought from around the globe to prolong availability, it is often expensive and seldom tastes as good as fresh British produce grown in season.

Much less was imported in our grandparents' time. Instead, in summer and autumn they bottled all manner of local – often home-grown – fruit and vegetables and used them to brighten up their winter menus.

Spiced fruit Cinnamon sticks and cloves add a delicious flavour to bottled yellow plums.

The process of bottling is relatively modern – a little over a hundred years old – and is based on the principle of sterilisation.

All the equipment needed can be found in your kitchen, apart from bottling jars, which you can buy from kitchenware shops or by mail order.

Rules for sterilising

Early summer is the start of the annual bottling season. Only fresh, undamaged fruit should be used.

Before sterilising, all equipment including jars, rubber sealing rings, screw bands and clips must be washed in soapy water and rinsed with boiling water. Leave the jars upside-down to drain until they are needed. If re-using rubber screw bands from a previous year, check they have not perished.

The recipes given here sterilise the produce using the oven method. Pack the fruit or vegetables into the jars leaving a 2cm (¾in) gap below the rim and cover them with sugar syrup or water, leaving a space so it doesn't boil over. Put the jars on a baking tray in the centre of the oven with the lids closed but not tight. Secure the seals after cooling or the produce won't keep well.

and vegetables

BASIC RECIPE FOR BOTTLING

This recipe is for pears but it can be used for most types of fruit. The amount of sugar varies according to the sweetness of the fruit, and sterilising times depend on the fruit's texture. This recipe makes about three 1 litre (1¾ pint) jars.

2kg (4lb 8oz) pears
3 litres (5¼ pints) water
200-500g (7oz-1lb 2oz)
   caster sugar

Wash the jars. Peel, halve and core the pears. Pour 1 litre (1¾ pints) of the water into a pan and boil. Add the pears and blanch for 2-3 minutes, then remove and dip them in iced water. Leave to drain in a sieve. Pack the fruit in layers into the jars, leaving a gap of 2cm (¾in) below the rim.

Pour the remaining water and the sugar into a pan and boil rapidly for 5 minutes until it forms a syrup. Pour the syrup over the pears so that they are completely covered. Wipe clean the rim of each jar, then put on the lid but do not screw or clip on.

Sterilise the jars of fruit in the oven at 150°C (300°F, gas mark 2) for 1 hour 15 minutes. Seal each jar with a screw band or clip and leave to cool.

GOOSEBERRIES

Choose large, under-ripe fruit, as they retain their shape better. Makes about three 1 litre (1¾ pint) jars.

2kg (4lb 8oz) gooseberries
1 litre (1¾ pints) water
800g (1lb 12oz) caster sugar

Top and tail the gooseberries. Prick the skins with a cocktail stick and put in a bowl. Put the water and sugar into a pan and boil for 2-3 minutes. Pour it over the fruit. Leave for about 5 minutes for the gooseberries to turn yellow.

Remove the fruit from the liquid and pack into glass jars. Boil the liquid again and pour over to cover the fruit. Place the lids on top of the jars and sterilise in the oven for 45 minutes at 150°C (300°F, gas mark 2). Seal each jar and cool.

Cherry stoner

Cherry stoners, indispensable gadgets for making jam in our grandparents' day, are still invaluable. A thick shaft pierces the cherry and forces out the stone.

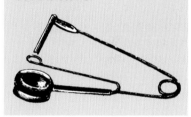

Nature's harvest If you don't grow your own produce you can still buy it in season, when it is great value.

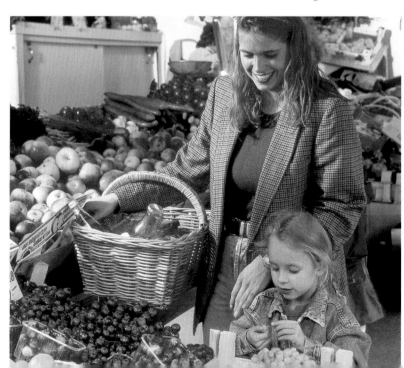

APPLES WITH PEPPERMINT

Mint and vanilla add a fresh flavour to apples. The quantities below fill about three 1 litre (1¾ pint) jars.

2kg (4lb 8oz) small dessert apples
juice of 2 lemons
1 litre (1¾ pints) water
500g (1lb 2oz) sugar
1 vanilla pod
small bunch fresh peppermint leaves

Peel, halve and core the apples. Fill a pan with water, add half the lemon juice and bring to the boil. Blanch the apples for 2 minutes, drain, then dip in ice-cold water.

Put the water and sugar into a pan and boil until they form a syrup. Split the vanilla pod in half lengthways and scrape out the seeds. Add the seeds and the remaining lemon juice to the syrup.

Wash the mint, then tear it into small pieces. Arrange the mint and apples in alternate layers in glass jars, leaving a 2cm (¾in) gap below the rim. Cover with the hot syrup and sterilise for an hour in the oven at 150°C (300°F, gas mark 2). Seal tightly when cool.

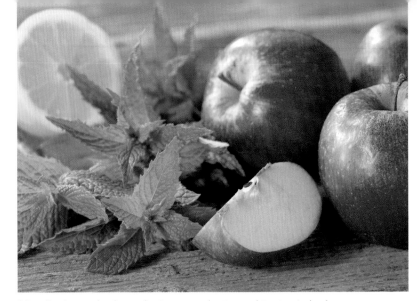

Mint freshness Apples and mint are a classic combination in both sweet and savoury dishes. Peppermint leaves create a clean, tangy taste.

The quick method to bottle soft fruit

This is a quick method of bottling. If done correctly, it will preserve the fruit just as well as sterilising in the oven. This time the fruit is cooked in the sugar solution, left to simmer until just tender and then put into hot jars, which are sealed and left to cool. The cooked fruit should not be too soft as it continues softening in the jar.

CHERRIES & REDCURRANTS OR BLACKCURRANTS

Large cherries and berries are best. Makes three 1 litre (1¾ pint) jars.

1kg (2lb 4oz) cherries
1kg (2lb 4oz) redcurrants
   or
1kg (2lb 4oz) blackcurrants
1 litre (1¾ pints) water
600g (1lb 5oz) sugar

Remove the stalks and stones from the cherries and the stalks from the currants. Pour the water into a pan with the sugar and boil until they form a syrup. Add the cherries and boil for 5 minutes, then add the currants and boil for 2 minutes. Transfer the fruit and syrup to hot glass jars and seal immediately.

RASPBERRIES IN SYRUP

Store bottled dark fruit such as raspberries and blackberries in a cool, dark place. This recipe makes about three 1 litre (1¾ pint) jars.

2kg (4lb 8oz) raspberries
1 litre (1¾ pints) water
600g (1lb 5oz) sugar

Wash the raspberries and gently pat them dry with kitchen paper. Pour the water and sugar into a pan and boil until they form a syrup. Add the raspberries and simmer for 2-3 minutes.

Remove the fruit from the syrup with a slotted spoon and pack it into glass jars. Boil the syrup and pour it over the fruit. Seal the jars immediately and leave to cool.

Apple-corer

This useful tool removes the core with all the pips, while leaving the fruit whole. Antique corers would have had wooden handles.

Bottling equipment

- **You can buy bottling jars in different sizes from 250ml (9fl oz) to 3 litres (5¼ pints). They have spring clips or screw tops.**

- **Spotlessly clean pots, pans, jars and equipment are absolutely essential. Wash the jars thoroughly and rinse in hot water. Leave to drain rather than drying with a tea towel which might leave behind lint or bacteria.**

- **Do not touch the jars during the sterilising process. If necessary, wrap a cloth around the jar.**

Bottling fruit

- **As an alternative to boiled sugar syrup, you can use hot fruit juice to preserve whole or halved fruit.**

- **Wash greengages, remove stalks and boil in water for 10 minutes. Remove with a slotted spoon and pack into bottling jars. Seal and sterilise for 10 minutes at 110°C (225°F, gas mark ¼).**

- **Before bottling soft fruit such as blackberries, redcurrants, blackcurrants, loganberries and raspberries, check for damaged or maggoty fruit. Also remove hulls and stalks.**

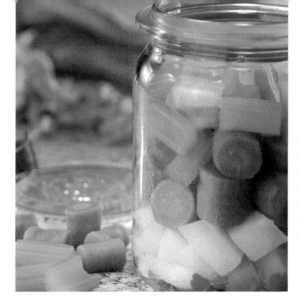

Tasty vegetables
Bottling in salted water helps vegetables to retain their flavour. They can be added to soups, casseroles or curries, or cooked and served in a creamy sauce as an accompaniment to other dishes.

Bottling fresh vegetables from your garden

Bottled vegetables provide an excellent substitute when fresh vegetables are not in season. But only the best should be bottled. Blemished vegetables should be used up immediately.

CHERRY TOMATOES WITH BASIL

This recipe will make enough to fill a 1 litre (1¾ pint) glass bottling jar.

1kg (2lb 4oz) cherry tomatoes
5 cloves garlic
fresh basil
1 teaspoon each salt and sugar

Wash the tomatoes and prick the skins with a cocktail stick. Peel the garlic. Pack the jar with the tomatoes, adding basil leaves, garlic, salt and sugar between the layers.

Line an oven tray with cardboard and stand the jar on it with the lid closed but not sealed. Sterilise in the oven at 120°C (250°F, gas mark ½) for 45 minutes, then seal and leave to cool.

VEGETABLES FOR SOUP

These bottled vegetables are excellent for making a quick soup. Makes two 1 litre (1¾ pint) jars.

500g (1lb 2oz) each carrots, baby turnips and celery
1 big bunch flat-leaf parsley
1 litre (1¾ pints) water
1 teaspoon salt

Peel and wash the vegetables. Cut them into 3cm (1¼in) chunks. Bring a large pan of salted water to the boil and blanch the vegetables in small batches, then refresh them in iced water and leave to dry.

Divide the parsley between the jars, then add layers of vegetables. Pour the water and the salt into a pan and boil for 30 seconds. Pour this over the vegetables until it is 1cm (½in) below the rim. Sterilise the bottled vegetables for 1 hour at 110°C (225°F, gas mark ¼).

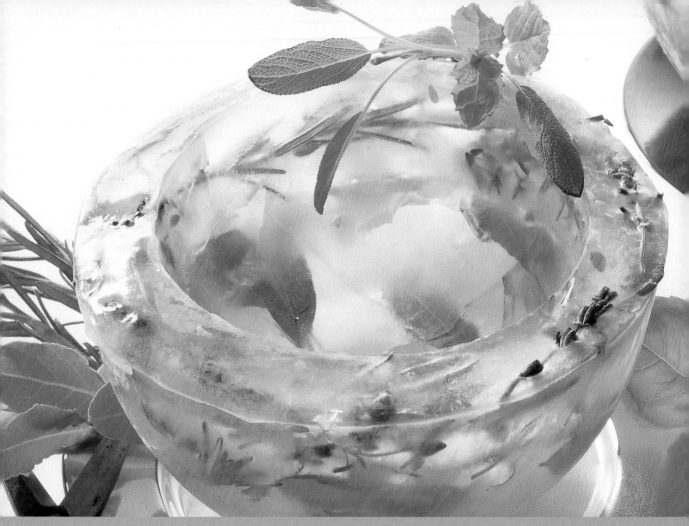

Floral ice bowl

This frozen table decoration will be the crowning
glory of any lunch or dinner party. It is ideal for
chilling a fruit salad or ice cream.

To make an ice bowl you will need two
freezerproof bowls. One should fit inside the
other, leaving a 2.5cm (1in) gap all round.

The flowers, leaves and herbs make an
eye-catching display once the water has
frozen. Use any small, delicate or colourful
flowers, petals or herbs.

Great care is needed when detaching the ice
from the bowls. Try not to splash any hot
water over the surface of the ice.

Keep your floral ice bowl in the freezer
until the table is laid and your guests are
seated. Place the bowl on an attractive plate
to catch any drips as the ice melts.

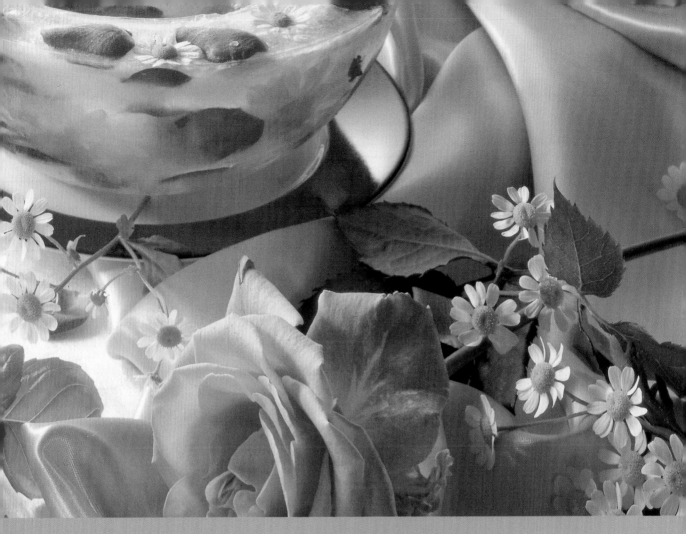

How to make a floral ice bowl
Makes one bowl

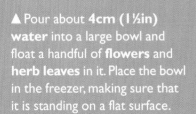

▲ Pour about **4cm (1½in) water** into a large bowl and float a handful of **flowers** and **herb leaves** in it. Place the bowl in the freezer, making sure that it is standing on a flat surface.

▼ Once the water has frozen, stand a smaller bowl on top of it and weight it down. Fill the space between the bowls with more water and float flowers and leaves all round. Put the bowls back in the freezer.

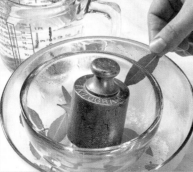

▲ Take the bowls out of the freezer when the water has frozen. Carefully swirl hot water around the small bowl. Use a cloth to detach the bowl from the ice. Run hot water over the outer bowl until it, too, can be removed.

Preserving with salt,

Combine the delicious taste of fresh fruit and vegetables with delicately flavoured vinegars and oils to make some of the best-loved pickles, chutneys and preserves.

The practice of preserving fruit and vegetables in salt, vinegar or oil dates back to ancient times.

The Romans, for example, brought back many fresh foods from the lands they conquered, including lemons, onions and peaches. They preserved them in large vases in a mixture of vinegar, oil and brine to ensure that they could be enjoyed over many months. Our grandparents also used salt and vinegar to preserve a wide range of foods.

In different ways, salt, vinegar and oil all prevent fruit and vegetables from decay by protecting against the micro-organisms that could rot them. Salt removes moisture and can prevent the growth of any living organism.

Vinegar preserves because it is acidic while oil coats food and prevents contamination from the air.

Today, salt and vinegar are still used for making pickles and chutneys and many foods are preserved in oil. Malt is the most economical vinegar to use: choose either brown or distilled (clear) varieties. Cider and wine vinegars are ideal for a milder flavour.

Seasonings including herbs, garlic, whole spices or dried chillies can be added to flavourless oils such as corn, sunflower or vegetable oil.

Salted beans Preserving runner beans in brine brings out their flavour so they taste almost as good as if they have just been freshly picked.

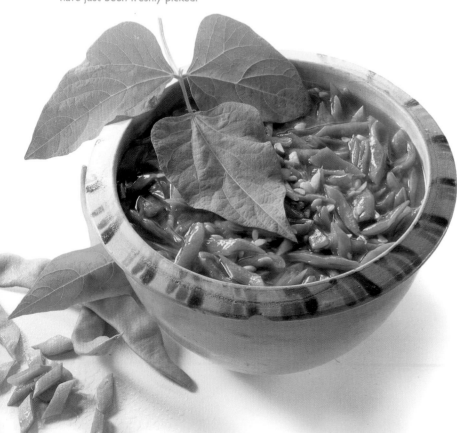

Bean slicer

In large houses where scullery maids had the task of slicing an entire harvest of beans, this gadget was a must.

vinegar and oil

Preserving with salt

Salt has been used to preserve food for thousands of years. It can be added directly to raw vegetables, or boiled with water to make brine.

Used in large quantities, salt prevents the build-up of bacteria and mould. When preserving vegetables in salt, it is best to use unglazed earthenware jars with airtight seals. Also, make sure that the contents are totally immersed in the brine.

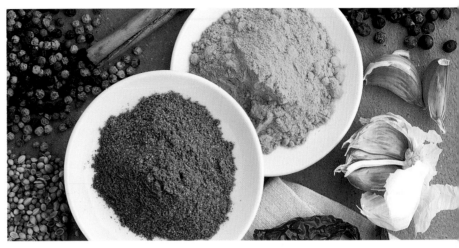

Fiery flavourings A wide range of spices can be used to flavour pickles and chutneys, so you can pick the ones you like best.

RUNNER BEANS

Enjoy a summer crop of beans during the winter months. This recipe will make about two 1 litre (1¾ pint) jars.

1 kg (2lb 4oz) runner beans
6 cloves garlic, peeled and chopped
1 litre (1¾ pints) water
1 teaspoon salt

Tail and string the beans, then slice them into thin strips. Bring a pan of salted water to the boil and blanch the beans for 2 minutes. Drain, then cool them under running cold water and pat dry.

Pack the beans into preserving jars, layering them with the garlic. Pour the water and salt into a pan. Boil for 30 seconds and pour over the beans to cover. Sterilise the jars for an hour at 110°C (225°F, gas mark ¼), then seal and cool.

Pickles – a treat for all the family

Sweet or savoury pickles to accompany meat or poultry were a firm favourite in our grandparents' time. Today, there are many different pickles available in the shops. But making your own allows you far more variety, both in your choice of main ingredients and of spices.

Pickling is not suitable for all fruit and vegetables, but it is ideal for preserving cucumbers, onions courgettes, and cabbage. For the best results, use only very fresh, crisp produce. Homemade spiced pickling vinegar (see right) preserves the food and adds a delicate flavour.

SPICED PICKLING VINEGAR

This vinegar can be used for vegetable and fruit pickles, or when making chutneys and relishes.

1 cinnamon stick, broken into short lengths
2 blades of mace
1 tablespoon coriander seeds
1 tablespoon mixed white and black peppercorns
1 teaspoon dried chilli flakes (optional)
1.2 litres (2 pints) vinegar

Put all the spices in a large 2 litre (3½ pint) sterilised glass jar. Pour in the vinegar, seal with a screw-top lid and shake. Store in a cool, dark place for at least one month before using so that the spices have time to flavour the vinegar.

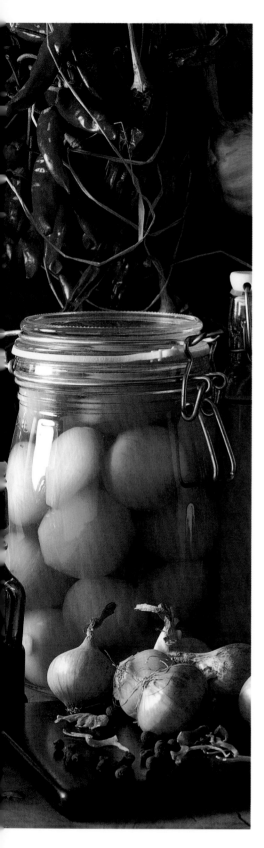

PICKLED CAULIFLOWER AND CARROTS

This colourful vegetable pickle can be served with cold meats or cheese. The recipe makes three or four 1 litre (1¾ pint) jars.

2 cauliflowers
2 large carrots
150g (5½oz) salt
900ml (1 pint 12fl oz) water
1 tablespoon allspice
    or
1 tablespoon dried juniper
    berries
900ml (1 pint 12fl oz)
    strained spiced
    pickling vinegar

Trim the cauliflowers and cut them into small florets, discarding the tough stalks. Peel and thinly slice the carrots. Place both vegetables into a large plastic or ceramic bowl. Dissolve the salt in the water and pour it over the vegetables. Place a weighted plate on top to ensure that they remain immersed in the salty water and leave to soak for 24 hours.

Drain the vegetables and rinse them under cold running water. Pat dry and pack into sterilised jars. Add a few allspice or juniper berries to each jar. Pour over the spiced vinegar, ensuring that each vegetable is covered. Seal the jars, label and keep in a cool, dark place for three months to mature.

Pickled onions Small silverskin or pickling onions are the usual choice. But pickled shallots and whole cloves of garlic make a tasty alternative.

Take care

Avoid using unlined metal lids on jars that contain pickle or chutney. The vinegar will corrode and rust the seals. Instead, put a cellophane disc over the top of the jar and screw on a plastic lid. You can also buy preserving jars with rubber-sealed spring-clip lids.

PICKLED ONIONS

Occasionally yellow spots appear on pickled onions. Although they detract from the appearance of the onions, they are harmless and have no adverse effect on the taste. This recipe makes about three 1 litre (1¾ pint) jars.

1kg (2lb 4oz) pickling onions
    or
1kg (2lb 4oz) shallots
100g (3½oz) salt
1.2 litres (2 pints) water
750ml (1¼ pints) spiced
    pickling vinegar

Peel the onions and place them in a large plastic or ceramic bowl. Dissolve the salt in the water and pour it over the onions. Cover the bowl and leave for 24 hours, stirring occasionally.

Drain the onions and rinse under cold running water. Drain again and pat dry. Pack the onions into sterilised jars until they are about 2.5cm (1in) from the rims. Pour over the spiced vinegar so that the onions are covered. Tap the jars to dislodge any trapped bubbles. Seal the jars and label. Keep in a dark place for one month before using.

• **Vegetables for preserving in vinegar need 'brining' with salt water first to draw out excess moisture that would otherwise seep into the vinegar and dilute it.**

• **Use coarse sea salt as it contains none of the anti-caking agents added to table salt.**

• **The brining time varies with vegetable texture. Dense vegetables such as carrots or cauliflowers will need longer than runner beans or cucumbers.**

• **When brining vegetables always use a plastic, earthenware, ceramic or glass bowl – never a metal one or the salt will 'pit' it.**

• **Avoid using aluminium, brass or copper pans when preserving food in vinegar. The acetic acid in the vinegar corrodes these metals and releases potentially harmful substances into the food. Use stainless steel instead.**

• **To ensure that vegetables stay submerged in vinegar or oil, place a piece of crumpled greaseproof paper or a special plastic 'plug' (available from kitchenware shops) at the top of the jar.**

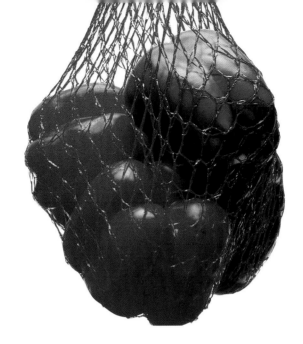

Instant colour
Sweet red and green peppers are excellent preserved in vinegar or oil and keep their appetising rich colours.

PICKLED RED CABBAGE

This is an excellent accompaniment to cold roast meats, especially pork or turkey. Makes two or three 1 litre (1¾ pint) jars.

1 red cabbage, weighing about 1.2kg (2lb 10oz)
85g (3oz) salt
1 teaspoon sugar
300ml (½ pint) spiced pickling vinegar

Remove any discoloured outer leaves and cut the cabbage into quarters. Cut away the stalk and finely shred the cabbage leaves. Layer the cabbage with the salt in a large plastic or ceramic bowl, put a weighted plate on top and leave for 24 hours.

Rinse the cabbage well, drain, then pack into sterilised glass jars, sprinkling a little sugar into each. Pour over the vinegar to cover the cabbage and tap the jars to disperse any air pockets. Seal and label. Keep in a dark place for two to three weeks before eating.

PICKLED CUCUMBER AND PEPPERS

Serve this relish with cheese or pork pies. Makes about two 1 litre (1¾ pint) jars.

1 each large red, orange and yellow pepper
½ cucumber
1 red onion
175g (6oz) salt
400ml (14fl oz) spiced pickling vinegar
55g (2oz) caster sugar

Wash, halve and deseed the peppers, then slice thinly. Peel the cucumber, if preferred, and slice thinly. Peel and finely chop the onion. Layer the vegetables in a plastic or ceramic bowl with the salt. Cover and leave for 1 hour.

Rinse the vegetables under cold running water. Drain and pat dry. Heat the vinegar and sugar in a pan, stirring until the sugar has dissolved. Leave to cool. Pack the vegetables into sterilised jars and cover with the vinegar. Seal, label and store for one month before eating.

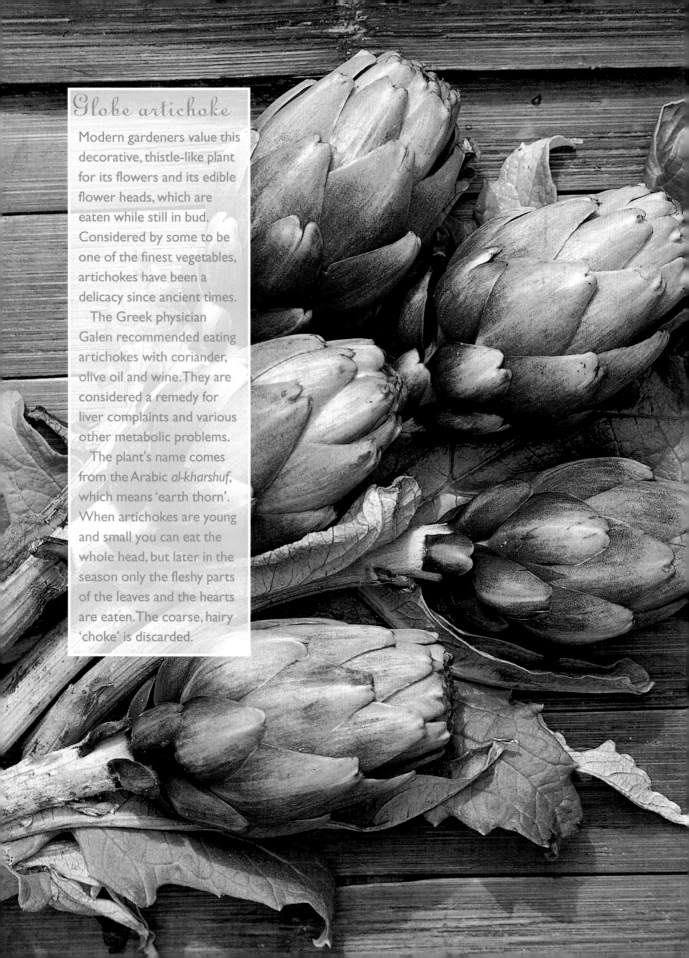

Globe artichoke

Modern gardeners value this decorative, thistle-like plant for its flowers and its edible flower heads, which are eaten while still in bud. Considered by some to be one of the finest vegetables, artichokes have been a delicacy since ancient times.

The Greek physician Galen recommended eating artichokes with coriander, olive oil and wine. They are considered a remedy for liver complaints and various other metabolic problems.

The plant's name comes from the Arabic *al-kharshuf*, which means 'earth thorn'. When artichokes are young and small you can eat the whole head, but later in the season only the fleshy parts of the leaves and the hearts are eaten. The coarse, hairy 'choke' is discarded.

Preserving culinary delights in oil

In warm Mediterranean countries oil has been used for preserving food since Greek and Roman times. In the colder climes of northern Europe, animal fat was used in a similar way to exclude the air and prevent food from deteriorating.

With the greater availability of a whole range of oils, preserving in oil has become increasingly popular in Britain. Use virgin olive oil, which is milder and less costly than extra virgin olive oil, and flavour it with herbs and spices.

ARTICHOKES IN OIL

Use very young, slender globe artichokes and cold pressed olive oil. Makes two 1 litre (1¾ pint) jars.

5-8 globe artichokes
juice of 3 lemons
3 tablespoons salt
1 tablespoon black
**   peppercorns**
2 bay leaves
500ml (18fl oz) white
**   wine vinegar**
500ml (18fl oz) water
1 unwaxed lemon
1 litre (1¾ pints) olive oil

Trim the artichokes, cut off the stalks and scrape out the hairy 'choke'. Chop them into quarters. Fill a bowl with water, add the lemon juice and immerse the artichoke pieces in the liquid to prevent them from discolouring.

Place the salt, pepper, bay leaves, vinegar and water in a pan. Drain the artichokes and add them to the pan. Simmer for 20 minutes, drain and leave to cool.

Squeeze the liquid from the artichokes. Wash and slice the lemon. Layer the artichokes and lemon in a sterilised glass jar. Cover with the olive oil and seal. Store for 4-6 weeks before eating.

TOMATOES IN OIL

It is rarely hot enough in Britain to sun-dry tomatoes. Instead, dry them in the oven as in the recipe for Apricots, peaches and plums (see page 201). You can preserve the tomatoes with or without the herbs. The recipe makes two 1 litre (1¾ pint) jars.

2kg (4lb 8oz) ripe, firm,
**   cherry tomatoes**
250ml (9fl oz) white
**   wine vinegar**
250ml (9fl oz) water
1 garlic bulb
herbs such as basil, sage,
**   thyme, parsley**
1 litre (1¾ pints) cold pressed
**   olive oil**

Wash and pat dry the tomatoes, then cut them into halves. Mix the vinegar with the water in a bowl and add the tomatoes. Peel the garlic cloves. Wash and pat dry a few sprigs of basil, sage, thyme and parsley, according to taste. Drain the tomatoes and pack into a sterilised glass jar with the garlic and herbs. Pour over the olive oil and seal. Refrigerate once the jar is opened.

Olive oil

At harvest time, all the small traditional olive mills in the Mediterranean are so busy that their grindstones are turning almost nonstop.

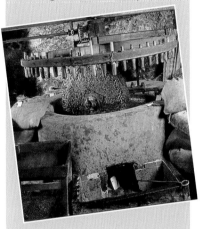

After the olives have been crushed, the resulting paste is squeezed by a press. The first cold pressing produces the highest quality oil, known as extra virgin olive oil. This fine oil, which is produced in relatively small quantities, is mechanically cleaned and filtered, but not otherwise refined in any way.

Making fruit and vegetable chutneys

Chutney originated in India. It became popular in Britain when expatriates living on the sub-continent during the days of the Raj returned home, bringing chutney, curry and kedgeree recipes with them.

The name is an anglicisation of the Hindu word *chanti*, meaning 'highly spiced'. Nowadays, it also encompasses sweet-sour relishes of fruit, vegetables and spices.

Although mango chutney was the original flavoured chutney imported from India, the recipe was soon adapted for all kinds of fruit and vegetables. Our grandparents would have made chutneys and relishes from surplus garden produce. They are an excellent way of using up windfall apples and pears, unripened green tomatoes or a glut of any fruit that has become too ripe for making jam. Always remove bruised or diseased parts of fruit and discard those that are very soft and squashy.

Chutneys can be eaten as soon as they are made but their flavour improves greatly if the sealed jars are stored for a couple of months in a cool, dark place. Once opened, chutney should be stored in the fridge. Half-used jars stored for too long need a good stir before serving.

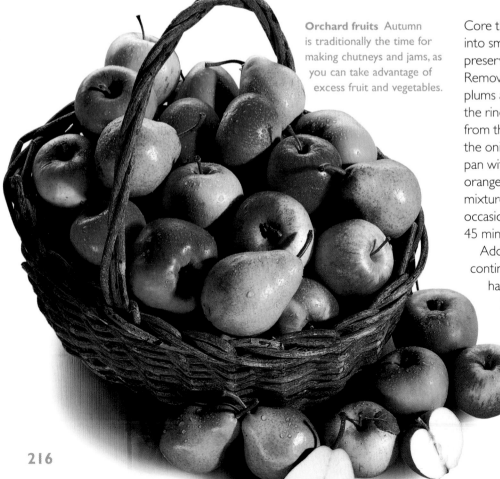

Orchard fruits Autumn is traditionally the time for making chutneys and jams, as you can take advantage of excess fruit and vegetables.

AUTUMN FRUIT CHUTNEY

Any variety of apples and pears can be used. The plums can be replaced with apricots, peaches or quinces if you prefer. This recipe makes about 1.5kg (3lb 5oz).

500g (1lb 2oz) pears
500g (1lb 2oz) cooking apples
400g (14oz) dark-skinned plums
1 orange
250g (9oz) large onions
250g (9oz) pitted dates, chopped
600ml (1 pint) malt vinegar
350g (12oz) soft dark brown sugar
1 teaspoon ground ginger

Core the pears and apples, cut into small chunks and place in a preserving pan or large saucepan. Remove the stones from the plums and chop coarsely. Grate the rind and squeeze the juice from the orange. Peel and slice the onions, then add them to the pan with the plums, dates, vinegar, orange zest and juice. Bring the mixture to the boil, stirring occasionally, then simmer for 45 minutes or until the fruit is soft.

Add the sugar and ginger and continue to stir until the sugar has dissolved. Simmer for 1-1½ hours or until most of the liquid has evaporated and the chutney has reduced and thickened. Spoon into sterilised glass jars, seal and label.

Tried & Trusted

Added sweetness

- Any kind of sugar can be used for making chutneys. White and brown sugars are suitable, as are the new 'golden' sugars. The colour of the chutney may vary according to the sugar used.

- The sugar can also be mixed with a little honey, golden syrup, molasses or maple syrup. Only use a small quantity, as these sweeteners may crystallise if stored in a cool place.

The right pan

- Aluminium pans should not be used for making chutneys as the vinegar will discolour and corrode the metal. Potentially health-damaging substances may be leaked into the food.

- Whatever type of pan you use, it needs to be wide at the top and not too deep. This shape allows the liquid to evaporate easily and the chutney to thicken quickly.

Ready for the jar

- Lift one side of the pan to test if the chutney is cooked. Very little liquid should run across the surface.

- Use wide-rimmed glass jars and preferably a jam funnel to pour the chutney into the jars cleanly.

TOMATO AND RED ONION CHUTNEY

Peeling tomatoes is rather tedious but it is necessary as the skins would give the chutney a coarse texture and bitter flavour.

1.3kg (3lb) ripe tomatoes
675g (1lb 8oz) red onions
1kg (2lb 4oz) cooking apples
500ml (18fl oz) cider vinegar
350g (12oz) demerara sugar
175g (6oz) raisins
1 teaspoon salt
1 teaspoon ground coriander
1 teaspoon mustard seeds
1 teaspoon Worcestershire
   sauce

Place the tomatoes in a heatproof bowl, cover with boiling water and leave for 30 seconds. Drain the tomatoes, cool under cold running water then peel off the skins. Roughly chop the tomatoes and place them in a preserving pan or large saucepan.

Peel and finely chop the onions. Core, peel and chop the apples. Add them to the pan with the onions and all the remaining ingredients and stir thoroughly. Bring the mixture to the boil, stirring until the sugar has dissolved. Simmer for 1½ hours or until the vegetables and fruit are soft and the mixture has reduced and thickened.

Spoon the chutney into sterilised jars and seal. Label when cold and store in a cool, dark place for one month before eating.

Take care

Glass chutney jars should be scrupulously cleaned to prevent mould growth during storage. Wash them in hot soapy water, then submerge in boiling water for five minutes. Drain and dry them upside down in a low oven for 20 minutes before filling.

BEETROOT CHUTNEY

Beetroot was a popular crop grown in our grandparents' vegetable plot. It makes a dark, richly flavoured chutney. This recipe makes about 2.5kg (5lb 8oz).

900g (2lb) raw beetroot
450g (1lb) onions
700g (1lb 9oz) apples
   or
700g (1lb 9oz) quinces
250g (9oz) pitted prunes,
   roughly chopped
200g (7oz) raisins
1 litre (1¾ pints) malt vinegar
900g (2lb) granulated sugar
1 teaspoon ground allspice
1 teaspoon ground cinnamon
½ teaspoon ground cloves

Peel and grate the beetroot. Peel and chop the onions. Core and chop the apples or quinces, leaving on the skins. Put all the ingredients in a preserving pan or large saucepan and bring to the boil. Stir until the sugar has dissolved.

Simmer the mixture over a moderate heat for about 1 hour until thick and pulpy. Pour the chutney into sterilised jars and seal.

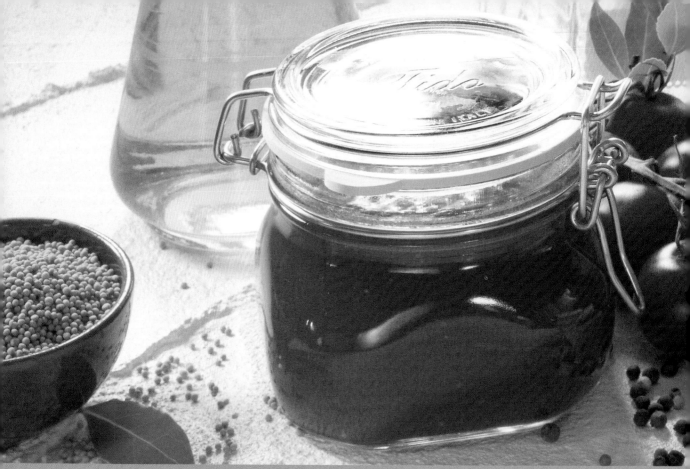

Tasty tomato ketchup

Homemade tomato ketchup is spicier and not as sweet
as the ready-made variety. Use home-grown or local
fresh tomatoes to make your own sauce: the flavour is
simply mouth-watering.

Ketchup comes from the Chinese
word *koetsiap*, meaning 'pickled fish sauce'.
Today, it describes a slightly sharp sauce
consisting of tomatoes, spices and vinegar.

The recipe for tomato ketchup came from
Asia to Europe in the 18th century. Later, a
version of the sauce was made in the United
States, where it has now become the most
popular ready-made sauce of all time.

There are many different recipes for tomato
sauce. Other vegetables and fruit can also be
incorporated, as well as a variety of spices.

Vinegar gives ketchup the familiar, slightly
sharp taste, but a more subtle flavour can be
achieved by using red wine instead. Before
preparing large quantities, all bottling jars
must be sterilised. The ketchup will then
keep for 4–5 months.

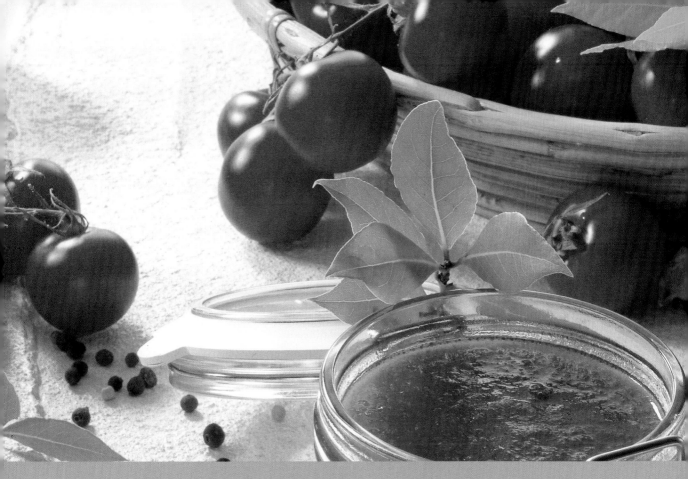

How to make tomato ketchup
Makes about 1.2 litres (2 pints)

▼ Put **4 bay leaves**, **6 black peppercorns**, **1 teaspoon each mustard seeds** and **caraway seeds** in a pan. Pour over **250ml (9fl oz) cider vinegar**. Heat just to simmering point, then strain the liquid through a fine sieve.

▼ Pour the sieved tomatoes and the onion purée into a pan, then bring to the boil, stirring constantly. Stir in the flavoured vinegar and leave the mixture to simmer for about 30 minutes until pulpy. Pour into sterilised glass jars and seal.

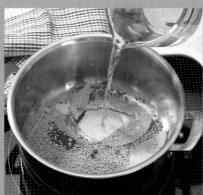

▲ Chop **4.5kg (10lb) tomatoes**. Cook gently for 2-3 minutes then press through a sieve. Chop **500g (1lb 2oz) onions** place in a pan with a little water and cook until soft, then purée. Simmer **500g (1lb 2oz) sugar**, **150g (5½oz) salt** **200ml (7fl oz) sunflower oil** and **200ml (7fl oz) vinegar** in a pan until the sugar has dissolved.

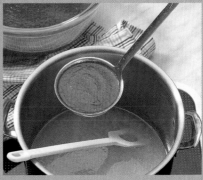

Homemade juices

In our grandparents' day homemade fruit juices and syrups were considered a real treat. Rediscover their exquisite taste with the help of traditional recipes.

Start your day with a glass of homemade freshly squeezed fruit juice. As well as tasting delicious, it will provide you with plenty of important nutrients and long-lasting energy.

Juices and syrups are rich in vitamins and fructose, a natural sugar. To gain the most from the vitamins, fresh juices should be drunk as soon as possible.

Fruit syrups and heated juices can be stored for four weeks in the fridge because the large amount of sugar in them acts as a preservative.

Some juices aid the immune system and help to prevent illness. Elderberry and redcurrant, for example, can help to relieve colds and fevers, while cranberry is used to treat cystitis and may help to prevent its recurrence.

Homemade fruit juices and syrups are also perfect to offer at summer parties. Serve them alone, diluting syrup with mineral water, or in cocktails. Your guests will be delighted and impressed.

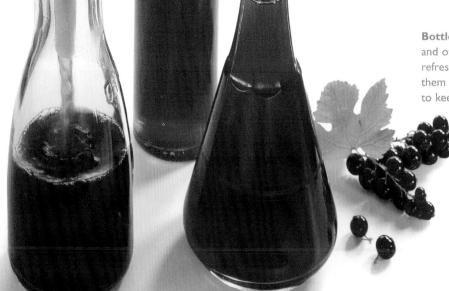

Bottled berries Redcurrants and other soft berry fruits make refreshing fruit juices. Store them in the fridge to help them to keep for longer.

and fruit syrups

Making your own fruit juices

The simplest way to make large quantities of homemade juice is in a juicer. For small quantities, you can pulp the chopped fresh or cooked fruits in a blender or food processor. Unripe fruit is unsuitable for use as it will contain only a small amount of juice.

You then need to press the fruit purée through a fine sieve or a jelly bag – a nylon mesh bag suspended on a stand – to extract the juice from the pulp. If you don't have a jelly bag you can improvise by putting the pulp in a piece of muslin or cheesecloth and suspending it over a bowl.

Make sure that all your juicing equipment is spotlessly clean. If left for more than two or three days, non-heated juices may begin to ferment.

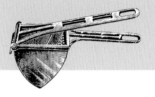

Fruit press

In the past apples, pears and quinces were cored and then the firm fruit was pushed through a press which resembled a large garlic press.

Pain for gain Picking wild blackberries can be a painful experience because of the thorns, but worth the effort for the intense flavour of the fruit.

BLACKBERRY JUICE

Use a jelly bag or muslin to strain the juice. Makes 1.5 litres (2¾ pints).

2kg (4lb 8oz) blackberries
peel of ½ unwaxed lemon
250g (9oz) caster sugar
1 cinnamon stick
3-4 cloves

Wash the blackberries and put them in a pan without water. Cook over a low heat until the juice runs out of the berries. Do not let it boil. Strain the juice through a jelly bag or muslin cloth into a bowl. Leave to drip for several hours. Do not squash the fruit with a spoon to extract more juice or the liquid will turn cloudy.

Pour the juice into a pan. Add the lemon peel, sugar and spices and simmer for 30 minutes. Cool, then strain into bottles and seal.

SOUR REDCURRANT JUICE

This bright red refreshing juice is excellent for flavouring cocktails and sauces. The berries have three times as much vitamin C as citrus fruit. This recipe makes about 2.5 litres (4½ pints).

2kg (4lb 8oz) redcurrants
2 litres (3½ pints) water
40g (1½oz) cream of tartar
150g (5½oz) caster sugar

Wash the redcurrants, remove the stalks with a fork and place the fruit in a bowl. Pour the water into another bowl and dissolve the cream of tartar. Pour this over the currants. Leave overnight, then strain the juice through a jelly bag.

Transfer the strained juice to a pan and add the sugar. Heat gently, stirring until the sugar has dissolved. Leave the juice to cool, then pour it into bottles and seal.

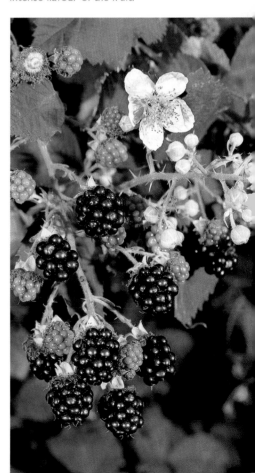

ELDERBERRY JUICE

The purple-black berries of the elder tree make a richly flavoured juice. Collect the fruit when it is ripe in September or October.

3kg (6lb 8oz) elderberries

Carefully strip the berries from the stems with a fork. Place them in a sieve set over a bowl. Place the bowl in a pan of simmering water or in a steamer. Cover with a lid and steam the berries for at least 1 hour. Remove the lid and leave to cool a little before pouring the juice into bottles. This juice is excellent poured over ice cream.

BERRY PUNCH

Make a non-alcoholic punch with fresh strawberries, raspberries and homemade juices. Makes 15-20 small glassfuls.

1kg (2lb 4oz) raspberries
**   and strawberries**
juice of 1 lemon
1.5 litres (2¾ pints) mixed
**   fruit juices**
1-2 bottles sparkling mineral
**   water**

Put the fruit and juices into a glass bowl and leave them to stand for 2-3 hours. Top up with mineral water just before serving.

Fresh is best Like most soft fruit, raspberries deteriorate quickly, so use them soon after picking or buying.

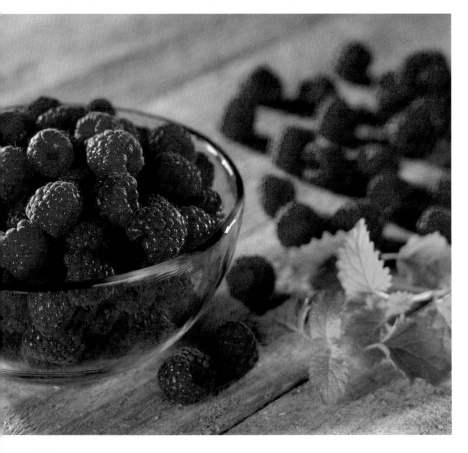

Tried & Trusted

Juicing aid

• **Juice can be gently extracted with the help of steam. The steam makes the fruit burst and the juice can be collected in a bowl. Bottle the juice immediately after cooling.**

Vegetable juices

• **You can make some very tasty and healthy juices with vegetables. However, if the juices are to be kept, they must be sterilised (see Basic recipe for bottling, page 205).**

• **For tomato juice, halve ripe tomatoes and cook until tender, then press through a fine sieve. For every 500ml (18fl oz) of tomato pulp add 100ml (3½fl oz) water, 15g (½oz) sugar, ½ teaspoon salt and ½ teaspoon ground black pepper. Bring the juice to the boil, cool slightly, then pour it into bottles.**

• **Wash and finely grate 2kg (4lb 8oz) young carrots. Sprinkle with 1 tablespoon orange juice and transfer to a juicer. Strain the juice through a muslin cloth or jelly bag, then pour it into a bottle and keep refrigerated. Use within one day.**

Homemade fruit and herb syrups

Syrups are a concentrated blend of fruit or vegetable juice and sugar. Currants and berries are suitable for syrups, but they must be really ripe and unblemished.

Herbs, such as peppermint, lemon balm and rosemary, can also be used. You can extract the juice from raw fruit and herbs and leave it to ferment in a warm place.

Alternatively, fruit can be cooked first and strained through a muslin cloth or jelly bag. The high sugar content of these syrups means they will keep for a couple of months.

RASPBERRY SYRUP

A dash of syrup in sparkling mineral water makes a cooling drink.

**1.2kg (2lb 10oz) raspberries
1kg (2lb 4oz) caster sugar
15g (½oz) citric acid**

Put the raspberries into a bowl and crush them with a potato masher. Strain the juice through a jelly bag or muslin cloth for several hours. Transfer the juice to a pan and stir in the sugar and citric acid. Simmer for 10 minutes, cool, then pour into bottles and seal.

RHUBARB SYRUP

Rhubarb tastes less sharp if you add some ginger to the juice.

**15 sticks rhubarb
1 litre (1¾ pints) water
caster sugar
pinch of ground ginger**

Wash the rhubarb and cut it into chunks. Place in a pan with the water and boil for 6-8 minutes. Strain the juice through a jelly bag or muslin cloth for several hours. Measure the juice and pour it into a pan. Add an equal amount of sugar and the ginger. Cook for 15 minutes. Pour the juice into bottles and seal.

PEPPERMINT SYRUP

Peppermint syrup diluted with water is a favourite with children.

**1 bunch fresh peppermint
leaves
1.2 litres (2 pints) water
350g (12oz) caster sugar
few drops green food
colouring (optional)**

Wash the peppermint, place the leaves in a pan, cover with the water and bring to the boil. Simmer for 10 minutes, then leave to stand for 30 minutes. Strain the juice through a fine sieve. Mix 500ml (18fl oz) of the juice with the sugar.

Pour this mixture into a pan and simmer for 15 minutes, stirring until the sugar has dissolved. When cool, pour the syrup into bottles and seal.

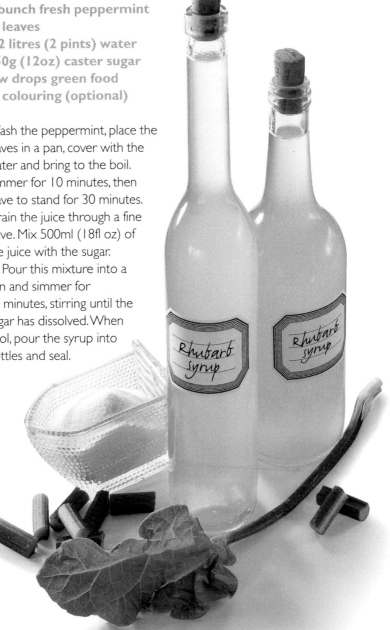

Springtime delicacy Originally from Asia, rhubarb is technically a vegetable rather than a fruit. Its juice is cheering in winter, giving a foretaste of spring.

Marmalade, jellies

There is immense satisfaction to be gained from stocking your larder with a wonderful selection of your own homemade preserves – just as our grandmothers once did.

For many people, breakfast without marmalade or tea without jam would be unthinkable.

It is now possible to buy expensive conserves that taste almost as good as the homemade variety. But making your own is more economical and an excellent way of using up a bumper crop if you grow or pick your own fruit. It also allows you to adjust the flavour to your own taste.

Nostalgia may also add to the appeal, as homemade jam is a feature of the rosy picture we call the 'good old days'.

Certainly jam-making was very important a hundred years ago as preserves were not readily available in the shops. At the beginning of the 20th century, most housewives would prepare a fresh stock of fruit marmalades, jellies, jams and purées each year.

Certain types of fruit, such as quinces and rowans, were mainly preserved as jellies. Other types, such as plums, were mostly puréed.

The word marmalade comes from the Portuguese *marmelada*, meaning 'quince jam', but in English it is used largely for jams made from citrus fruit, especially Seville oranges. Whole-fruit varieties of jam are often called preserves and conserves.

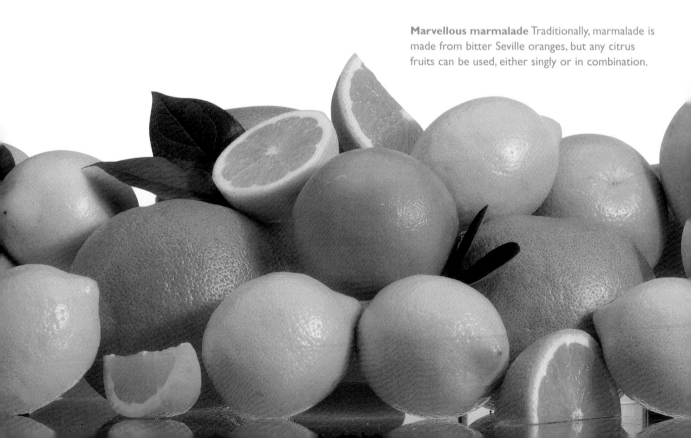

Marvellous marmalade Traditionally, marmalade is made from bitter Seville oranges, but any citrus fruits can be used, either singly or in combination.

and jams

Making your own fruit jams and preserves

It is easy to make your own jam. You will probably already have most of the equipment you need. If you are intending to make large amounts on a regular basis, a preserving pan is a good investment. Otherwise, use a large saucepan with a heavy base to prevent the jam from scorching on the bottom.

A sugar thermometer is useful, though not essential, for judging the setting point of your jam.

Successful setting

To get the fruit mixture to set, you may need extra pectin (a natural coagulant found in unripe fruit) or preserving sugar which contains pectin. Follow the instructions on the bottle or packet when using pectin or preserving sugar.

DAMSON JAM

This is a good old-fashioned favourite on toasted crumpets. Makes about 2.5kg (5lb 8oz).

2.7kg (6lb) damsons
2kg (4lb 8oz) preserving
    sugar

Wash the damsons and remove any stalks and leaves. Put the fruit and sugar in a preserving pan or saucepan. Place over a low heat and slowly bring to the boil, stirring until the sugar has dissolved. Boil for about an hour until thick and sticky, removing the stones with a slotted spoon as they rise to the surface. Pour into warm, sterilised glass jars and leave to cool. Seal with screw-top lids.

RASPBERRY CONSERVE

Ripe raspberries are full of flavour. Makes about 3kg (6lb 8oz).

3kg (6lb 8oz) raspberries
3kg (6lb 8oz) granulated
    sugar

Place the raspberries in a pan without water and heat gently, then simmer until soft. Add the sugar, stirring until it has dissolved. Boil the mixture to a set.

To test whether setting point is reached, cool a saucer in the freezer for 5 minutes. Take the jam off the heat and spoon 1 teaspoon of jam onto the saucer and leave it to cool slightly. If a skin forms on the surface which wrinkles when pushed, it is ready. If not, boil the jam and test again. Pour into glass jars and seal.

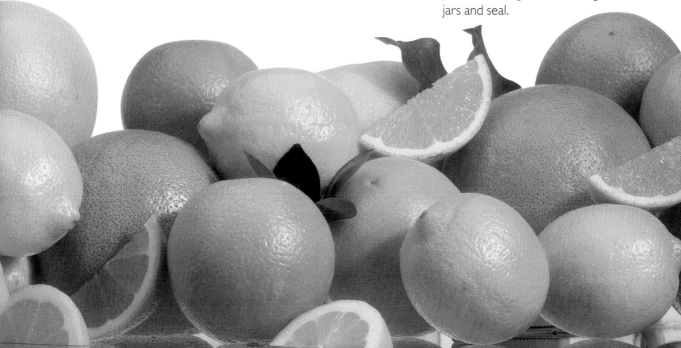

BLACKBERRY JAM

Wild blackberries have the best flavour, but cultivated varieties can also be used. Makes 3kg (6lb 8oz).

3kg (6lb 8oz) blackberries
200ml (7fl oz) water
3kg (6lb 8oz) granulated
sugar

Wash and dry the blackberries and put them in the pan with the water. Simmer gently over a low heat until the blackberries soften.

Add the sugar and stir until it has dissolved. Boil the mixture until setting point is reached (see Raspberry conserve, page 225). Pour the jam into glass jars and seal with screw-top lids.

PEACH PRESERVE

Sweet cicely adds a subtle flavour. Makes about 750g (1lb 10oz).

1kg (2lb 4oz) peaches
450g (1lb) granulated sugar
juice of 2 lemons
3 fresh sweet cicely leaves

Immerse the peaches in boiling water for 30 seconds, drain and peel off the skins. Remove the stones and cut the flesh into segments. Place the peaches and sugar in a pan and simmer, stirring constantly until the sugar has dissolved.

Add the lemon juice and boil the mixture until setting point is reached (see Raspberry conserve, page 225). Put a sweet cicely leaf in each glass jar, pour in the preserve and seal with screw-top lids.

STRAWBERRY PRESERVE

A classic jam to serve with fresh scones and cream. Makes about 1.25kg (2lb 12oz).

1kg (2lb 4oz) strawberries
1kg (2lb 4oz) granulated
sugar
3 tablespoons lemon juice

Hull the strawberries and place in a preserving pan. Sprinkle them with 500g (1lb 2oz) of the sugar and leave for a few hours to encourage the juice to flow. Simmer for 15 minutes.

Slowly add the remaining sugar and lemon juice, stirring constantly. Boil the mixture until setting point is reached (see Raspberry conserve, page 225). Pour into glass jars; seal with screw-top lids.

Covering up If using jars with screw-top lids, close them immediately after filling with hot jam. Leave jars without lids to cool completely, then seal with cellophane covers.

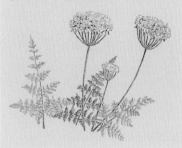

Sweet cicely

This herb grows along hedgerows, in woods and fields. Its aromatic leaves have a flavour similar to anise and can be used to add sweetness to homemade jams and stewed fruit.

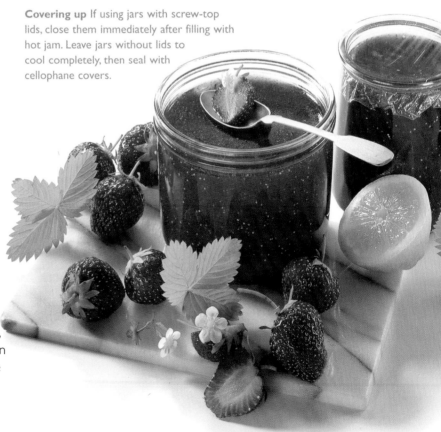

- There's no need to buy special preserving jars for jams. Just keep old glass jars with their lids.

- Wash the jars thoroughly before use. Warm them in a preheated oven, 110°C (225°F, gas mark ¼), to prevent them from cracking when they are being filled with hot jam.

- To stop mould from growing on the surface of a low-sugar jam, place a cellophane disc on the hot preserve and pour on a teaspoon of rum or brandy. Double the amount for large 500g (1lb 2oz) jars.

- Re-use metal lids that can be screwed onto jars tightly. They should have no dents and should be lined with a non-corrosive material. Plastic clip-on lids are also suitable.

If things go wrong

- If jams or jellies don't set after several attempts, the pectin content is probably too low. Add a little more preserving sugar, return the mixture to the heat and boil again until setting point is reached.

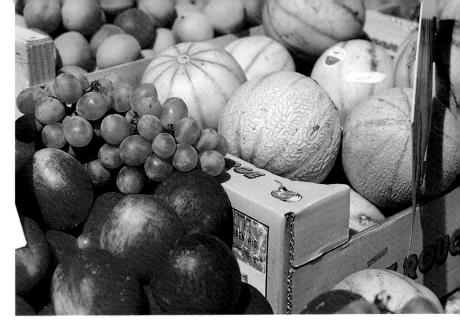

Spoilt for choice In late summer and autumn there's a feast of seasonal fruits on offer, just waiting to be made into jams and jellies.

Making traditional fruit jellies

Jellies are made from the juice of the fruit. This means that you have to extract it, either by putting raw fruit in a juicer or by straining the cooked fruit through a jelly bag.

The amount of juice that is obtained depends on the ripeness of the fruit and, if you are using a jelly bag, how long the pulp is left to drip. To get the jelly to set successfully, you will need to measure the fruit juice and calculate the quantity of sugar carefully as stated in the recipe.

Jellies should be clear and firm enough to be cut with a spoon. Pectin-rich fruits do not require extra gelling agents. Sharp apples, redcurrants and unripe quinces have a particularly high pectin content. Sugar alone needs to be added before the juice is boiled.

BRAMBLE JELLY

Use this jelly for making tarts and steamed sponges. Makes about 2kg (4lb 8oz).

1.8kg (4lb) blackberries
juice of 2 large lemons
400ml (14fl oz) water
caster sugar

Rinse the blackberries and put them in a pan with the lemon juice and water. Simmer for an hour or until the fruit is soft. Strain the juice through a jelly bag or muslin cloth. Leave it overnight for all the juice to drip through.

Measure the blackberry juice and return it to the pan, adding 450g (1lb) sugar for each 600ml (1 pint) juice. Stir the mixture over a low heat until the sugar has dissolved, then boil until setting point is reached (see Raspberry conserve, page 225). Spoon off any froth and pour the jelly into sterilised glass jars. Seal with lids.

APPLE JELLY WITH ROSE PETALS

Use petals from unsprayed roses. Makes about 500g (1lb 2oz).

**30 strongly scented
   rose petals
500ml (18fl oz) freshly
   pressed apple juice
250g (9oz) granulated sugar**

Strip the rose petals from the flowers and place in a bowl. Pour boiling water over them. Drain immediately, dip the petals into ice-cold water, then place them on a cloth to dry.

Put the apple juice and sugar in a pan and bring to the boil, stirring until the sugar has dissolved. Boil for 5 minutes, skimming off any froth. Add the rose petals and continue cooking for another 4 minutes or until setting point is reached (see Raspberry conserve, page 225). Pour the jelly into glass jars and seal with lids.

BLACKCURRANT JELLY

Blackcurrants create a richly flavoured jelly high in vitamin C. Makes about 2kg (4lb 8oz).

**2kg (4lb 8oz) blackcurrants
1 litre (1¾ pints) water
granulated sugar**

Rinse the blackcurrants and strip them from their stalks with a fork. Put in a pan with two-thirds of the water and simmer until soft.

Strain the juice through muslin cloth or a jelly bag into a bowl. Reserving the liquid, return the pulp to the pan with the remaining water and boil for 5 minutes. Strain the juice again, leaving the pulp overnight to drip through.

Pour the juice into a pan, bring to the boil and stir in 1kg (2lb 4oz) sugar for each 1 litre (1¾ pints) of juice. Boil the jelly until setting point is reached (see Raspberry conserve, page 225). Pour the jelly into glass jars and seal with lids.

The refrigerator

The first household refrigerators appeared in Britain in the 1920s, but they were luxury items. Until the 1950s most families made do with an ice box or a 'safe' that was kept on a cold slab in the pantry.

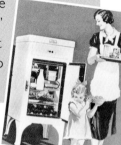

SEVILLE MARMALADE

Most of the pectin in oranges is in the pips and membranes. Makes about 4.5kg (10lb).

**1.3kg (3lb) Seville oranges
juice of 2 large lemons
3.6 litres (6 pints) water
2.7kg (6lb) granulated sugar**

Wash and halve the oranges, then squeeze out the juice and pips. Pare the peel and slice thinly. Put the peel in a preserving pan with the juices and water. Tie up the pith and pips in a small square of muslin and add to the pan.

Simmer the mixture for 2 hours until the peel is soft and the liquid has reduced by half. Remove the muslin bag and squeeze between two plates so the juice goes back into the pan. Add the sugar and stir until dissolved. Boil until setting point is reached (see Raspberry conserve, page 225). Leave to stand for 30 minutes. Stir, then pour into glass jars and seal.

Versatile preserve Blackcurrant jelly can be served with both sweet and savoury food.

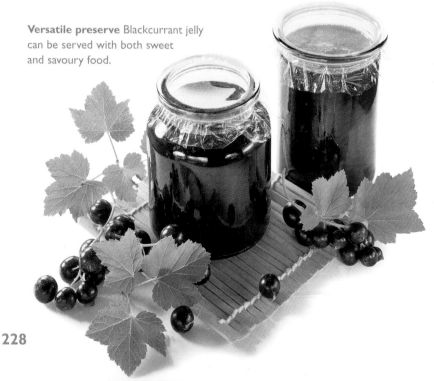

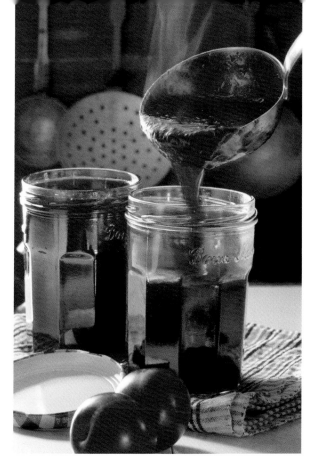

Pure purée
Making your own purées and preserves allows you to decide the ingredients. As a result you'll have a natural product free from additives and artificial colourings.

Making delicious purées from ripe fruit

Sweet purées are delicious both in tarts and served as sauces with old-fashioned steamed puddings. They are made by cooking ripe fruit with a little sugar until all the liquid has evaporated and the mixture turns into a thick, mushy pulp. Fruits suitable for puréeing include fleshy apples and pears, stone fruit such as plums and apricots or berries.

Store purées in preserving jars, filling them to 2cm (¾in) below the rim. Because of their low sugar content, fruit purées do not keep well and should be used within a few months.

To prevent a purée from going off too quickly, you can brush the surface of the mixture with rum after filling the jars. Once opened, keep fruit purées in the fridge.

PLUM PURÉE

Damsons can also be used in this recipe. Makes 2.5kg (5lb 8oz).

2.5kg (5lb 8oz) plums
1 litre (1¾ pints) water
2 sticks cinnamon
3kg (6lb 8oz) granulated sugar

Wash and dry the plums. Place the fruit in a pan with the water and cook gently until soft and mushy, stirring occasionally. Remove the stones with a slotted spoon then add the cinnamon and sugar.

Simmer and stir the purée until the sugar has dissolved, then boil until the mixture is really thick. Remove the cinnamon sticks and pour it into glass jars. Seal with lids.

ELDERBERRY PURÉE

Freshly made elderberry purée was very popular during the Second World War and is delicious spread on rolls or as a dessert. Makes about 1kg (2lb 4oz).

500g (1lb 2oz) elderberries
250g (9oz) plums
 or
250g (9oz) damsons
250g (9oz) pears
85ml (3fl oz) water
55g (2oz) granulated sugar
½ teaspoon ground cloves
½ teaspoon ground cinnamon

Strip the elderberries from the stalks with a fork, then wash and drain them. Stone and halve the plums or damsons. Quarter, peel and core the pears.

Put all the fruit in a pan with the water, sugar and spices. Place over a moderately high heat until the sugar dissolves, stirring continuously, then simmer for 10 minutes, mashing the pears with a fork. Pour into glass jars and seal.

Take care

Prevent micro-organisms from contaminating purées by sterilising jars after they have been sealed. This is vital for preserving purées.

Place the jars on a trivet in a deep pan and pour in hot water up to their necks. Cover the pan, bring the water to the boil and simmer for 5 minutes. Spoon out a little water, carefully remove the jars and leave to cool.

Soups and sauces

In our grandparents' time soups and sauces were all homemade. These traditional recipes remain favourites today and are as delicious as ever.

The secret of a good soup is to start with a well-flavoured stock. If you do not have time to make your own, buy good quality cubes, bouillon powder or ready-made fresh chilled stock.

When making a vegetable soup, start by 'sweating' the vegetables for 10 minutes in a pan with butter to bring out their flavour. Use a low heat, cover the pan so the vegetables don't start to brown and shake or stir occasionally.

Soups can be light and clear, such as consommé, or hearty, one-pot meals in their own right. When thickening a soup, flour or cornflour can be used but mashed potato makes a tasty alternative.

For extra interest and colour, plain soups can be garnished with fresh chopped herbs. Cream, sour cream or croutons also look attractive.

Traditional garnishes for consommés include small herb leaves and tiny pasta shapes. To garnish a creamy vegetable soup, grate or chop a little of the vegetable from which it is made and scatter over the surface.

Soup of the day In most large households, soup was served in a large flat, lidded dish called a tureen. They ranged from functional white dishes to ornate pieces of crockery with raised gold designs as part of a dinner service.

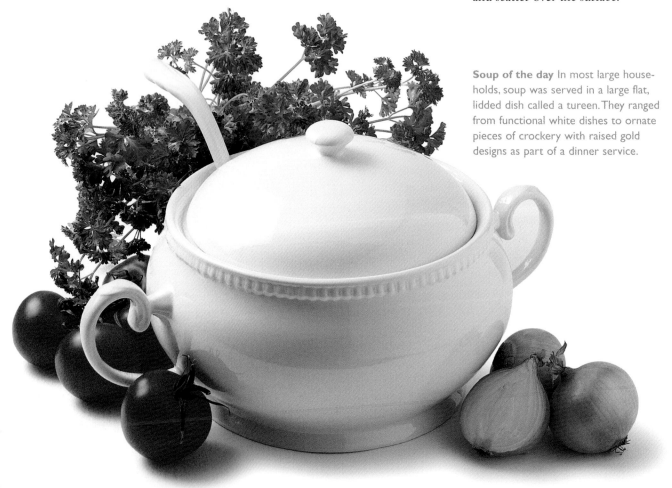

- **Before puréeing, allow a soup to cool, then purée it in small batches in a liquidiser. Avoid overfilling the machine as it could overflow. Pour the puréed soup into a clean pan and dilute it to the desired consistency with extra stock or water.**

- **Many hot winter soups are delicious served chilled in summer. Examples include leek and potato, watercress, tomato and orange or green pea and mint.**

- **As a starter, allow about 200ml (7fl oz) per serving of thick soup. For a main course, allow 300ml (½ pint) per serving with plenty of crusty bread.**

- **'Sweating' the vegetables over a low heat helps to start the cooking process and draws out their flavour. Remember that browning the vegetables will affect the look and flavour of the finished soup.**

- **Thick soups can be garnished with crunchy croutons. Cut sliced bread into 5mm (¼in) dice and fry them in hot oil until golden and crisp. Drain on kitchen paper before scattering them on the soup.**

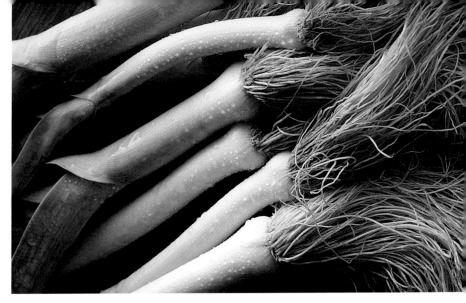

The hardy leek Easy to grow and resistant to the most severe winter weather, leeks make a delicate flavouring for soups.

THICK TOMATO AND CELERIAC SOUP

Sieve the tomatoes to remove the bitter pips. Serves four.

1 medium onion, peeled
2 medium carrots
225g (8oz) celeriac, peeled
1 tablespoon sunflower oil
25g (1oz) butter
900g (2lb) tomatoes, quartered
300ml (½ pint) vegetable stock
150ml (¼ pint) tomato juice
1 teaspoon sugar
zest and juice of 1 orange
salt and pepper

Chop the onion, carrots and celeriac into small dice. Heat the oil and butter in a pan. Add the diced vegetables, cover and sweat for 10 minutes. Add the remaining ingredients, cover again and simmer for 45 minutes. Sieve the soup and return it to the pan. Dilute the soup to the desired consistency with stock or water. Season to taste and reheat.

COCK-A-LEEKIE

This hearty broth dates back to the reign of James I. Serves four.

2 chicken legs, skinned
1.2 litres (2 pints) water
3 large leeks, trimmed and washed
1 fresh bay leaf
2 tablespoons short grain rice
2 teaspoons dark brown sugar
8 pitted prunes
salt and pepper
4 tablespoons chopped fresh parsley

Put the chicken legs in a pan with the water. Chop the leeks and add to the pan with the bay leaf, rice and sugar. Cover the pan and simmer for 30 minutes.

Add the prunes, re-cover and cook for 20 minutes or until the rice is tender. Remove the chicken, cut the flesh into small pieces and return it to the pan. Reheat the soup uncovered for 5 minutes. Season and garnish with parsley.

POTATO AND PARSLEY SOUP

A classic winter soup. Serves six.

55g (2oz) butter
2 leeks, trimmed and washed
2 sticks celery
350g (12oz) potatoes, peeled
1 litre (1¾ pints) chicken stock
150ml (¼ pint) double cream
salt and pepper
3 tablespoons chopped fresh parsley
fried bread croutons

Heat the butter in a pan. Slice the leeks then add them to the pan. Cover and cook for 10 minutes until the leeks have softened. Chop the celery and potatoes, add to the pan, re-cover and cook for a further 5 minutes. Pour in the stock, cover the pan and simmer for 30 minutes.

Liquidise the soup until smooth, return to the pan and stir in the cream, seasoning and parsley. Dilute to the desired consistency with stock or water, reheat and serve garnished with croutons.

CREAM OF CARROT SOUP

Serve this soup garnished with croutons and finely shaved carrot curls. Serves four.

500g (1lb 2oz) carrots
1 onion
55g (2oz) butter
40g (1½oz) long grain rice
850ml (1½ pints) vegetable stock
1 teaspoon fresh thyme leaves
½ teaspoon caster sugar
salt and pepper
4 tablespoons double cream

Peel and thinly slice the carrots and onion. Heat the butter in a large pan. Add the carrots and onion, stir to coat in the butter, then bring to the boil. Cover and cook gently for 15 minutes. Stir in the rice, stock, thyme and sugar.

Cover the pan and simmer gently for 30 minutes until the vegetables and rice are tender. Purée in a liquidiser, season to taste and reheat when needed. Add the cream just before serving.

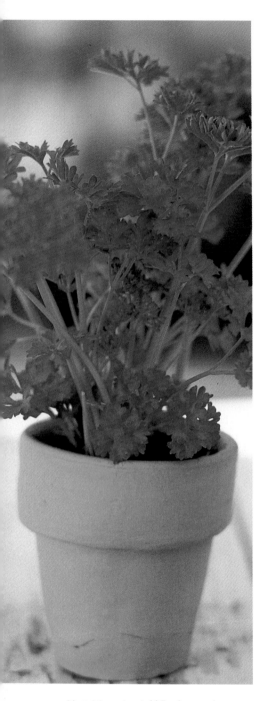

Nutritious herb Whether curly or flat-leaved, parsley adds flavour and colour to soups. It is also rich in iron and vitamin C.

Allotments

The Allotment Movement began in the early 1800s in response to the extreme hardship of the many agricultural workers who were leaving the land to find work in the newly industrial towns. What started as a local initiative to provide land for poor families to cultivate became a national requirement. By 1882, all parish authorities were obliged to provide allotments, as local councils are to this day.

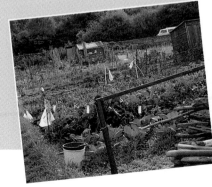

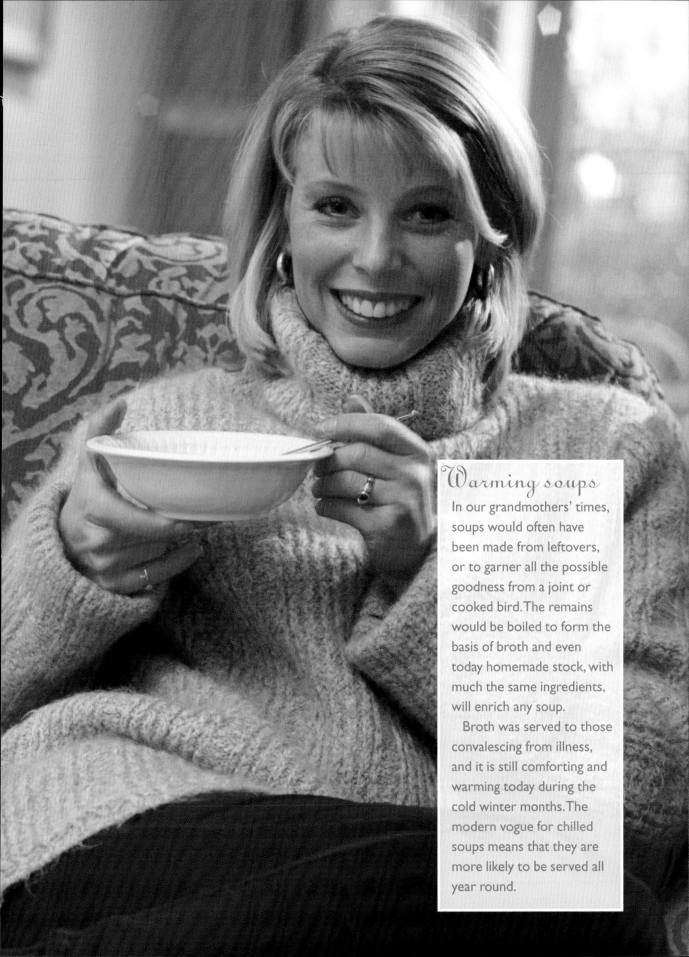

Warming soups

In our grandmothers' times, soups would often have been made from leftovers, or to garner all the possible goodness from a joint or cooked bird. The remains would be boiled to form the basis of broth and even today homemade stock, with much the same ingredients, will enrich any soup.

Broth was served to those convalescing from illness, and it is still comforting and warming today during the cold winter months. The modern vogue for chilled soups means that they are more likely to be served all year round.

Making traditional savoury sauces

Sauces have been used to add flavour and colour to plainly cooked food for centuries.

Savoury sauces can be as simple as the meat juices from a roasting tin. The classic savoury white sauce is based on a butter and flour 'roux', which is blended with milk and heated until thick. It can then be flavoured with additional ingredients such as parsley, onions, cheese or mushrooms.

HOLLANDAISE SAUCE

Serve this egg-based sauce with salmon, white fish dishes or asparagus. Serves four.

2 tablespoons white wine
  or
2 tablespoons tarragon
  vinegar
1 tablespoon water
2 egg yolks
100g (3½oz) butter
salt and pepper

Put the wine or vinegar and water in a pan and boil until reduced to 1 tablespoon. Pour into a heatproof bowl with the egg yolks and place over a pan of simmering water. Stir until the mixture thickens.

Cut the butter into small pieces and whisk into the sauce. Season, then add more butter if the sauce is too sharp. The finished sauce should be thick enough to coat a spoon.

Classic combination The sharp taste of hollandaise sauce complements ham and eggs in the dish Eggs benedict.

BREAD SAUCE

A familiar accompaniment to roast turkey or chicken. Serves eight.

1 large onion
8 whole cloves
900ml (1 pint 12fl oz) milk
2 dried bay leaves
175g (6oz) fresh
  breadcrumbs
salt and pepper
1 teaspoon wholegrain
  mustard
3 tablespoons double cream

Peel the onion, stud it with the cloves and put in a pan with the milk and bay leaves. Simmer for 1 minute. Cover and leave to cool, then discard the bay leaves.

Finely chop the onion, discard the cloves, then stir the onion with the breadcrumbs back into the milk. Season the sauce, then add the mustard. Warm for 3-4 minutes and stir in the cream.

CAPER SAUCE

It is customary to serve caper sauce with boiled leg of lamb or mutton. Serves four.

25g (1oz) butter
2 tablespoons plain flour
300ml (½ pint) milk and
  lamb stock, mixed
1 tablespoon capers
2 teaspoons vinegar from
  the caper jar
  or
2 teaspoons lemon juice
salt and pepper

Melt the butter in a pan. Stir in the flour and cook for 2 minutes. Remove the pan from the heat and gradually stir in the liquid.

Return the pan to the heat and cook gently, stirring until the sauce thickens. Simmer for 1 minute, then stir in the capers and vinegar or lemon juice. Season with salt and pepper.

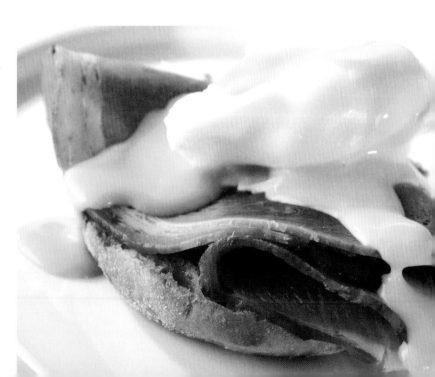

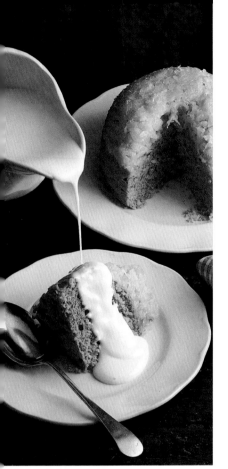

All-time favourite Custard is delicious served with many traditional baked and steamed puddings. It can be flavoured with grated citrus zest or vanilla or almond essence.

Sweet sauces

Sweet sauces can be made from a basic white sauce (béchamel) with sugar or honey added to sweeten them. Other good flavourings are mixed spice, melted chocolate, citrus zest and alcohol.

Adding egg yolks to a white sauce will turn it into custard, the favourite accompaniment to many British puddings through the ages.

A fruit sauce made by puréeing soft or stewed fruit and adding a liqueur, if liked, goes well with sponge puddings and ice cream.

TRADITIONAL CUSTARD

If you prefer a plain egg custard, omit the vanilla pod. Serves four.

1 vanilla pod
300ml (½ pint) milk
3 large egg yolks
1 tablespoon caster sugar
1 tablespoon cornflour

Halve the vanilla pod lengthways and scrape out the seeds. Put the milk, vanilla pod and seeds in a pan and heat gently until bubbles appear on the surface. Remove the pan from the heat and leave to infuse for 10 minutes.

Put the egg yolks, sugar and cornflour in a bowl and whisk until smooth. Remove the vanilla pod, then pour the milk onto the egg mixture and stir thoroughly.

Pour the mixture into a pan and stir constantly over a low heat until the sauce thickens. Simmer for 1-2 minutes. Serve hot.

BITTER CHOCOLATE SAUCE

Pour this sauce over stewed pears, profiteroles or steamed chocolate pudding. Serves four.

100g (3½oz) plain chocolate
 with 70% cocoa solids
15g (½oz) butter
3 tablespoons strong
 black coffee

Break the chocolate into small pieces and heat in a heavy pan with the butter and coffee. Stir continuously until the chocolate and butter have melted and the sauce is smooth. Serve warm.

Flavoured vinegars

Vinegars and oils absorb the flavours of herbs, spices, soft fruit and flowers. Use nature's seasonings to make subtly flavoured condiments that add interest to dressings, marinades and sauces.

Many old cookery books contain recipes for vinegars made with spices, herbs and fruit.

Flavoured vinegars and oils are easy to make. Most culinary herbs can be used, including rosemary, thyme, tarragon, marjoram, fennel, savory, sage and basil. The herbs are left in to impart their aroma, then the vinegar or oil is strained. You can repeat the process until you have the desired taste. Decant the vinegar or oil into a clean bottle and add fresh herbs for decoration.

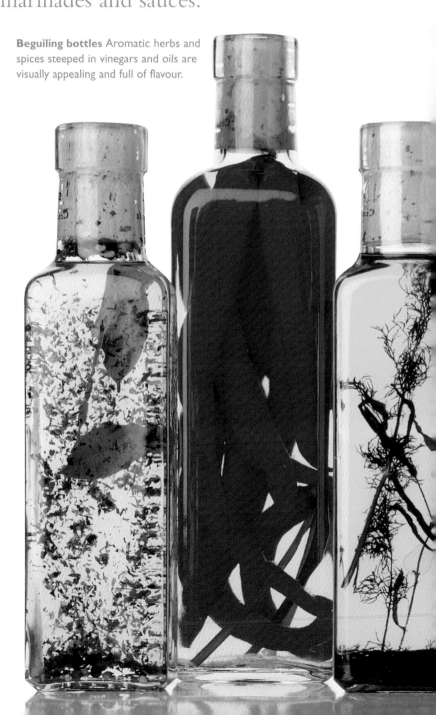

Beguiling bottles Aromatic herbs and spices steeped in vinegars and oils are visually appealing and full of flavour.

Mezzaluna

Called a 'half moon' because of the shape of the curved blade, this double-handled knife was invented in the early 20th century. It is ideal for chopping herbs quickly.

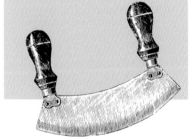

and oils

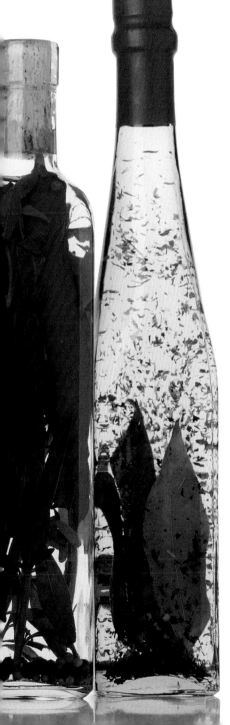

A selection of flavoured vinegars

A clear, mild vinegar such as white wine vinegar or cider vinegar is best for making flavoured vinegars as it doesn't overpower the herbs.

All the equipment used in the preparation of the vinegar must be spotlessly clean. Bottles must be dry when they are filled and clean corks should be used to seal them.

You will need a pan, a bowl, a fine sieve or muslin and a funnel. Don't forget to label and date your bottles. These vinegars will keep for about three months.

LEMON AND LIME VINEGAR

This vinegar flavoured with citrus fruit will add a tang to Hollandaise sauce (see page 234). The recipe makes 600ml (1 pint).

1 unwaxed lime
2 unwaxed lemons
600ml (1 pint) white
   wine vinegar

Pare the zest from the lime and one of the lemons. Place the zest in a bowl. Pour the vinegar into a pan and bring to the boil. Pour the boiling vinegar over the zest. Cover with a cloth or plate and leave to infuse for three days.

Pare the zest from the second lemon. Strain the vinegar through a fine sieve and pour it into a glass bottle. Add the fresh lemon zest and seal with a cork.

TARRAGON VINEGAR

Use long sprigs of tarragon for this vinegar. Makes 1 litre (1¾ pints).

sprigs and leaves of
   fresh tarragon
1 litre (1¾ pints) white
   wine vinegar

Half fill a 1 litre (1¾ pint) glass jar with the tarragon. Top up with the vinegar, seal with a cork or lid and leave to infuse for four weeks.

Strain the vinegar through a fine sieve into a bowl. Place a sprig of tarragon in a clean jar. Pour over the flavoured vinegar and seal.

ROSEMARY VINEGAR

This vinegar is ideal for salad dressings. Makes 600ml (1 pint).

7 large sprigs fresh rosemary
600ml (1 pint) white wine
   or cider vinegar

Strip the leaves from six sprigs of rosemary. Chop them finely and place them in a bowl. Pour the vinegar into a pan and bring to the boil, then pour over the rosemary.

Cover the bowl with a cloth or plate and leave to infuse for three days, then strain the vinegar. Put the remaining sprig in a glass bottle and pour over the flavoured vinegar. Seal with a cork.

PEPPERMINT VINEGAR

This vinegar adds a minty fresh flavour to salad dressings. Makes 1 litre (1¾ pints).

1 litre (1¾ pints) white wine vinegar
2 handfuls fresh young peppermint leaves

Pour the vinegar into a pan and bring to the boil. Rinse and dry the peppermint and place in a bowl. Pour the boiling vinegar over the leaves. Cover with a cloth or plate and leave to infuse for 2 hours. Strain the vinegar through a fine sieve and pour into glass bottles. Seal with a cork or cap and leave for at least a week before using.

CHILLI VINEGAR

Drizzle a little chilli vinegar to perk up bland food. Makes 1 litre (1¾ pints).

55g (2oz) fresh red chillies
1 litre (1¾ pints) red wine vinegar

Wash the chillies, split them in half lengthways and place in a bowl. Pour over the vinegar, cover with a cloth or plate and leave to infuse for four to six weeks. Strain the vinegar, pour it into glass bottles and seal.

Mediterranean flavours Rosemary oil makes a tasty salad dressing to accompany barbecued lamb, as well as stimulating blood circulation.

RASPBERRY VINEGAR

Use this deep pink vinegar in meat sauces, on salads or lightly sprinkled over fresh raspberries.

500g (1lb 2oz) raspberries
2 litres (3½ pints) red or white wine vinegar

Carefully pick over the raspberries, put in a bowl and mash with a fork. Pour on the vinegar. Cover the bowl and leave for 12-14 days in a warm place. Strain the vinegar through muslin or cheesecloth, then bottle.

ROSE-PETAL VINEGAR

Rose petals give this vinegar a sweet fragrance. Makes 1 litre (1¾ pints).

unsprayed flower heads from dark red roses
1 litre (1¾ pints) white wine vinegar

Strip the petals from the flower heads. Half fill a 1 litre (1¾ pint) glass jar with the petals. Top up with the vinegar, cover and leave to infuse for three weeks. Strain the vinegar then bottle and cork.

Tried & Trusted
Flavoured vinegars

- **Use organic vinegar and fruit or herbs for a product that is completely natural.**

- **To make dill vinegar, follow the recipe for Tarragon vinegar (see page 237), substituting dill. Strain the vinegar after 14 days.**

Flavoured oils

- **For rosemary-flavoured oil, place a sprig of fresh rosemary in a glass bottle. Top it up with mild olive oil and leave to infuse for 14 days. Strain the oil through a fine sieve.**

- **Never keep flavoured olive oil in the fridge, as it will thicken and turn opaque in the cold.**

- **Always remove the herbs from the oil once infused or the herb can turn mouldy and taint the oil. Use the oil within one month if you add a herb for decoration.**

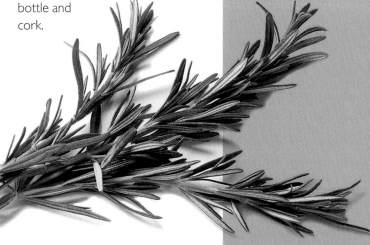

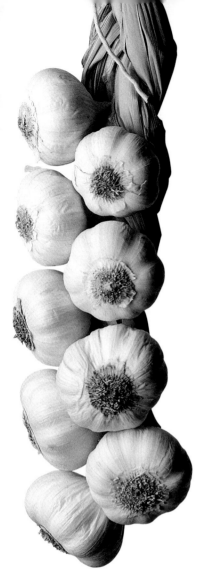

Instant flavour Use garlic oil to give added flavour to grilled and roasted meat and vegetable dishes.

Take care

Handle raw chillies with caution. They can cause severe irritation to the eyes, nose and other sensitive areas. When chopping chillies, either wear thin disposable gloves to avoid getting chilli on your fingers, or make sure you wash your hands immediately afterwards.

Homemade flavoured oils

By steeping herbs in oil you can incorporate subtle flavours into your meals.

Making your own spiced oils is easy. Use only high-quality and neutral oils such as mild olive, sunflower or soya oil. These oils go well with herbs and spices because they act as carriers for both the flavours and aromas of the added ingredients. Extra virgin olive oil has too strong a flavour for many aromatic herbs, so if you use olive oil, chose a lighter refined oil or an oil that is a mixture of refined and virgin oils.

You will need the same equipment for making flavoured oils as for flavoured vinegars (see page 237).

GARLIC OIL

Use fresh, plump cloves of garlic for this versatile oil.

**2 cloves garlic
1 sprig each of fresh thyme
    and rosemary
1 small dried red chilli
500ml (18fl oz) olive oil**

Peel the garlic and bruise it with the blade of a knife until moisture is extracted. Transfer it to a glass bottle. Add the thyme, rosemary and chilli. Pour over the oil and seal the bottle with a cork. Leave to infuse for one week before use.

BASIL OIL

The only way to preserve the flavour and scent of basil is by steeping it in olive oil.

**150g (5½ oz) fresh basil leaves
1 litre (1¾ pints) olive oil**

Wash and dry the basil. Place in a 1 litre (1¾ pint) glass bottle and push down with the handle of a wooden spoon. Pour the oil into a pan and heat to 40°C (75°F). Pour the oil over the basil, seal the bottle with a cork and leave to infuse for 3-4 weeks. Use the oil within a few weeks.

Basil oil will keep for longer if the leaves are removed, as they will quickly become slimy and taint the oil. Strain the oil through a fine sieve, transfer it to a clean glass bottle and seal with a cork.

THYME OIL

Use this oil to flavour salads or as a bath oil to help relieve a cold.

**200g (7oz) sprigs fresh thyme
1 litre (1¾ pints) olive
    or
1 litre (1¾ pints) sunflower oil**

Wash and pat dry the thyme. Strip the leaves from the stems, place on a wooden board and bruise them with a rolling pin. Place the leaves and oil in a bowl and cover with a cloth or plate. Leave to infuse for two weeks. Strain the oil and pour it into glass bottles. Seal with corks.

Wines, punch and

Alcohol has been a basis of drinks for centuries, although mixed cocktails have only become popular in the 20th century. Fruit soaked in alcohol also makes a tasty dessert.

Fermenting grapes to make wine goes back to Neolithic times and the mountains of Iran where wine was first made more than 7000 years ago. Later the ancient Greeks and Romans cultivated grapes, enjoyed wine and had their own gods – the Greek Dionysus and the Roman Bacchus – devoted to wine and pleasure.

Fruit beverages and alcoholic desserts, such as peach wine and prunes in Armagnac, are also part of a long tradition. In the 9th century, monks and apothecaries realised that alcohol prolonged the use of the fruit and herbs that they made into medicinal remedies.

Soon the monks were treating themselves to a glass of their own liqueurs and not just for medicinal purposes. Sugar was added to soften the bitter taste of many of the herbs, and thus liqueurs and distilled drinks were invented.

To create your own festive drinks and desserts, start planning at least two or three months in advance, in order to allow the fruit and alcohol to infuse.

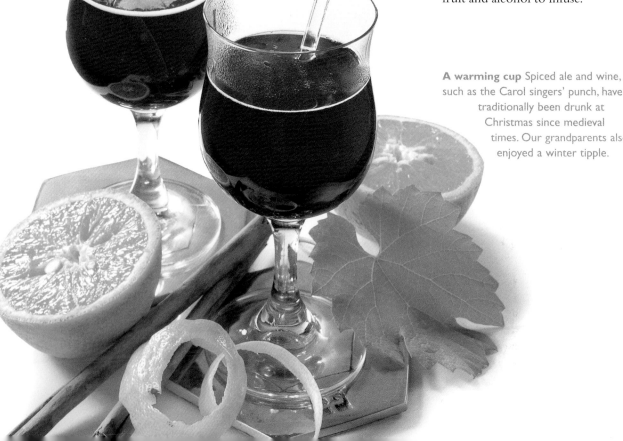

A warming cup Spiced ale and wine, such as the Carol singers' punch, have traditionally been drunk at Christmas since medieval times. Our grandparents also enjoyed a winter tipple.

liqueurs

Homemade wines and punch

If you want to make quality fruit wines yourself, it is important to use fresh fruit and spices as well as a good wine. Start by making small quantities and experiment to see which recipes you prefer.

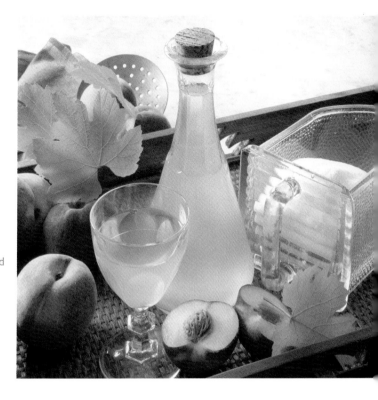

Dessert wine
Peach wine is delicious with a pudding. It is sweet, perfumed and cleans the palate.

PEACH WINE

This wine should be kept in the fridge and will last for two weeks. Makes 1.3 litres (2¼ pints).

6 peaches
1 litre (1¾ pints) white wine
200g (7oz) caster sugar
175ml (6fl oz) brandy

Peel, halve and stone the peaches. Pour the wine into a pan with the fruit and simmer until the peaches are soft. Cover with a lid and leave to infuse overnight. Remove the peaches, pour the wine through a coffee filter into a bowl. Stir in the brandy, then bottle and seal.

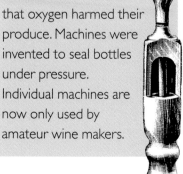

Corking machine

Wine makers realised that oxygen harmed their produce. Machines were invented to seal bottles under pressure. Individual machines are now only used by amateur wine makers.

BLACKCURRANT WINE

In this recipe the blackcurrants are left to infuse in the wine.

2kg (4lb 8oz) blackcurrants
1 litre (1¾ pints) red wine
150g (5½oz) caster sugar
2-3 liqueur glassfuls (45ml)
   fruit brandy

Wash the blackcurrants and strip the fruit from the stalks with a fork. Put the currants in a bowl, mash gently with a wooden spoon, then add the wine. Cover with a cloth or plate and leave to infuse for 3-4 days. Strain the liquid through a fine sieve into a bowl. Dissolve the sugar in the wine, then add the fruit brandy. Pour the wine into glass bottles and seal.

CAROL SINGERS' PUNCH

On long winter evenings this punch can be enjoyed at full strength or diluted with soda water.

175g (6oz) caster sugar
300ml (½ pint) water
zest of 1 lemon and 1 orange
2 cinnamon sticks
6 cloves
1 bottle white wine
1 bottle red wine
3 liqueur glassfuls (45ml)
   brandy

Heat the sugar, water and citrus zest with the spices in a pan, stirring constantly until the sugar has dissolved. Simmer the mixture for 15 minutes over a low heat. Pour in the wine and brandy and serve the punch hot.

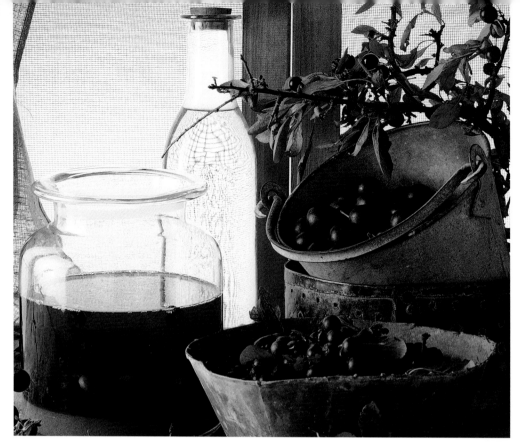

Fruity tipple
Sloe gin makes a wonderful winter aperitif. Pick the sloes in autumn when they are fully ripe and steep them in gin. It will be ready to drink or give as a gift at Christmas.

Fruit liqueurs and fruit soaked in alcohol

Brandy, gin and whisky are all good bases for flavoured liqueurs. The drinks are best prepared in wide-necked jars.

For soaking fruit in alcohol, choose rum, fruit brandy or Armagnac as they absorb additional flavourings easily.

Take care

If you use clear glass pots or jars for preserving fruit in alcohol, store them in a dark place because daylight will affect the colour of the fruit. In Germany, rum-soaked fruit was traditionally stored in an earthenware pot called a 'Rumtopf' (see right).

SLOE GIN

Sloes – fruits of the blackthorn – give the gin a distinctive taste. Makes 1 large or 2 small bottles.

450g (1lb) sloes
85g (3oz) sugar
few drops almond essence
1 bottle gin

Remove the stalks from the sloes, then wash and pat dry. Prick the sloes all over with a darning needle or cocktail stick and put them in a large screw-top jar. Add the sugar and almond essence. Pour in the gin, seal tightly and leave in a cool, dark place for three months, shaking occasionally.

Strain the gin through a coffee filter paper or muslin until clear. Pour into bottles, cork and label.

APRICOT LIQUEUR

Flavoured liqueurs need warmth in order to mature well.

500g (1lb 2oz) apricots
1 litre (1¾ pints) dry
**   white wine**
500g (1lb 2oz) caster sugar
700ml (1¼ pints) gin

Wash, halve and stone the apricots. Reserve the stones. Place the apricots, wine and sugar in a pan and boil, stirring until the sugar has dissolved. Pour into a bowl, then add the gin.

Crack the stones with a hammer, then add the kernels to the bowl. Cover with a cloth or plate and leave to infuse for 3-4 days. Strain the liquid, pour into bottles and seal.

PRUNES IN ARMAGNAC

Use plump Agen prunes for this classic recipe. Makes one large jar.

250ml (9fl oz) lime-flower tea
4 fresh vervain leaves
1kg (2lb 4oz) prunes
2 tablespoons water
200g (7oz) icing sugar
1 litre (1¾ pints) Armagnac

Make a strong lime-flower infusion, then add the vervain. When cool, add the prunes and leave to soak overnight. Remove the prunes and pat dry with kitchen paper.

Pour the water and sugar into a pan and boil to a syrup. When cool, stir in the Armagnac. Put the prunes in a jar and cover with the syrup. Seal with a screw-top lid and store for a couple of months.

Delicious dessert
Preserve the season's fruits in alcohol to produce an intoxicating mixed fruit dessert with a wonderfully sweet liqueur.

FRUITS IN RUM

For this recipe you need an earthenware jar that holds about 3 litres (5¼ pints). The seasonal fruit is added as it ripens. In Germany this recipe is known as 'Rumtopf'.

1kg (2lb 4oz) seasonal stone fruits and berries
1 litre (1¾ pints) rum
1kg (2lb 4oz) icing sugar

Wash and dry the fruit. Stone, core and chop as necessary. Peel apricots, peaches and pears. Put a small amount of one fruit in the jar, adding the same quantity of sugar, cover with rum, then put on the lid.

Add each new fruit layer in the same way, storing the jar in a cool place. After adding the last layer, leave it to infuse for a month.

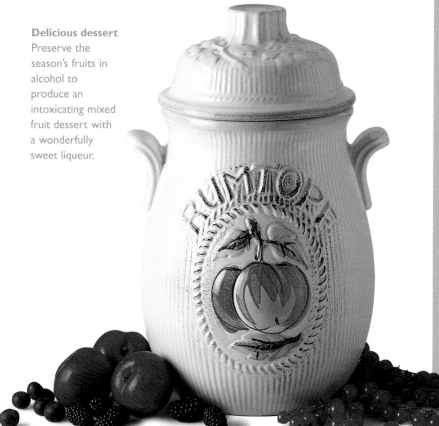

Tried & Trusted
Quick recipes

• **To make raspberry liqueur, put 250g (9oz) raspberries, 250g (9oz) caster sugar and a bottle of whisky or vodka into a large jar, cover with a lid and leave for four weeks. Strain and pour the liqueur into bottles. Blackberry and redcurrant liqueurs are made in the same way.**

• **Brandy flavoured with fruit and herbs is called ratafia. Simply add the fruit and herbs to the spirit and leave to mature in a warm place for four weeks.**

• **To make cherry brandy, remove the stalks from 450g (1lb) Morello cherries, wash and prick with a cocktail stick. Put in a jar, layering with 85g (3oz) caster sugar. Cover with 600ml (1 pint) brandy and leave for three months, shaking regularly. Strain and bottle.**

Medicinal uses

• **Juniper spirits such as gin are said to help build up a resistance against flu. Gin is also thought to provide relief from overeating.**

• **Herb liqueurs can be used as remedies for a variety of complaints. Rosemary liqueur can help to combat tiredness while peppermint liqueur aids digestion.**

Tempting delicacies

Crystallised fruits, children's lollies, sugared almonds and peanut brittle are just some of the long-loved sweets you can create at home. They make excellent gifts for all ages and party fare for children.

Homemade confectionery sounds like a lot of work, but in fact many sweets and other treats are much easier to make than you might think. It's certainly worth having a go, and even beginners should have success with the recipes on these pages.

The art of crystallising has largely been forgotten, no doubt because today's hectic lifestyles leave little time to pursue such skills.

Things were different in times past, when fruit was crystallised in order to preserve it. Flowers were crystallised as well – candied petals were once considered a delicacy.

If you are health–conscious but have a sweet tooth, fruit confectionery may appeal as a lower calorie alternative to other types of sweets. Dried fruit retains its nutrients and vitamins and contains fructose, so you don't need to add sugar.

Alternatively, you could make a selection of marzipan fruits, sugared almonds or fudge, just as our grandmothers would have done, to give as a present or to celebrate a special occasion.

Bite-size treats Chunks of fresh fruit retain their juicy characteristics when coated with crystallised sugar syrup.

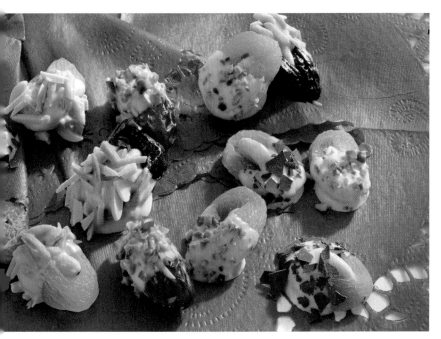

Something special Enjoy this delicious homemade fruit confectionery. No shop-bought variety can possibly compete.

Homemade fruit confectionery and sweets

Making fruit confectionery and sweets is inexpensive and a skill worth cultivating. It may appear fiddly, but it is mainly just a case of shaping, dipping or coating and a creative touch to add a final decorative flourish.

Very little special equipment is needed to make sweets. However, as the success of many recipes depends on boiling sugar to an exact temperature, a sugar thermometer, available from kitchenware shops, is essential.

Look for a thermometer that is easy to read and preferably has a protective mesh to prevent the glass from cracking, and a clip to attach it to a pan. After you have used the thermometer, stand it immediately in hot water to dissolve any syrup or sugar crystals that are sticking to it, then wash it gently but thoroughly.

To boil syrup, use a heavy-based pan, preferably made of stainless steel and without a non-stick surface. The high temperature of the syrup may damage the coating.

A dipping fork can be useful for coating sweets in melted chocolate or fondant coatings. However, it is not an essential piece of equipment as you can use a small fork or a skewer instead.

Confectionery recipes require constant attention during preparation and cooling. Set aside a time when you are unlikely to be disturbed. Avoid cooking other food at the same time, as sweets need a cool, airy kitchen to set.

Take care

When heating sugar-based mixtures to extremely high temperatures and handling them afterwards, be very careful not to get any on your skin; it will cause a deep burn. If you do, place the area immediately under cold running water and hold it there for 10 minutes. Seek medical help if necessary.

Hot favourite Wrapped in cellophane and decorated with ribbons, fruit lollies are sure to be popular at a children's birthday party.

CRYSTALLISED FRUIT

Be sure to heat the sugar syrup to the correct temperature.

fruits such as pineapple, strawberries, cherries, seedless grapes, nectarines
1 litre (1¾ pints) water
1 kg (2lb 4oz) caster sugar

Wash and dry the fruit. Remove any tough skins and cut large fruit into wedges. Prick grapes and cherries with a needle. Place the water and sugar in a pan. Boil until the liquid has reached 107°C (225°F) and forms threads.

Put the fruit in a fine metal sieve placed over a heatproof bowl. Pour the syrup over the fruit to coat it. Cover with a plate and leave for 24 hours.

Repeat four more times, ensuring that the fruit is coated and reheating the sugar solution to the same temperature. On the last coating, leave the fruit to dry on a wire rack.

FRUIT LOLLIES

Ready-prepared fruit juices can be used instead of orange juice, such as cranberry or blackcurrant.

100ml (3½fl oz) freshly squeezed orange juice
250g (9oz) caster sugar
1 tablespoon liquid glucose
½ teaspoon citric acid
8 small lolly sticks

Put the juice, sugar, glucose and citric acid into a heavy-based pan. Heat to 150°C (300°F), checking the temperature of the liquid with a sugar thermometer and stirring constantly.

As soon as the temperature is reached, plunge the base of the pan into a basin filled with cold water to stop the mixture from cooking further.

Grease a baking sheet, then drop spoonfuls of the mixture onto the surface. Push a stick into each sugar circle immediately and trickle a little more of the mixture over it to secure. Leave the lollies to cool and set.

Sugar towers

In the 16th century, sugar became more widely available and was refined into crystalline cones. Crystallised fruit, sweetmeats and syrups were all popular.

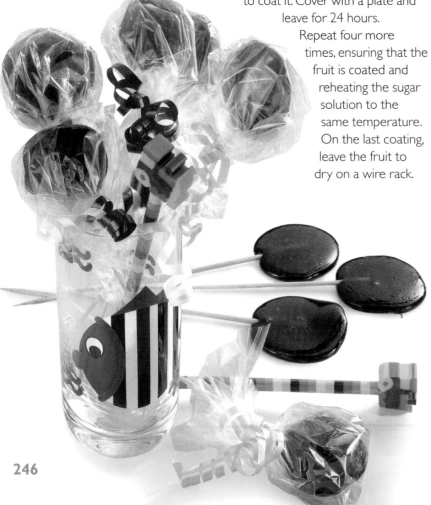

WHITE CHOCOLATE FRUIT

Store this confectionery in an airtight container lined with greaseproof paper.

300g (10½oz) dried fruit such
  as prunes, apricots
  and dates
1 tablespoon orange liqueur
40g (1½oz) roasted whole
  almonds
roasted almond slivers
  roughly chopped
pistachio nuts, chopped
grated chocolate
100g (3½oz) white chocolate

Line a tray with non-stick baking parchment. Cut each fruit lengthways but do not slice through completely as you need to create a pocket. Remove any stones as necessary. Sprinkle the fruit with a few drops of liqueur and stuff with a roasted whole almond.

Put the almond slivers, chopped pistachios and grated chocolate on separate plates. Melt the white chocolate in a bowl set over a pan of simmering water. Pick up each fruit, dip the bottom half in the melted chocolate and let the excess drip back into the bowl.

Roll the chocolate end of the sweet in either the nuts or grated chocolate. Place them on the tray and leave to set. Put the sweets into petit four cases and store in a sealed container.

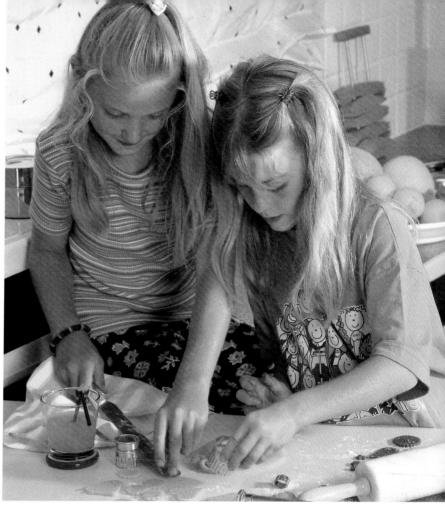

Safe sweets Children love making sweets. Marzipan is perfect because it is simple to mould and cut into shapes.

Moulding marzipan fruits

These moulded fruits make an attractive gift or they can be served with coffee after a meal.

White marzipan was once always homemade, but now it is readily available from delicatessens and supermarkets in 250g (9oz) packs – a convenient size to use when experimenting with moulding sweets.

Divide the marzipan into small pieces. Add a few drops of food colouring to each piece and gently knead the marzipan to obtain a uniform colour. Add only a tiny amount of colour at a time and dust your hands with icing sugar to prevent the marzipan from becoming too sticky.

To make oranges and lemons, roll small balls of marzipan. 'Pit' their surface by rolling the marzipan against a fine grater.

Make fruit stalks for apples and pears from short pieces of crystallised angelica. Brush the marzipan fruits with diluted food colouring to add a 'blush'.

Paint brown lines down yellow marzipan to make bananas. Leave the sweets to 'set' for 24 hours. Store in a cool, dry place.

Tantalising treats for a sweet tooth

When making chocolates or chocolate-flavoured candies, it is important to use a good quality chocolate with at least 70% cocoa solids. Cheaper chocolate has a higher proportion of vegetable fats and sugar and won't give the same concentrated flavour.

Once the sweets have cooled, store them in an airtight container lined with greaseproof paper to prevent sugar or chocolate coatings from getting sticky. Make sure that the confectionery is completely cold as warm sweets will create condensation on the lid and make them soggy. Put an extra sheet of greaseproof paper between the layers of sweets to prevent them sticking together.

Crunch toffee Often associated with bonfire night, toffee apples taste delicious with their crunchy sweet coatings and fruity insides.

TOFFEE APPLES

Use medium-sized, crisp eating apples. Makes four.

4 apples
4 wooden lolly sticks
4 tablespoons caster sugar
400g (14oz) cube sugar
50ml (2fl oz) water
1 teaspoon red food
    colouring
1 teaspoon vanilla essence
1 teaspoon vinegar

Wash and dry the apples, then twist out the stalks and replace them with lolly sticks. Sprinkle the caster sugar on a plate. Put the rest of the ingredients in a pan and boil to the hard crack stage (see Sugar boiling, page 245).

Plunge the base of the pan into cold water. Dip each apple in the syrup until thickly coated. Place on the sugared plate and leave to set.

CHOCOLATE NUT SQUARES

Fudge is a rich mixture of sugar, butter and milk. In this recipe it is flavoured with dark chocolate and walnuts. Makes 700g (1lb 9oz).

450g (1lb) caster sugar
150ml (5fl oz) milk
150g (5½oz) butter
100g (3½oz) dark chocolate,
    chopped
55g (2oz) honey
55g (2oz) chopped walnuts

Grease a shallow 18cm (7in) square tin. Place the sugar, milk, butter, chocolate and honey in a large, heavy-based pan and stir over a gentle heat until melted.

Boil the mixture steadily to the soft ball stage (see Sugar boiling, page 245). It is important to stir the mixture from time to time to prevent it sticking. Do not let it boil too rapidly or the sugar will burn on the bottom of the pan.

Remove the pan from the heat and leave to cool for 5 minutes, then add the walnuts. Beat the mixture until it is thick and creamy and beginning to look grainy.

Pour the fudge into the greased tin, mark it into squares and leave to set for 3-4 hours or until hard. Cut up when cold.

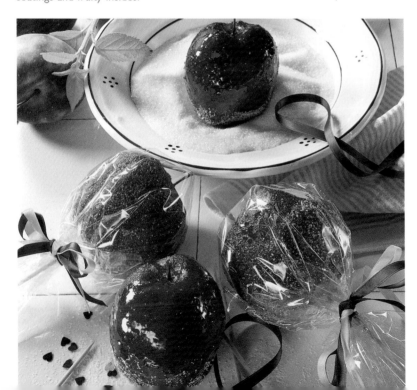

SUGARED ALMONDS

Roasting the almonds before they are sugared gives them a warm, toasted flavour.

250g (9oz) unblanched
   almonds
250g (9oz) cube sugar
5 tablespoons water
½ teaspoon ground cinnamon

Roast the almonds on a baking tray in an oven preheated to 200°C (400°F, gas mark 6) until the skins start to come off.

Grease a second baking tray. Put the sugar and water in a heavy-based pan and stir over a low heat until the sugar has dissolved. Increase the heat and boil until the hard crack stage is reached (see Sugar boiling, page 245).

Skin the almonds and add them to the pan. Stir over the heat with a wooden spoon until they are coated with syrup. Remove the pan from the heat, add the cinnamon and stir until the almonds are dry.

Tip the almonds onto the greased tray and separate them with a fork. Leave to cool.

PEANUT BRITTLE

Leave the brittle to set and break it into pieces with a toffee hammer. Makes 900g (2lb).

250g (9oz) unsalted peanuts
   without skins
400g (14oz) demerara sugar
175g (6oz) light soft
   brown sugar
175g (6oz) golden syrup
150ml (5fl oz) water
55g (2oz) butter
1 teaspoon baking soda

Chop the peanuts and place them in the oven to warm, but not brown. Grease a tin measuring about 30×10cm (12×4in). Put the sugars, syrup and water in a pan and heat, stirring continuously, until the sugar has dissolved.

Add the butter and boil steadily, but not fiercely, to the hard crack stage (see Sugar boiling, page 245). Add the soda and nuts. Pour into the tin. Break up when cold.

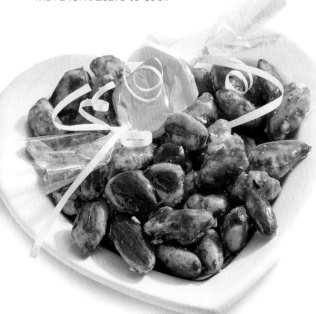

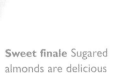

Sweet finale Sugared almonds are delicious served with coffee at the end of a meal.

Tried & Trusted
More sweet recipes

- **To make chocolate-flavoured marzipan sweets, roll small balls of marzipan in cocoa powder mixed with a little icing sugar.**

- **For peppermint creams, heat 450g (1lb) sugar and 150ml (¼ pint) water in a pan to softball stage. Sprinkle a worktop with water, then pour on a little of the syrup and leave to cool. When a skin forms, knead the mixture with a spatula. Continue until it becomes firm. Knead in a few drops of peppermint essence and roll out to 5mm (¼in) thick and cut into 2.5cm (1in) rounds.**

- **To make almond nibbles, toast 100g (3½oz) roughly chopped almonds. Melt an equal amount of chocolate, mix in the almonds, then spoon small nuggets onto foil and leave to cool.**

Sweet success

- **Buy paper or foil petit four cases to dress up your confectioneries.**

- **Sweets don't store well in a warm environment. Keep them in a cool place.**

- **Use crystallised fruit or petals as cake decorations or as a topping for dinner-party desserts.**

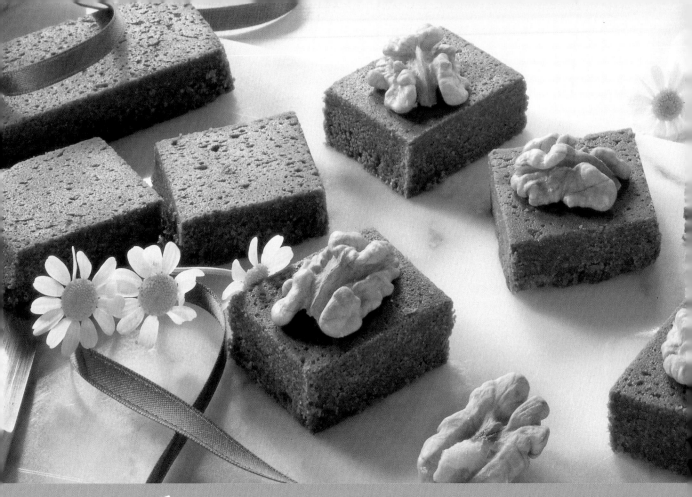

Walnut squares

Caramel, fudge and toffee have long been popular with both young and old. In this recipe tasty walnuts make a decorative topping.

These mouth-watering goodies are easy to make and fun to cook during the winter holidays, when fresh walnuts are at their best. The finished caramels can be packed in cellophane bags, tied attractively with coloured ribbons and given as gifts to friends.

When you are making the caramel, heat the ingredients in a heavy-based pan so the chocolate doesn't burn.

Pour the hot caramel into a shallow greased tin measuring about 28×18cm (11×7in) and leave it in a cool place.

As soon as the walnut caramel is firm enough, cut it into rectangles and decorate each one with a walnut half. Leave the caramels to cool completely, then remove them from the tin with a palette knife. Store in an airtight container.

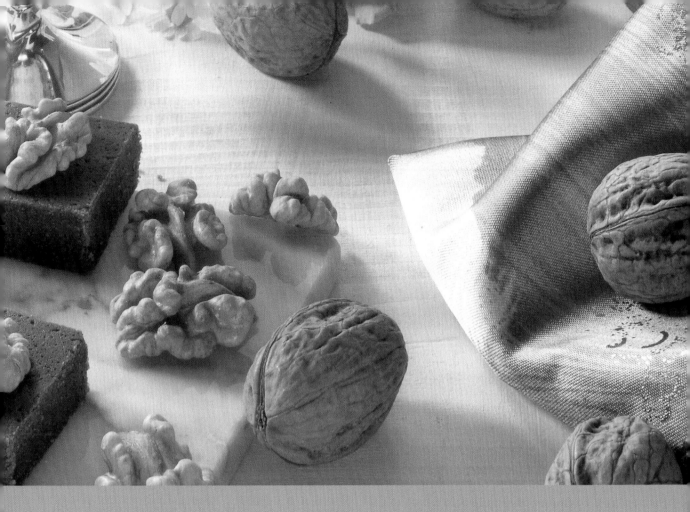

How to make walnut squares
Makes about 500g (1lb 2oz)

▼ Warm **200g (7oz) condensed milk** in a pan over a gentle heat for 2-3 minutes, stirring continuously.

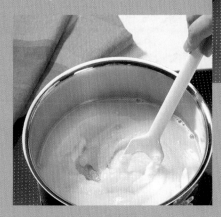

▲ Add **350g (12oz) grated plain chocolate** and **25g (1oz) soft butter** and heat until the chocolate has amalgamated well. Stir the mixture all the time.

▼ Remove the pan from the heat and pour into a shallow greased tin. Leave to cool slightly then mark into squares and decorate with **walnut halves**.

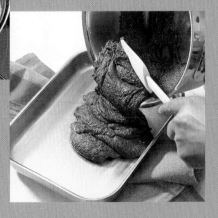

Baking at its best

In many households in the early 20th century making bread was a necessary part of a day's work. Today, we no longer have to bake our own, but the results make it well worth the effort.

There are few things more appetising than the smell of freshly baked bread or more satisfying than a loaf of bread you have baked yourself.

You can use fresh or dried yeast for bread-making. Fresh yeast can be hard to obtain unless you have a friendly baker who will sell it to you, so the traditional recipes here give amounts for dried yeast.

Originally dried yeast had to be mixed with water and a pinch of sugar to activate it, but most dried yeast sold in supermarkets these days comes in individual sachets and is termed 'easy blend dried yeast'. The contents of the sachet should be sprinkled over the flour and stirred in thoroughly before any liquid is added.

To test if a loaf is cooked, tip it out of the tin onto a clean tea towel and tap the base. If the loaf sounds hollow it is cooked through. You can use the same method to check that rolls and scones are cooked. Take care not to burn your hands.

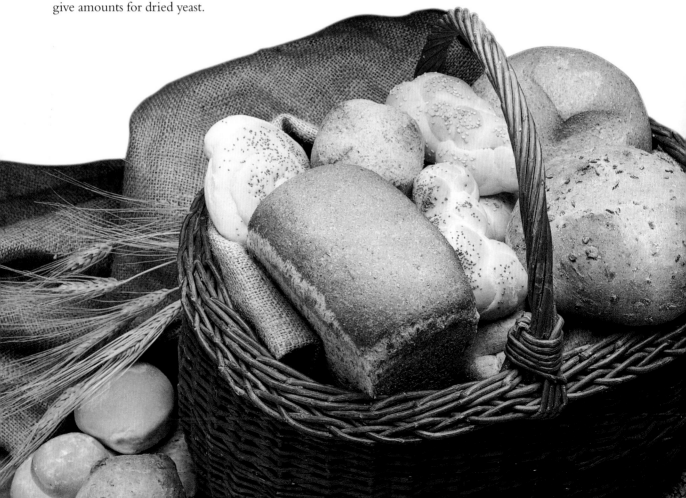

Making traditional unleavened bread

Not all breads are leavened with yeast. Many regional breads and flat breads are made without it.

Soda bread, the famous bread of Ireland, was made quickly with flour, baking soda and buttermilk. The bread was then cooked on a griddle or bakestone on top of the stove. The soda and buttermilk acted as raising agents to produce a sour-tasting loaf.

Take care

Whatever type of bread you are making, it is important to start with a dough that has the right consistency. If it seems very wet, add a little more flour; if it feels dry, add more liquid.

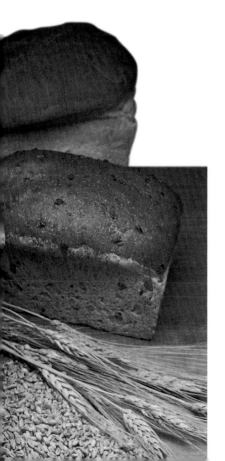

SODA BREAD

This modern version of the classic recipe uses yoghurt instead of buttermilk and the loaf is baked in a conventional oven. The recipe makes one large loaf.

700g (1lb 9oz) plain flour
1 teaspoon cream of tartar
1 teaspoon salt
1 teaspoon baking soda
1 teaspoon caster sugar
300ml (½ pint) milk
150g (5½oz) natural yoghurt

Preheat the oven to 190°C (375°F, gas mark 5). Sieve the flour, cream of tartar, salt and soda into a bowl. Stir in the sugar and make a well in the centre.

Whisk together the milk and yoghurt and pour most of it into the well. Mix to make a slack but not wet dough, adding a little more milk if the dough is too stiff.

Turn out onto a lightly floured surface and flatten into a round about 4cm (1½in) thick with the heel of your hand. Lift the dough onto a greased baking sheet and cut a deep cross in the top using a floured knife. Bake for 45 minutes.

To find out if the loaf is cooked through, push a skewer into the centre and if it comes out clean the bread is ready.

Bread basket Whatever shape it takes, there is nothing to beat freshly baked, homemade bread eaten while it is still warm.

Tried & Trusted
Working the dough

• For bread recipes that use yeast, kneading the dough and letting it rise are essential to produce a loaf with a light, even crumb.

• Once the dough is mixed, turn it out onto a floured surface and knead for about 10 minutes until it is smooth and elastic.

• To begin with, the mixture will seem heavy and quite wet. As you knead, the dough will gradually become drier as the water it contains is absorbed.

• When the dough is soft and springy, shape into a ball and place in an oiled bowl. Cover the bowl with a damp tea towel and leave to rise at room temperature until doubled in size. The time this takes will vary with the type of dough and the warmth of the room.

• Knock the risen dough down with your fist, transfer to a floured surface and knead again for about 5 minutes. Shape the dough as required.

• Re-cover with a damp tea towel and leave to rise again until doubled in size. Glaze and bake according to the recipe instructions.

Soft or crisp crusts on risen breads

Before you put the dough in the oven sprinkle it with flour or glaze it. The type of glaze used will determine the crust on the baked loaf or rolls. For a crisp crust, brush with a little beaten egg or milk.

For a soft crust, glaze with single cream and when you take the bread out of the oven, leave it to cool on a wire rack with a clean, dry tea towel on top.

Wood-fired oven

In rural areas of Europe the most common type of bread oven was semi-circular and deep. It was made of stone or fireproof bricks, which were heated by burning wood in the oven hours before baking.

Shortly before the bread went into the oven, the embers were removed. The bread was put in on a long-handled wooden shovel called a peel. Straw was added for moisture, giving the bread a golden colour.

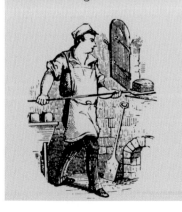

WHITE BREAD

You will need one 450g (1lb) loaf tin for this recipe.

375g (13oz) strong white bread flour
1 teaspoon salt
1 sachet easy blend dried yeast
pinch of caster sugar
200ml (⅓ pint) lukewarm water

Sieve the flour and salt into a mixing bowl. Sprinkle over the yeast and sugar and stir in. Make a well in the centre and add the water. Mix to a dough and knead until the texture is smooth.

Shape the dough into a ball, dust with flour and leave in a warm place to rise for 30-40 minutes. Turn the dough onto a floured surface, flour your hands and knead for 5 minutes. Rest for a few minutes, then knead again for 5 minutes.

Preheat the oven to 200°C (400°F, gas mark 6). Grease the loaf tin, press in the dough and brush the top with lukewarm water. Cover and leave to rise for 15 minutes.

Bake in the centre of the oven for 10 minutes, then lower the temperature to 180°C (350°F, gas mark 4). Bake for a further 35 minutes, or until the loaf is well risen and sounds hollow when tapped on the bottom. Cool on a wire rack.

Take care

To get good results with dried yeast, first check its sell-by date as it has a limited shelf life. It is important that the liquid you add is 'tepid' or 'blood heat' – it should feel the same temperature as a finger dipped into it. If the liquid is too hot it will kill the yeast.

MILK BREAD

This pleasant-tasting milk bread is a variation of the basic white bread recipe. Makes two 450g (1lb) loaves or one 900g (2lb) loaf.

500g (1lb 2oz) strong white bread flour
1 teaspoon salt
25g (1oz) butter
1 sachet easy blend dried yeast
25g (1oz) caster sugar
150ml (¼ pint) milk

Sieve the flour and salt into a mixing bowl. Rub in the butter, sprinkle over the yeast and sugar and stir in. Make a well in the centre and add the milk. Mix to a dough with a wooden spoon, then work together with your hands.

Knead until the dough feels smooth, then leave to rise, re-knead and bake as for White bread (left).

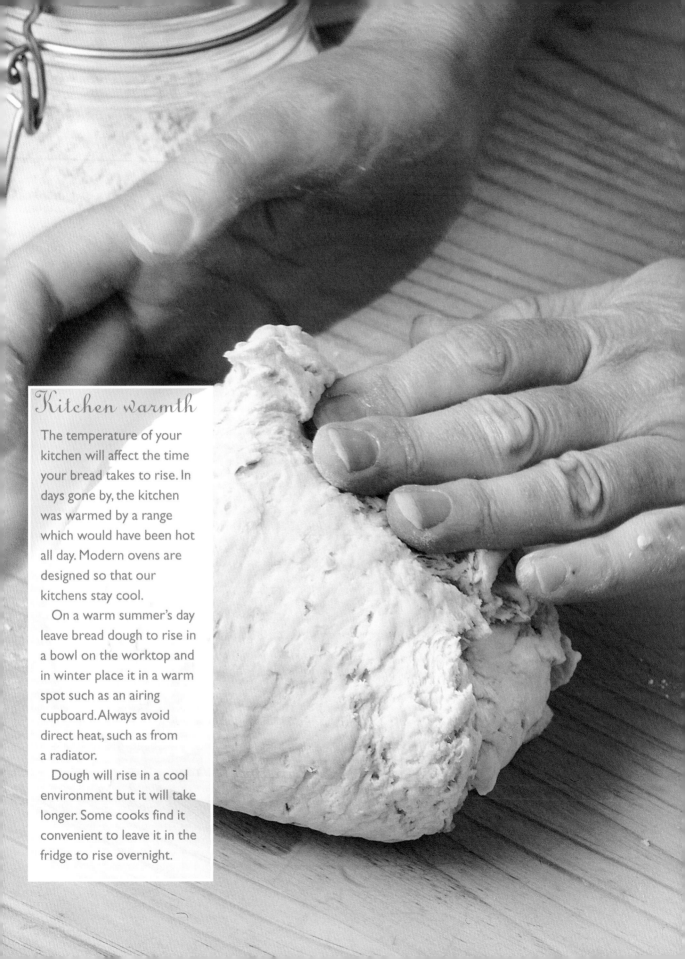

Kitchen warmth

The temperature of your kitchen will affect the time your bread takes to rise. In days gone by, the kitchen was warmed by a range which would have been hot all day. Modern ovens are designed so that our kitchens stay cool.

On a warm summer's day leave bread dough to rise in a bowl on the worktop and in winter place it in a warm spot such as an airing cupboard. Always avoid direct heat, such as from a radiator.

Dough will rise in a cool environment but it will take longer. Some cooks find it convenient to leave it in the fridge to rise overnight.

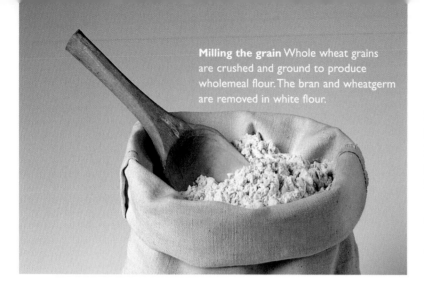

Milling the grain Whole wheat grains are crushed and ground to produce wholemeal flour. The bran and wheatgerm are removed in white flour.

WHOLEMEAL BREAD

This loaf is dense with a chewy crust. Makes one large loaf.

700g (1lb 9oz) stoneground wholemeal bread flour
2 teaspoons salt
1 sachet easy blend dried yeast
425ml (15fl oz) tepid water
2 teaspoons sunflower oil

Mix together the flour, salt and yeast. Add the water and sunflower oil and mix to a dough. Turn the dough out onto a floured surface and knead for 10 minutes. Leave to rise until doubled in size.

Transfer to a floured surface and knead again. Shape into a ball on a greased baking sheet. Re-cover with a damp tea towel and leave to rise again until doubled in size.

Preheat the oven to 220°C (425°F, gas mark 7). Slash the top of the loaf with a floured sharp knife and bake for 15 minutes, then lower the temperature to 190°C (375°F, gas mark 5) and bake for a further 20-25 minutes or until the loaf sounds hollow when tapped on the base. Cool on a wire rack.

HAZEL NUT BREAD

Nuts are good for us as they contain plenty of B vitamins. The recipe makes one 900g (2lb) loaf or two 450g (1lb) loaves.

200g (7oz) strong white bread flour
200g (7oz) rye flour
70g (2½oz) ground hazelnuts
1 teaspoon salt
1 sachet easy blend dried yeast
250ml (9fl oz) lukewarm milk
3 tablespoons walnut oil
100g (3½oz) whole hazelnuts

Combine the flours, ground hazelnuts, salt and yeast in a bowl. Make a well in the centre, pour in the milk and oil and mix to a dough. Turn out onto a floured surface and knead until smooth.

Leave to rise in a warm place for 2-3 hours. Knead well on a floured surface, working in the whole nuts. Grease a 900g (2lb) loaf tin, put in the dough and leave to rise for 45 minutes. Preheat the oven to 200°C (400°F, gas mark 6) and bake for 1 hour until cooked.

BARA BRITH

Similar to the Irish 'Barm Brack', the name 'Bara Brith' means 'speckled bread' in Welsh. Serve it sliced and spread with butter for afternoon tea. Makes one large loaf.

450g (1lb) strong plain white flour
½ teaspoon salt
1 teaspoon ground mixed spice
55g (2oz) butter
1 sachet easy blend dried yeast
55g (2oz) light soft brown sugar
225g (8oz) mixed dried fruit
1 large egg, beaten
225ml (8fl oz) tepid milk

Sieve the flour, salt and spice into a bowl. Rub in the butter. Sprinkle over the yeast and stir in the sugar and dried fruit. Add most of the egg and all of the milk, then mix to a dough. Turn out and knead on a floured surface for 10-15 minutes.

Transfer to an oiled bowl, cover and leave in a warm place for 2 hours or until doubled in size. Knead again. Shape into an oblong and press into a 900g (2lb) loaf tin.

Cover with cling film and leave to rise until the dough reaches the top of the tin. Preheat the oven to 200°C (400°F, gas mark 6). Brush the top of the loaf with the rest of the egg and bake for 45 minutes, covering with a piece of foil after 25 minutes if the top is browning too much. Cool in the tin for 10 minutes, then turn out onto a wire rack to cool completely. The loaf is best eaten fresh but it also freezes well.

POTATO BREAD

Potatoes are healthy, nutritious and rich in vitamins and minerals. Use a floury variety such as King Edwards for this loaf.

1kg (2lb 4oz) floury potatoes
500g (1lb 2oz) plain flour
1½ teaspoons salt
1½ teaspoons caster sugar
2 sachets easy blend
    dried yeast
125ml (4fl oz) lukewarm milk

Wash, peel and grate the potatoes. Leave to drain in a colander, pressing out any remaining liquid with the back of a spoon. Mix the flour, salt, sugar and yeast in a bowl. Add the potatoes and the lukewarm milk and mix to a dough. Knead well. Cover and leave in a warm place to rise.

Flour the work surface and knead the dough for 5 minutes. Preheat the oven to 150°C (300°F, gas mark 2). Grease a 900g (2lb) loaf tin and press in the dough. Cover and leave to rise in a warm place for about 15 minutes.

Bake in the oven on a low shelf for 20 minutes, then increase the temperature to 200°C (400°F, gas mark 6) and bake for a further 40 minutes. Leave the bread in the tin for 10 minutes then turn out and leave to cool on a wire rack.

Full of goodness Made from unrefined, whole grain flour, wholemeal bread has a robust, malty flavour and is high in fibre and vitamins.

WHITE ROLLS

These rolls will keep for four days or for one month in the freezer. Makes 24 rolls.

700g (1lb 9oz) white
    bread flour
1 tablespoon salt
1 sachet easy blend
    dried yeast
425ml (15fl oz) tepid water
milk to glaze

Mix the flour, salt and yeast in a bowl. Add the water and mix to a dough. Knead for 10 minutes, then put in a greased bowl, cover and leave until doubled in size.

Knock back the dough and cut into 24 pieces. Shape into smooth balls and place well spaced on greased baking sheets. Cover with a damp cloth and leave to rise until almost doubled in size.

Preheat the oven to 220°C (425°F, gas mark 7). Glaze the tops with milk and bake for 20 minutes.

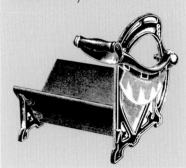

Bread cutter

Bread cutters like this first appeared in the 1880s. Bakeries now have automatic machines so that you can have your freshly baked loaf sliced while you wait.

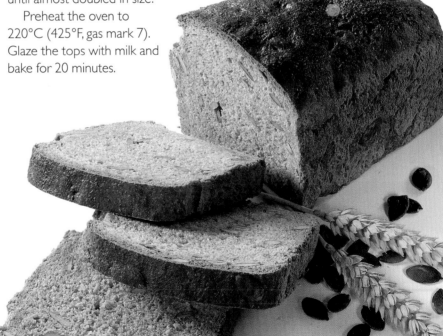

Making buns, scones and savoury cakes

A wide range of sweet and savoury buns and cakes can easily be made at home, with or without yeast.

Where yeast is included in a recipe, it is normally used with a strong white flour, which has a higher gluten content than ordinary plain flour. Gluten is the substance that makes the dough stretch and expand, necessary for bread, rolls and buns.

For Scotch pancakes and scones an ordinary plain flour is best. This gives a lighter texture, which can be made lighter still by adding a little baking powder.

As with most baking, the results are best when they are fresh. Herb cakes, Scotch pancakes and currant buns are especially delicious when they are still warm from the oven.

SCOTCH PANCAKES

Traditionally these were cooked on a griddle but a heavy-based frying pan will do. Makes 15 pancakes.

175g (6oz) plain flour
1½ teaspoons baking powder
85g (3oz) butter
55g (2oz) caster sugar
1 medium egg, beaten
milk to mix

Sieve the flour and baking powder into a bowl. Rub in the butter and mix in the sugar. Add the egg and enough milk to mix to a pastry-like dough. Knead until smooth, roll out 5mm (¼in) thick and cut into 6.5cm (2½in) rounds. Cook for 3-3½ minutes on each side in a dry hot pan until browned.

CURRANT BUNS

Don't over-cook these buns or any currants on the outside will burn. Makes 12-16 buns.

500g (1lb 2oz) strong
    white flour
1 teaspoon salt
1 teaspoon caster sugar
1½ sachets easy blend
    dried yeast
3 tablespoons sunflower oil
200-250ml (7-9fl oz)
    lukewarm milk
2 medium eggs
250g (9oz) currants
milk to glaze

Put the flour, salt and sugar into a bowl and stir in the yeast. Beat together the oil, milk and eggs, and pour into the flour mixture. Mix in the currants. Knead well until the dough comes away from the sides of the bowl. Cover the dough and leave for 30 minutes.

Knead the dough for about 5 minutes, then shape into a roll and divide into 12-16 pieces. Flour your hands and roll each piece into a bun. Line two baking sheets with baking parchment, place the buns on the sheets and brush with milk.

Leave the buns in a warm place for 30 minutes. Meanwhile preheat the oven to 180°C (350°F, gas mark 4). Bake in the centre of the oven for 25-30 minutes, until golden brown.

Simple pleasures Currant buns taste best fresh from the oven and served warm with butter.

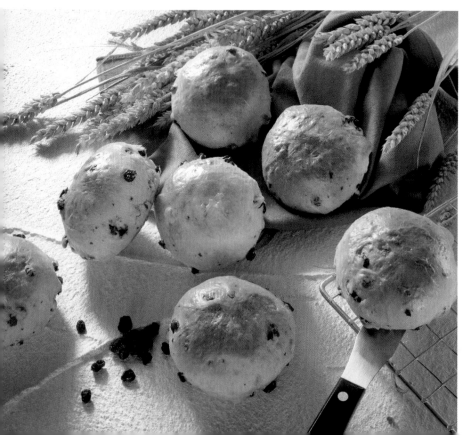

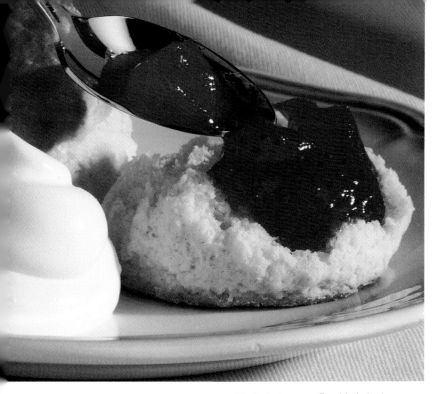

Made in heaven Freshly baked scones melt in the mouth. No shop-bought scone tastes as good.

DEVON FRUIT SCONES

Serve with strawberry jam and clotted cream. Makes 8 scones.

225g (8oz) plain flour
2 teaspoons baking powder
55g (2oz) butter
25g (1oz) caster sugar
55g (2oz) sultanas
150ml (5fl oz) milk
beaten egg to glaze

Preheat the oven to 230°C (450°F, gas mark 8). Grease a baking sheet. Sieve the flour and baking powder into a bowl, rub in the butter and stir in the sugar and sultanas.

Add all the milk and mix to a soft dough. Knead briefly on a floured surface until smooth. Roll out to 1cm (½in) thick and cut into 6.5cm (2½in) rounds. Brush the tops with beaten egg. Bake for 7-10 minutes. Tap the scones on the base. If they sound hollow they are done. Cool on a wire rack.

OATCAKES

Historically, oatcakes were toasted on a peat fire. Makes about 8 triangular cakes.

125g (4½oz) medium oatmeal
pinch of salt
pinch of baking soda
2 teaspoons butter
4 tablespoons boiling water

Mix the dry ingredients in a bowl, then make a well in the centre. Melt the butter in the water and pour it into the well. Mix to a stiff dough.

Turn out onto a floured surface and knead lightly. Roll out very thinly and cut into eight triangles. Cook on a hot griddle or in a dry, heavy frying pan until the edges curl up and the cakes are firm. Store in an airtight container and reheat in the oven before eating.

Shortbread

Easy to make and deliciously melt-in-the-mouth, shortbread biscuits are excellent served with coffee and tea or packed into a pretty tin and given as a gift to someone special.

Although usually considered a Scottish speciality, shortbread is enjoyed all over the world.

In Spain, fingers of Polvorones Sevillanos (almond shortbread) are wrapped in twists of coloured paper and traditionally passed around with sherry after Christmas dinner. In the Middle East, recipes have been passed down through the generations since the ancient Persian empire and include savoury varieties such as chickpea shortbread.

To make a savoury shortbread that tastes delicous with cheese omit the sugar from the recipe and flavour the dough with 75g (3oz) finely grated Parmesan and a pinch of ground coriander.

How to make shortbread
Makes six large biscuits

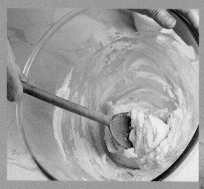

▲ In a mixing bowl, cream together **175g (6oz) butter** with **75g (3oz) caster sugar** until light and fluffy. Sieve in **175g (6oz) plain flour** and **75g (3oz) ground rice**.

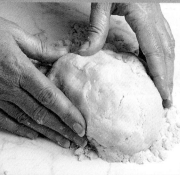

▼ Stir with a wooden spoon until the mixture resembles breadcrumbs. Press it together lightly with your fingers until the dough sticks together.

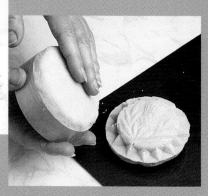

▼ Divide the dough into six and press each portion into a 7.5cm (3in) shortbread mould. Turn out onto a greased baking sheet. Chill for 30 minutes, then bake for 20 minutes at 170°C (325°F, gas mark 3). Dust with caster sugar and leave to firm up for 15 minutes. Cool on a wire rack.

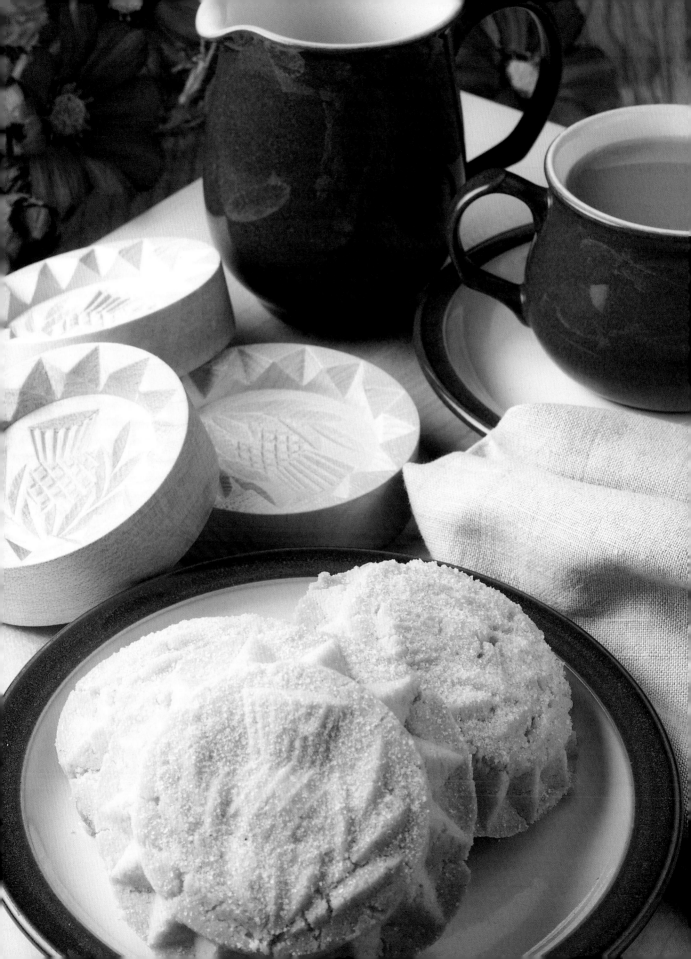

Mouth-watering cakes for special occasions

Cake mixes can be flavoured with many different ingredients, including cocoa, orange and lemon zest, coconut, coffee and sweet spices. Nuts, dried fruits, chocolate chips, candied peel, dried fruit and poppy seeds all add extra texture as well as flavour.

Modern appliances such as mixers and food processors have taken the hard work out of creaming and mixing but, if you

have the time, the old-fashioned way of beating the ingredients together in a bowl with a wooden spoon is still very satisfying.

Heavy fruit cakes need to be made several weeks before you intend to serve them to allow time for their flavours to develop. Storing them also makes them easier to cut – an important consideration if the cake is intended for a formal occasion.

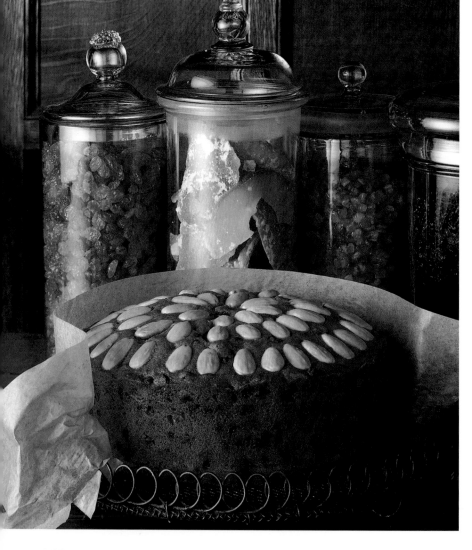

DUNDEE CAKE

This almond-topped cake recipe dates from the late 18th century.

225g (8oz) plain flour
1 teaspoon baking powder
175g (6oz) butter
175g (6oz) light brown sugar
3 large eggs, beaten
2 tablespoons coarse cut marmalade
55g (2oz) ground almonds
350g (12oz) mixed dried fruit
55g (2oz) chopped mixed peel
2 tablespoons milk
115g (4oz) whole almonds

Grease and line a 20cm (8in) round deep cake tin. Preheat the oven to 150°C (300°F, gas mark 2). Sieve together the flour and baking powder. In a separate bowl, cream the butter and sugar until light. Add the eggs a little at a time.

Stir in the marmalade, ground almonds, mixed fruit and peel. Fold in the flour, then add the milk, mixing lightly. Spoon into the tin, level the surface, then decorate with the halved almonds.

Bake for 2½-3 hours. Cool in the tin for 30 minutes, then turn out onto a wire rack. When cold, wrap in greaseproof paper and foil. Keep for one week before cutting.

Teatime treat A homemade Dundee cake transforms a high tea into a special occasion. Indeed, it is often given as a christening, wedding or Christmas gift.

Tried & Trusted
Cake-making tips

• To test if a fruit cake or tea loaf is cooked, push a skewer into the centre. If it comes out clean, the cake is ready. To test if a sponge is cooked, press the surface lightly with your finger; it should spring back.

• Once a cake is cooked, leave it in the tin to cool and firm up before turning out. Light sponge layers only need 5 minutes, but a heavy fruit cake should be left for 30 minutes as it may crack if you turn it out too quickly.

• Brush the inside of the cake tin with melted butter or a flavourless oil and line with greaseproof paper. Cakes will stick to old tins with a damaged surface.

• Alternatively, grease the tin and dust with caster sugar before spooning in the mixture.

• Sponge cakes need to be light, airy and eaten as fresh as possible. A light hand is needed when creaming the butter and sugar together.

• If you are adding flour to a whisked sponge, fold it in carefully until the ingredients are just combined. If you beat it in, all the air will be pushed out and the end result will be a flat, heavy cake.

Take care

In our grandparents' day one of the delights of cake-making was scraping the bowl and eating the left-over mixture. Today, some people are more wary, as we now know that raw egg can contain the salmonella bacterium, which causes food poisoning and is a particular threat to young children, pregnant women and the elderly.

CHOCOLATE FROSTED VICTORIA SANDWICH

A versatile cake that can be served as a dessert or at teatime.

175g (6oz) soft margarine
175g (6oz) caster sugar
3 medium eggs
150g (5½oz) self-raising flour
25g (1oz) cocoa powder
1 teaspoon baking powder
For the frosting:
325g (11½oz) icing sugar
25g (1oz) cocoa powder
175g (6oz) soft margarine
extra cocoa powder to dust

Preheat the oven to 190°C (375°F, gas mark 5). Grease and line two 18cm (7in) sandwich tins. Beat the ingredients together until smooth. Divide the mixture between the tins and bake for 20-25 minutes until springy. Turn out and cool.

For the frosting, sieve the icing sugar and cocoa together then beat into the margarine. Use half to sandwich the layers together, then spread the rest over the top and sides. Dust with cocoa powder.

MALTED TEA LOAF

Serve the loaf sliced, either plain or spread with a little butter.

350g (12oz) wholemeal self-raising flour
25g (1oz) malted milk drink powder
55g (2oz) dark muscovado sugar
175g (6oz) raisins
4 tablespoons thick honey
300ml (½ pint) milk

Preheat the oven to 160°C (325°F, gas mark 3). Grease and line a 900g (2lb) loaf tin. Mix together the dry ingredients and raisins. Add the honey and milk and beat until combined. Spoon the mixture into the tin, spread level and bake for 1¼ hours. Cool in the tin for 30 minutes, then remove and cool on a wire rack.

Tiered cakes

Commonly baked for formal celebrations, the exquisitely decorated tiered wedding cake originated in the 18th century, when Mr Rich, a pastry cook in Fleet Street, London, began making wedding cakes modelled on the elegant spire of St Bride's church.

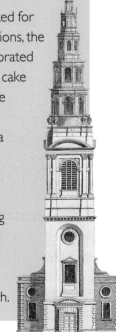

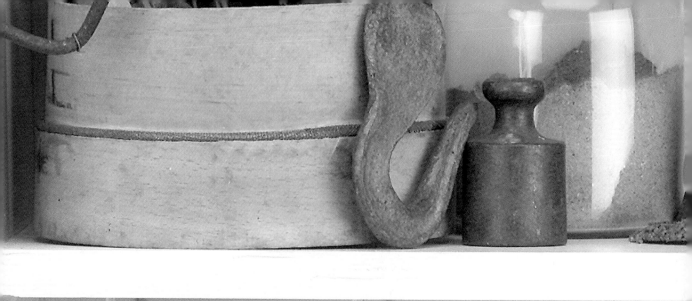

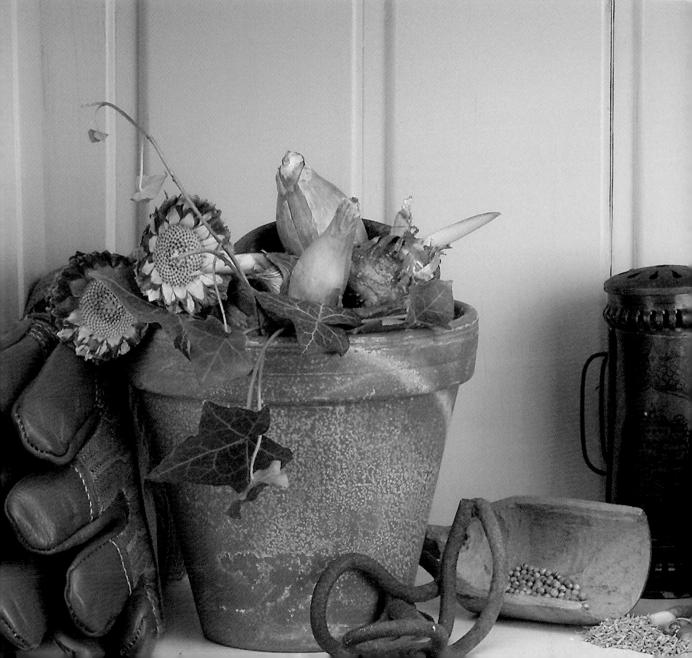

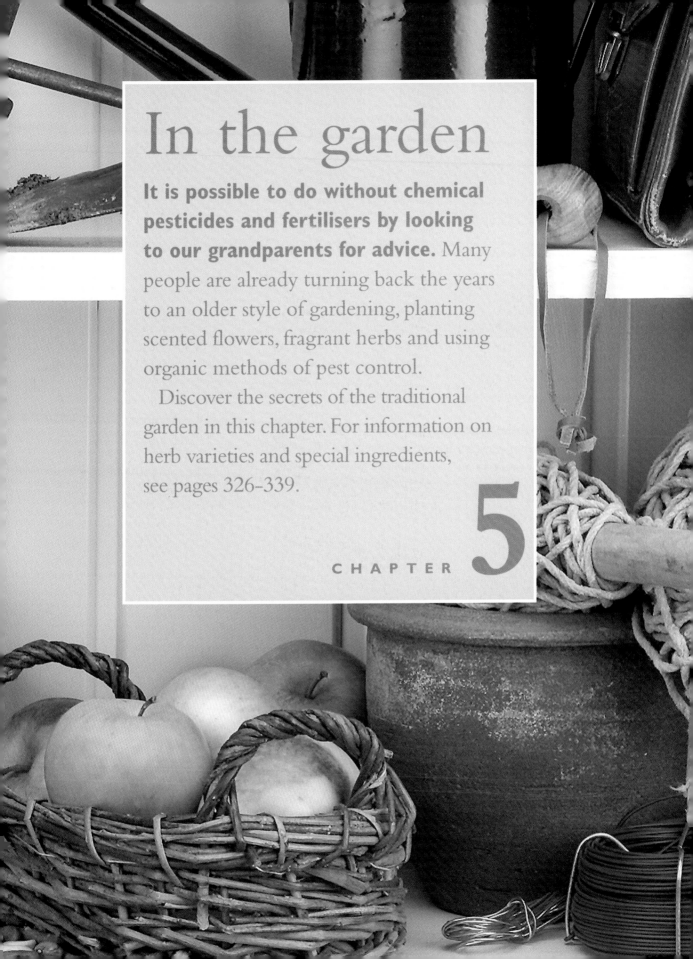

In the garden

It is possible to do without chemical pesticides and fertilisers by looking to our grandparents for advice. Many people are already turning back the years to an older style of gardening, planting scented flowers, fragrant herbs and using organic methods of pest control.

Discover the secrets of the traditional garden in this chapter. For information on herb varieties and special ingredients, see pages 326–339.

CHAPTER 5

Start with the basics:

How successfully plants grow in your garden depends largely on the richness of your soil. Even if you are not blessed with naturally fertile ground, take heart as there are plenty of ways to improve it.

There are rich soils and poor soils – a fact that all gardeners learn sooner rather than later, often when plants die or fail to thrive.

Not all earth is suitable for gardening. Many of the edible and decorative plants we cultivate place higher demands on the soil than those which grow naturally, such as wild flowers. For example, you won't usually get good crops of fruit or vegetables from trees or plants growing in soil that has not had manure or fertiliser added.

Fertile soil is light and crumbly and contains plenty of beneficial humus – a dark brown, spongy substance formed by decomposing plant materials. Without improvement, dense clay soil and sandy soil are not naturally suited to intense cultivation.

You can discover what type of garden soil you have by carrying out a simple soil test.

If you find that you need to enhance the quality of the soil, there are two methods: mulching and green manuring. Both have been used since medieval times, when they were practised in monastery gardens, and rely on natural plant and garden waste.

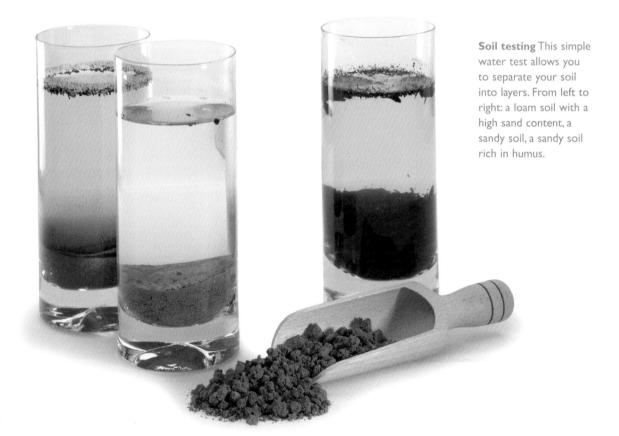

Soil testing This simple water test allows you to separate your soil into layers. From left to right: a loam soil with a high sand content, a sandy soil, a sandy soil rich in humus.

a healthy soil

What type of soil do I have in my garden?

Soil contains three types of mineral particles in varying proportions – sand, silt and clay.

To determine the properties of the soil in your garden, you need to examine its texture. If it is a light, open soil with clearly visible, coarse-grained particles, it is likely to have a high proportion of sand. If it is a heavy, sticky soil with an oily sheen and a fine texture, it will be mainly clay.

An ideal soil for most gardens is a mixed, or loam, soil. This is well aerated and free-draining, and contains an easily workable blend of sand, silt and clay, as well as plenty of humus to encourage your plants to grow.

A loam soil will store the right balance of rainwater and nutrients. In soil with a high level of clay, the fine particles become compacted, so that it cannot easily soak up water or release sufficient nutrients to the plants it supports.

Soil that contains too much sand cannot retain water and nutrients for long. Sandy soil can be improved by digging in humus, while heavy earth rich in clay can be lightened by adding sand.

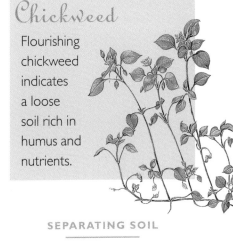

Chickweed

Flourishing chickweed indicates a loose soil rich in humus and nutrients.

SEPARATING SOIL

This easy method will help you to find out the constituents of your soil and their proportions.

I glass water
I handful soil

Add a handful of soil from your garden to a glass of water and stir thoroughly. Leave to stand for about 12 hours, until the individual soil components have settled. Then examine the mixture.

Sand is made of large grains, so it will settle at the bottom of the glass, followed by silt. Clay is considerably lighter and finer, so it will settle on top of the sand and silt. Humus, being the lightest component, will form the top layer. Some of it may even float to the top of the glass (see far left).

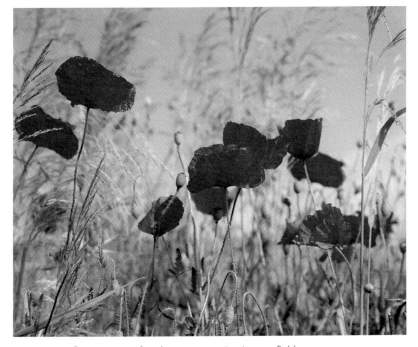

Lime lover Poppies can often be seen growing in cornfields. They indicate a fertile soil that contains lime and sufficient amounts of nitrogen – an important plant nutrient.

Clues from plants

Take a closer look at the weeds and other plants that grow naturally in your garden. As plants all have individual soil preferences, they will give you a good indication of the type of soil you have.

Dry soil, for example, will only support plants that either have deep roots or are exceptionally good at storing water or minimising its loss. Moist soil supports plants that have poor water-storage capacity and roots that will withstand rotting in damp conditions.

Tansy, meadow buttercup, broad-leaved plantain and dandelion indicate a loam soil, while wild thyme and knotweed are happy in sandy soil.

Chickweed, fumitory and fat hen prefer a loose soil with plenty of humus. Stinging nettles and black nightshade indicate that the soil contains a high level of nitrogen. Camomile thrives in lime-deficient soil while bindweed loves a soil rich in lime.

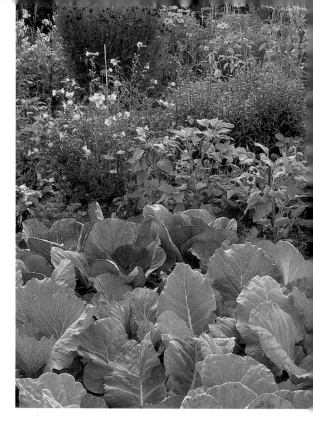

Garden paradise
Behind every gorgeous garden lies hard work. You will need to spend time manuring and mulching before you can achieve a result like this.

Coltsfoot

Coltsfoot flourishes in soil that contains a high proportion of clay and silt. It is a very robust plant that is difficult to eradicate where it grows as a weed.

Improving your soil the natural way

Once you have determined what type of soil you have, you can set about improving its quality and supplementing it with nutrients.

As nutrients are continually taken up by plants, most cultivated soil needs regular treatment. You do not need to use commercial fertilisers. Instead, you can rely on traditional methods by using homemade organic compost or green manure.

Nature's green fingers

The green manure technique involves sowing specific foliage plants such as clover and beans, then digging them back into the soil to provide nutrients.

This method has several advantages. While the plants are growing, the soil is protected from major fluctuations in temperature, from drying out and from weeds.

As the plants' roots make their way through the soil, they also help to loosen and aerate it.

Once the plants have reached about 20cm (8in), or have matured but are still soft and green, cut them down to ground level. Leave them lying on the surface of the soil for a day or two to wilt, then hoe or dig them back into the soil. They will produce humus, which bulks up your soil and supplies it with additional nutrients.

Green manure treatments are best carried out in between planting periods, for instance at the end of the summer or in early autumn, when most crops should have been harvested but before the first winter frosts.

Leguminous plants, such as clover, are best for green manure as they fix nitrogen in the soil and make it available for the next crop.

Other suitable plants include buckwheat, which is good for sandy soil. Sow the seeds in spring and summer, then dig the plants into the soil during late summer. Phacelia is also ideal for sandy soil and attracts beneficial insects.

Rye grass is an annual plant with a long bearded head. It makes one of the best green manures for improving soil structure.

Seeds for green manure plants are easily available from most major seed suppliers.

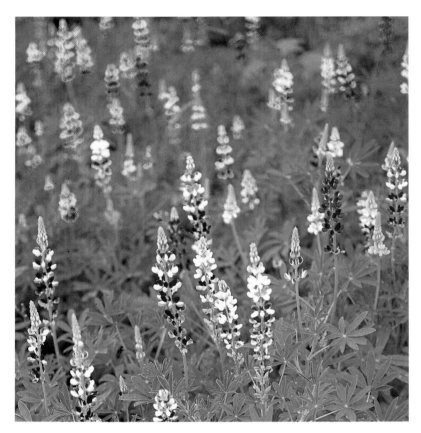

Colourful fertiliser Lupins are ideal green manure plants because they absorb nitrogen, which plants need for growth.

Protect your soil with plenty of mulch

Mulch is a top-dressing for your soil. It usually consists of organic material, such as lawn clippings, foliage or shredded green waste from the garden, but gravel is effective for covering small areas.

Spreading a layer of mulch on top of the soil has various benefits. It evens out extreme temperature fluctuations in the upper layers of the soil and helps prevent the earth from drying out.

Beneath a blanket of mulch, the soil will remain moist and crumbly. Weeds also have a hard time taking root in mulched soil as they become smothered by the top layer that conceals the sunlight.

Homemade compost

A well-maintained compost heap enables you to recycle vegetable and kitchen waste to create fertile humus that will enhance your soil. This totally organic practice should be a priority in every garden.

The best compost heap is one that contains a mixture of vegetable and plant waste collected from the kitchen and garden during the course of the year. However, you should not put diseased plants, such as blighted tomatoes, on the heap – these should be burned instead. By allowing the waste matter to rot down, you can recycle it and produce a nutritional treatment for your garden.

The process of decomposition is the work of billions of minuscule soil organisms and numerous earthworms, beetles and wood-lice. To ensure that they are able to work effectively, follow the basic principles of composting described opposite. At the end of the decomposition process, you'll be left with a humus rich in nutrients.

Compost is the most effective way of enhancing the quality of your soil. It can turn sterile sand or compact clay into fertile ground by improving the soil's structure and restoring its nutrients. A compost heap is, therefore, essential.

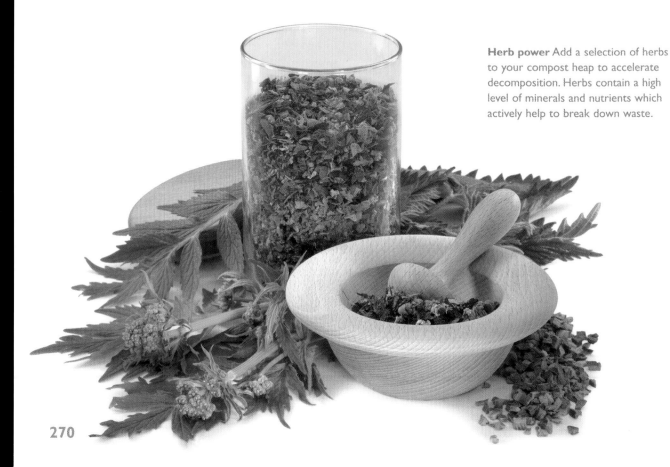

Herb power Add a selection of herbs to your compost heap to accelerate decomposition. Herbs contain a high level of minerals and nutrients which actively help to break down waste.

the organic way

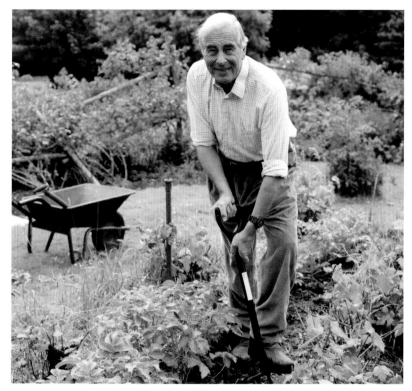

A good yield Vegetables are greedy growers. Add spadefuls of compost to your soil to help guarantee large, healthy crops.

Speed up decomposition

It can take up to two years for a compost heap to turn into a rich humus. If you want to accelerate the process, add the herb-based booster described below. By adding this booster, your compost may rot down in as little as six weeks in summer, three months in autumn or five months in winter.

HERBAL COMPOST BOOSTER

The quantities given for this recipe will be enough to treat a small compost heap for about a year.

7 teaspoons liquid glucose
I teaspoon each dried valerian, stinging nettle, camomile, dandelion and yarrow leaves
I teaspoon dried oak bark
450ml (16fl oz) rainwater

Pour the liquid glucose into a plastic bottle. Add all of the herbs and the oak bark, then shake thoroughly. Add 2 teaspoons of the mixture to the rainwater and leave to infuse for 24 hours.

Use a pole to make about five evenly spaced holes in your compost heap. Pour 6 tablespoons of the herb water into each hole. Refill the holes with fine soil and press it down. Repeat every six weeks until the compost has completely rotted down.

How to make a good compost heap

Ideally, set up your compost heap in a semi-shaded area, so it won't dry out in the sun. Start to build up the heap directly on the soil to enable earthworms to access it from beneath.

All organic, cooked or uncooked waste from the kitchen or garden (with the exception of meat scraps, which can attract vermin) can be thrown on the heap. Shred large or woody items, such as branches or hedge trimmings, to help speed their decomposition.

Compost heaps are traditionally turned, or mixed, twice a year to allow air to circulate and speed up the rotting process. In the past this was always done manually, but you can now buy rotary plastic bins which will keep your compost well aerated.

Soggy grass clippings and rotting stems tend to clump together, so it is a good idea to mix them with dry items. Your compost will be ready when it turns dark brown, crumbly and has a pleasant smell.

Feed your plants and

To keep your plants in top condition, make sure they are getting the right nutrients and not succumbing to pests or diseases. Organic brews and manures can fulfil both of these requirements.

Plants take in nutrients through their roots and leaves. If they don't get enough of what they need, they flower poorly, produce a low crop yield and become weak and stunted. This makes it easier for pests and diseases to take their toll, weakening the plants further.

The solution is to use fertilisers that supply plants with the extra nutrients they require to produce healthy growth. Garden centres offer a huge selection of fertilisers, both organic and inorganic.

Organic fertilisers are derived from vegetable or animal matter, while inorganic ones are based on mineral deposits or are produced synthetically. Some are designed to be applied as a liquid, others are available in powder form.

Nature's own resources

Before you resort to proprietary brands, think about creating your own organic fertilisers in the way that gardeners did in years gone by. A range of herbs produce extracts, infusions, brews or liquid manure, all of which make effective garden fertilisers or pesticides.

At a time when chemical pesticides and fertilisers were not so widely used, people had to encourage wildlife into their gardens to help to control pests. Ladybirds, hedgehogs and birds are all ideal helpers, since they devour insects. You can help to make your garden inviting to wildlife by setting aside a corner to create a natural habitat.

Garden treat Herbs are not just for culinary use. Infusions and extracts made from herbs and plants, such as nasturtiums and garlic, make effective treatments for both plants and the soil.

keep them healthy

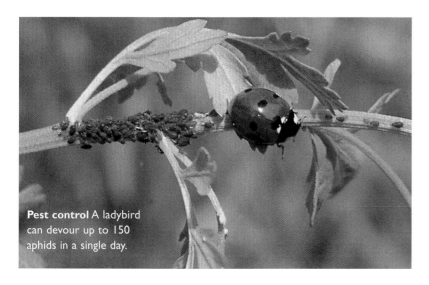

Pest control A ladybird can devour up to 150 aphids in a single day.

Extracts, brews, infusions and liquid manure

Four basic types of preparation will help to keep plants healthy: cold-water extracts, herbal brews, infusions and liquid manures.

The basic formulas for each type of herbal preparation are given in this book only once (see right and overleaf). Specific recipes give you the quantities and types of herbs required.

The finished liquid can either be sprayed onto your plants using a pump-action sprayer, or poured directly onto the ground around your plants.

Most of the preparations need to be diluted with water (1 part liquid to 10 parts water) before use. As these concentrated liquids do not contain preservatives or long-lasting chemicals they should all be used within one month.

BASIC COLD-WATER EXTRACT

Cold water is used in this preparation to allow the active plant enzymes to work. These would be destroyed if heated.

herbs as specified
1 litre (1¾ pints) cold water

Chop the herbs and place them in a bowl. Pour the cold water over them and keep them submerged by placing a weighted plate on top. Leave to infuse for 24 hours. Strain the liquid through a large sieve.

BASIC HERBAL BREW

To obtain every last drop of goodness from the herbs, squeeze them against the bottom of the sieve before discarding them.

herbs as specified
5 litres (8¾ pints) water

Chop the herbs and place them in a large bucket. Pour the cold water over them. Leave to infuse for 24 hours. Pour the mixture into an old cooking pan and simmer over a low heat for 15-30 minutes. Leave the brew to cool. Strain the liquid through a fine sieve, pressing the herbs through with the back of a wooden spoon.

BASIC PLANT INFUSION

While making an infusion, keep the bowl covered to prevent the aromatic substances in the herbs from evaporating.

herbs as specified
1 litre (1¾ pints) water

Chop the herbs and place them in a heatproof bowl. Boil the water and pour it over the herbs. Cover and leave to infuse for 15 minutes. Strain the liquid through a large sieve.

BASIC LIQUID MANURE

This liquid manure smells very pungent and should be stored away from the house.

herbs as specified
2 tablespoons fuller's earth
or
2 tablespoons talcum powder
10 litres (17½ pints) water

Chop the herbs and place them in a bucket. Add the fuller's earth or talcum powder, then pour in the cold water. Leave to infuse, stirring once a day. After three days fermentation should begin. The liquid manure will be ready to use after ten days, when the liquid darkens and the solids have settled at the bottom. Pour the liquid through a fine sieve into plastic bottles with caps.

STINGING NETTLE LIQUID MANURE

Nettle fertiliser provides plants with an extra helping of nitrogen. If possible, use stinging nettles that are about to flower. Always wear gardening gloves when handling nettles to avoid being stung.

1kg (2lb 4oz) fresh stinging nettle leaves

Prepare the liquid manure using the stinging nettles (see Basic liquid manure, above). Dilute the manure with water (1:10) and pour it on the soil around your plants. Use it every two weeks or more frequently if there is heavy rain.

The power of manure

Before artificial fertilisers were invented, manure was used to enrich the soil. The precise qualities of each type of manure – horse, cow, pig or chicken – were known in detail. In old gardening books, this was a subject to which extensive chapters were dedicated. Cattle dung was the most popular choice 20 or 30 years ago. It was said to make the earth mild, fresh and robust.

Nowadays, pelleted chicken manure and spent mushroom manure are more easily available and more pleasant to handle.

COMFREY MANURE

Tomato plants thrive with this potassium-rich preparation.

1kg (2lb 4oz) fresh comfrey leaves

Prepare the manure using comfrey (see Basic liquid manure, above). Dilute the manure with water (1:10). Pour it on the soil every two weeks.

DANDELION NOURISHER

Dandelion is not just a weed – it can give plants extra nourishment.

2kg (4½lb) fresh dandelion flowers and leaves

Prepare the nourisher using the dandelions (see Basic liquid manure, above). Spray undiluted nourisher onto the leaves of your plants every three weeks or pour it onto the soil once a fortnight.

HERB TEA FOR PLANTS

There are people who swear by camomile tea as a remedy for all manner of human ailments. But camomile can also help to give plants a boost.

25g (1oz) dried camomile flowers

Prepare the infusion using the camomile (see Basic plant infusion, page 273). Dilute the infusion with water (1:5) and spray it on the plants and surrounding soil every three weeks.

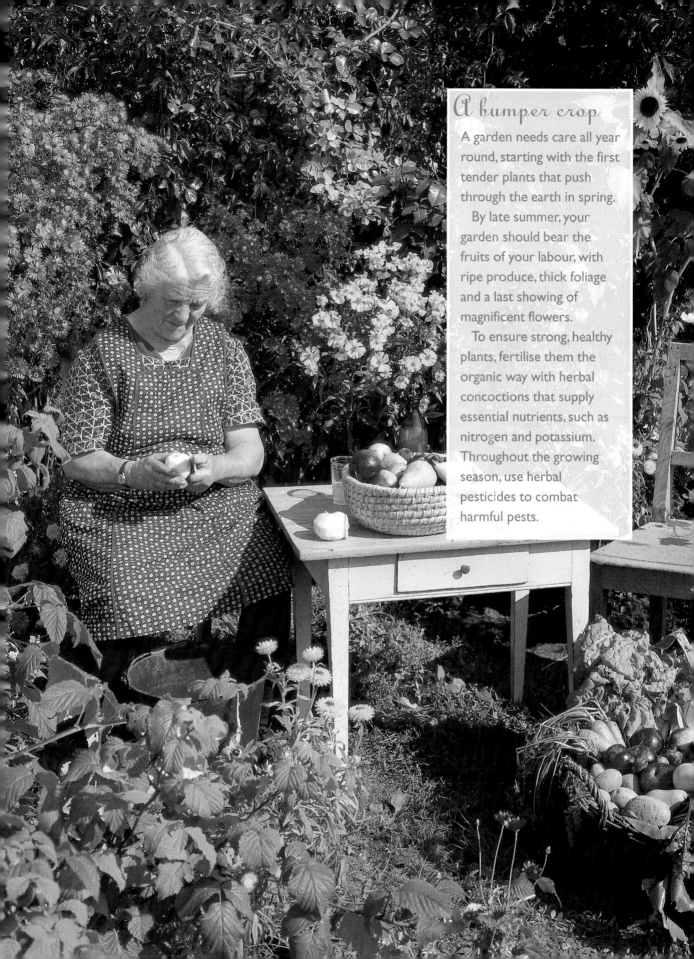

A bumper crop

A garden needs care all year round, starting with the first tender plants that push through the earth in spring.

By late summer, your garden should bear the fruits of your labour, with ripe produce, thick foliage and a last showing of magnificent flowers.

To ensure strong, healthy plants, fertilise them the organic way with herbal concoctions that supply essential nutrients, such as nitrogen and potassium. Throughout the growing season, use herbal pesticides to combat harmful pests.

YARROW EXTRACT

This mixture will help to protect your plants against fungi and insects.

200g (7oz) fresh yarrow flowers

Prepare the extract using yarrow (see Basic cold-water extract, page 273). Dilute the extract with water (1:10) and spray it on your plants at the first sign of pests.

HORSETAIL BREW

This brew will help ward off downy mildew – a disease that spreads quickly from plant to plant.

500g (1lb 2oz) fresh horsetail 'needles' and stems

Prepare the brew using horsetail (see Basic herbal brew, page 273). Dilute it with water (1:5). Spray your plants on three consecutive days.

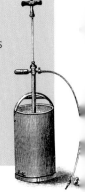

Spray pump
Gardeners from times past used galvanised tin pressure sprays, pumped by hand, to apply fertilisers and pesticides to plants.

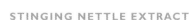

Fresh or dry
If you can't get hold of fresh stinging nettles to make a cold-water extract, use dried herbs instead. They contain the same amount of active substances.

NASTURTIUM INFUSION

Combat woolly aphids – a pest of apple trees – with nasturtiums.

200g (7oz) fresh nasturtium leaves and flowers

Prepare the infusion using nasturtiums (see Basic plant infusion, page 273). Apply the neat solution to the aphids with a brush. Repeat two weeks later.

HORSERADISH INFUSION

This infusion combats blossom rot and fungal diseases on stone fruits such as plums or cherries.

500g (1lb 2oz) fresh horseradish leaves

Prepare the infusion using horseradish (see Basic plant infusion, page 273). For blossom rot, dilute it with water (1:5) and spray on the flowers at the first sign of a problem. For fungal diseases, dilute it with water (1:1) and spray on the leaves every two weeks.

STINGING NETTLE EXTRACT

This cold-water extract is very effective for fighting aphids.

**200g (7oz) fresh stinging nettles
2 litres (3½ pints) water**

Prepare the cold-water extract with nettles (see page 273), using 2 litres (3½ pints) water. Leave to infuse in the sun. Dilute the extract with water (1:5) and spray on your plants as soon as you see tiny aphids appearing.

GARLIC INFUSION

An infusion of garlic helps to strengthen plant immunity against grey mould. It is particularly effective on strawberries.

25g (1oz) cloves garlic

Prepare the infusion using garlic cloves (see Basic plant infusion, page 273). Spray the garlic infusion undiluted on susceptible plants every two to three weeks.

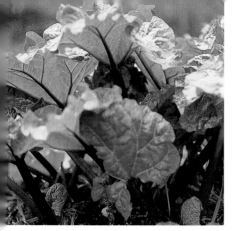

Rhubarb pesticide A brew made from rhubarb leaves will kill various plant pests, without harming useful insects and butterflies.

ANTI-MITE INFUSION

Tansy contains substances that can have a toxic effect on humans. Take care when handling it.

300g (10½oz) fresh tansy leaves and flowers

Prepare the infusion using tansy (see Basic plant infusion, page 273). Dilute it with water (1:3) and spray on the plants as soon as you see any mites on the leaves.

RHUBARB BREW

This brew will kill mites, caterpillars and various harmful larvae.

1kg (2lb 4oz) fresh rhubarb leaves

Prepare the brew using rhubarb leaves (see Basic herbal brew, page 273). Dilute it with water (1:10) and either spray it on your plants or pour it on the soil around the plant at the first sign of pests.

Tried & Trusted
Liquid manure tips

- Do not use a metal container when you are preparing liquid manure, as the fermented product will damage the surface.

- If you prefer, you can use dried herbs in place of fresh ones. For every 1kg (2lb 4oz) of fresh herbs, use 100g (3½oz) of dried.

- If possible, use rainwater to prepare liquid manure as it is 'softer' than tap water.

- When pouring liquid manure on the soil, ensure that the ground is not too dry, or the manure will drain away before the plant can take up the goodness.

- Do not apply liquid manure to your plants in the middle of the day as the sun will scorch the leaves through the liquid. The best time to use it is in the early morning or late evening, when the sun's rays are at their weakest.

- Liquid manure will ferment more quickly if left in a warm, sunny spot.

- Do not use a nettle manure on beans, peas or onions.

- For the following liquid manures use 1kg (2lb 4oz) of fresh vegetation to 10 litres (17½ pints) of water. Dilute the manure with water (1:10):

  Liquid manure prepared from tomato shoots can be used on beans, cucumbers, cabbages, leeks, parsley and onions.

  Prevent mildew on roses with liquid manure made from onions, deadnettles, birch leaves and the lateral shoots of tomatoes.

  To stimulate the growth of a newly sown lawn, water it with liquid manure prepared from beetroot leaves. Dilute this manure with water (1:5) and apply twice a week.

  Marigold leaf manure helps to boost disease resistance in vegetables and ornamental plants.

- Ingredients, such as sea bird dung (guano), fish blood and bone meal, can be added to herbal liquid manures to increase the quantities of phosphates, nitrogen and potassium.

Extracts

- A cold-water extract made from 200g (7oz) of fresh stag-horn sumach leaves (*Rhus typhina*) will kill aphids and potato beetle larvae. If you suffer from skin allergies, use protective gloves when making or using this extract.

Drying fresh herbs

Make sure you have a supply of herbs for making
liquid manure and other plant treatments by drying
your own fresh from the garden. You can also use
them in medicinal remedies or potpourris.

If you plan to dry your own herbs, pick
sprigs of them early on a dry, sunny
morning. Harvest them once any dew has
dried, but before the sun is too hot.

In the early 20th century, before herbs
were widely available in the shops or from
mail-order herbalists, many people had
herb gardens. Picked fresh herbs were tied
together in small, loose bundles, with raffia
bound around their stems. This allowed the
air to circulate around them and prevented
mould from growing. The herbs were then
hung upside-down near the kitchen range or
in an airing cupboard. You can also use this
method of drying herbs.

Alternatively, you can dry herbs very
quickly in a microwave (see Drying
aromatic herbs, page 203).

How to dry fresh herbs
Quantities vary according to types of herbs and amounts picked

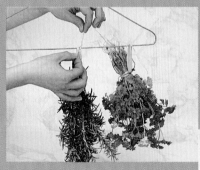

▼ Dry leaves and sprigs such as
sage, parsley and thyme on a
piece of **muslin** stretched
across a **wooden frame**. You
can also dry rosebuds and
lavender flowers in this way.

▼ After two weeks, the herbs
should be dry. Crumble each
sprig or leaf by hand or use a
pestle and mortar to crush
tough twigs. Store your dried
herbs in **airtight glass jars**.
Label each jar and keep it out
of direct sunlight.

▲ Pick **sprigs of herbs**. Group
them into bundles and remove
the leaves from the stems where
you are going to tie them
together. Secure each bundle with
raffia and attach it to a **wire
hanger** or **cane**. Hang up to dry.
Alternatively, tie the bundles onto
a clothes dryer.

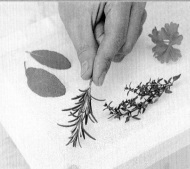

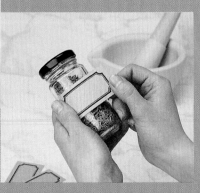

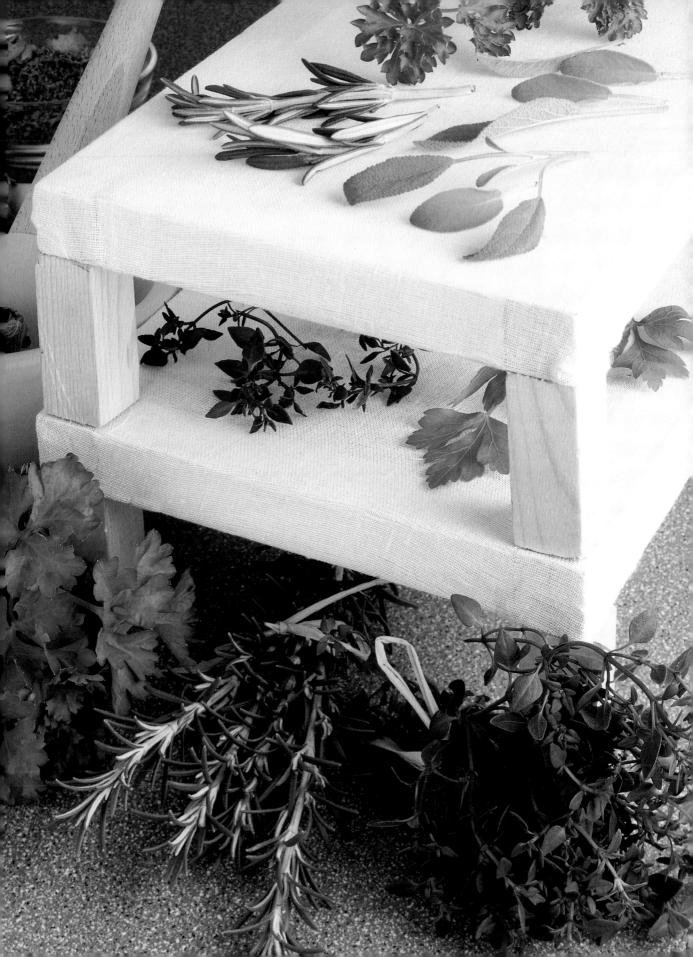

Companion planting

Over the centuries generations of gardeners have learned from their successes and failures with crops, gradually acquiring expertise. Apply their methods and benefit from their accumulated wisdom.

Through experience, gardeners and farmers in the past soon discovered that planting a field with the same crops year in and year out – a system now known as monoculture – was a sure way of causing soil 'fatigue' and producing poor yields. To counteract this effect, growers varied the crops that they planted in each location from year to year. Today, we have a scientific explanation for the benefits of crop rotation, or mixed plant culture.

Each plant takes up certain nutrients from the soil in different proportions. If the same type of plant is grown on a particular plot several years running, it will deplete the ground of the specific nutrients it needs; this imbalance provides an ideal environment for disease to flourish.

In planning a vegetable garden, you need to take account of the requirements of individual plants. You also need to be aware that some plants can be mutually beneficial, while others are not suitable for planting together.

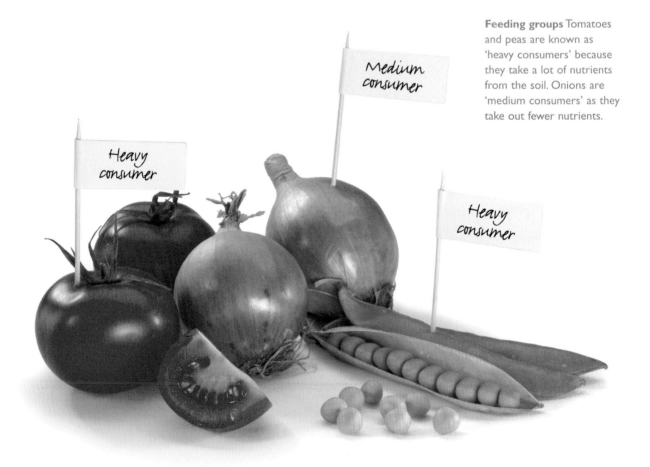

Feeding groups Tomatoes and peas are known as 'heavy consumers' because they take a lot of nutrients from the soil. Onions are 'medium consumers' as they take out fewer nutrients.

and crop rotation

Crop-swapping

To ensure a well-planned rotation of crops in your vegetable garden, keep a gardening diary. Note which crops you plan to cultivate in the coming year and when and where you plant them.

Divide your plot into three sections, so that each type of vegetable will be growing in the same section once in three years. To accommodate 'greedy' varieties such as peas, which should be planted on the same spot only once every six years, you may need to further divide your plot to provide more planting areas.

Group your vegetables

When planning your planting, group vegetables according to how quickly they take up nutrients from the soil. Some will be heavy nutrient consumers, some medium and others light consumers.

In the first year, plant 'gross feeders', the heavy consumers, on a well-fertilised plot. Replace them in the second year with medium consumers and in the third year with light consumers.

After this three-year period, the soil will need to be replenished with green manure and compost. The cycle can then begin anew.

A planned cycle of crop rotation is the best way to exploit the soil nutrients without exhausting the earth. It also helps to eradicate harmful soil fungus or nematode worms, which attack some plants.

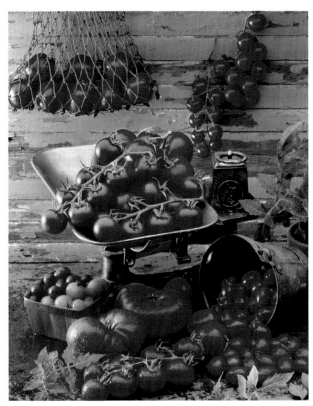

Top priority
To achieve a harvest as abundant as this one, give tomatoes priority in the crop rotation cycle and provide them with plenty of potassium.

Heavy consumers

This group of vegetables includes corn-on-the-cob, tomatoes, potatoes, celery, leeks, peas, beans, cucumbers, courgettes and pumpkins.

Start by preparing the plot in the autumn, enriching it with compost and organic fertilisers, such as a mixture of fish blood and bone or bone meal.

Medium consumers

This group includes onions, carrots, lettuces, radishes, turnips, spinach, spinach beet, peppers, beetroot and parsnips.

Add a little organic fertiliser or herbal liquid manure to the soil before planting.

Light consumers

These crops follow in rotation from the previous two groups and therefore require only small amounts of organic fertilisers and chalk or garden lime.

These vegetables include cabbages, broccoli, Brussels sprouts and cauliflowers. Turnips should follow crops that are harvested in early summer. Herbs can also be introduced into the cycle as they need very little manure to grow.

Companion planting – a friendly environment

Cultivating a variety of vegetables on the same plot is the best way of exploiting soil fertility and is known as companion planting.

This mixed culture method is in fact a form of precisely co-ordinated crop rotation within a single gardening year. It takes into account the ripening periods and harvesting times of the various crops, as well as their different nutrient uptakes and their root configurations, whether shallow, medium or deep.

There are also other advantages to companion planting. Some plants benefit from the substances that neighbouring plants deposit in the soil, allowing them to produce a more plentiful or superior yield, or protecting them from harmful pests and diseases. Cultivating a variety of vegetables ensures that the soil benefits from a mixture of both young and mature plants all year round. The shade from the foliage of mature plants can protect the soil from drying out and the ground cover they supply should help to prevent too many weeds from springing up.

The best and worst partners

Vegetable combinations can be beneficial or harmful. Lettuces, for instance, can be planted alongside most types of vegetable, although they will not do well if planted with parsley or celery. Beans, peas and brassicas (including cabbages, Brussels sprouts, swedes, turnips and cauliflowers) should not be planted with garlic or onions.

Potatoes need plenty of space to spread and are poor companions – the only vegetables they can be planted beside are French beans and turnips. Runner beans thrive when planted near cucumbers, turnips, radishes and celery. Tomatoes can be planted with French beans, garlic, lettuces, leeks, carrots and radishes. Carrots and leeks are good companions for most vegetables.

DOUBLE HARVEST

Lamb's lettuce, which also grows in the wild, is an ideal salad vegetable to plant after harvesting onions and carrots.

onions
carrots
lamb's lettuce

In spring, plant alternate rows of onions and carrots. In late summer, after harvesting the onions and carrots, sow lamb's lettuce which germinates and matures quickly and needs very few nutrients.

FOUR IN ONE

This cultivation plan combines plants that are heavy, medium and light nutrient consumers.

turnips
peas
endives
leeks

In spring, plant one row of turnips and one row of peas. In July, after harvesting each vegetable, plant endives in place of the turnips and leeks in place of the peas.

Alternation is the best medicine

Traditional books from the 1900s describe a gardening method known as alternate cropping. Without the knowledge of nutrient depletion by plants, gardeners could not explain why a particular crop would thrive one year and be a total failure the next. It was simply put down to soil 'fatigue'. An example used to illustrate the failure of monoculture was the growth of celery on the same patch for three years. In the first year the soil was fresh, in the second and third the celery had caused it to become poor. Alternate cropping ensured that the soil did not become depleted.

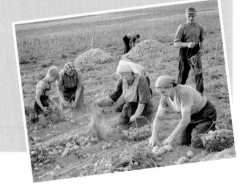

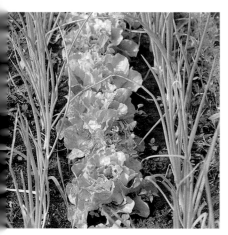

Well planted Lettuces can be planted with onions which, in turn, make good companions for carrots.

FIVE TO A PLOT

This is an example of how your vegetable garden can be occupied for the entire growing season and give you produce all year round.

radishes
lettuce (such as Tom Thumb)
runner beans
leeks
winter spinach

In spring, plant well-spaced rows of radishes. A few weeks later, plant lettuces between these rows and harvest them during the summer. In May, after the radishes have been picked, plant runner beans in their place.

In early autumn, harvest the beans and plant leeks. Plant winter spinach in the rows that were occupied by the lettuces.

Tried & Trusted

Good neighbours

- For a bumper crop of broccoli, companion plant it with spinach. The roots of the spinach secrete a growth-enhancing hormone into the soil which does wonders for many vegetables grown nearby.

- Plant caraway in your potato patch to enhance their flavour.

- Savory has a smell which deters black bean aphids.

- Dill is a good neighbour for cucumbers. Its feathery leaves protect fledgling plants from the sun. Once the cucumbers mature, it can be used in salads.

- Plant garlic among roses to help strengthen the bushes' resistance to disease.

- Lavender may stop aphids from attacking rose bushes.

- Plant garlic or leeks between rows of strawberries to help protect the fruits from grey mould.

- Planting a mixture of tall and low-growing vegetables in the same patch is an ideal way of making the most of the available space. For example, plant French beans with tomatoes or round-headed garden lettuces with leeks.

Crop rotation

- Extend a three-year planting cycle to a four-year cycle by growing green manure on a fourth plot of ground. You can then plant heavy nutrient consumers on this plot the following year.

- As long as they are free of blight, tomatoes can be cultivated on the same plot for several years if you feed them regularly.

- Ideally, carrots, new potatoes, parsley, cucumbers and peas should only be re-grown on the same spot every six years.

- Members of the mustard family don't grow well with related species, such as cruciferae, and should be separately rotated. Do not rotate brassicas, such as radishes, winter radishes and turnips, with each other.

- Make a detailed record of the cultivars grown, sowing and planting dates, treatments given, problems and results for each year. This will provide an invaluable guide for improving your garden's performance next year.

Traditional growing and harvesting

Many gardeners follow a traditional timetable for growing their plants, favouring specific days of the year for sowing and harvesting particular vegetables. Often, these methods have been handed down within families or by professional gardeners to their young apprentices.

Some people, for instance, always sow their broad beans and sweet peas on Boxing Day – because early sowings are said to be less prone to aphid attacks. Garlic cloves were traditionally planted on the shortest day of the year and harvested on the longest.

In the past, cultivation according to the phases of the moon and the stars was popular in the countryside.

There are still some people today who faithfully follow lunar guidelines when planting up their gardens. Due to the effect of the moon on the earth's atmosphere, it is more likely to rain just after a new moon. So traditionalists would advise you to plant at this time so that your seedlings get a good watering.

Another tenet of gardening by the moon is that plants with edible parts above the ground should be sown when the moon is rising. Similarly, root vegetables, with their edible parts below ground, should be sown as the moon sets.

There are also other garden tasks that can be carried out according to the lunar cycle, including

hoeing and preparing the ground for sowing vegetables and flowers, as well as pruning, earthing up potatoes, thinning carrots and planting out seedlings.

You can experiment with this ancient and mystic way of gardening by sowing a quick-growing vegetable, such as radishes, at different times during the lunar cycle. Take note of the differences in the way the seeds respond and the plants grow.

There are annual almanacs and lunar gardening books published for moon plantings, available from 'New Age' shops. However, remember that the times and phases will need to be adjusted to compensate for local time zones.

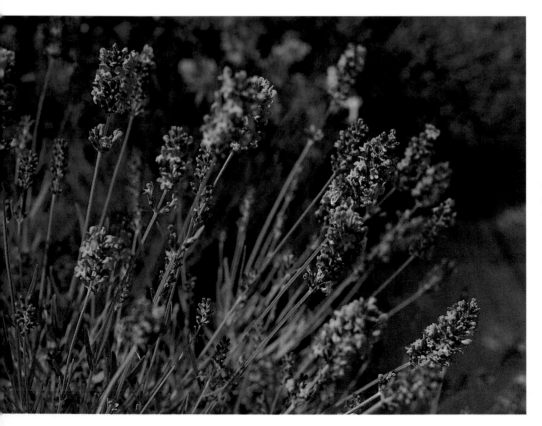

Helpful herb Lavender can benefit other plants growing nearby. It has a strong scent that deters pests but encourages helpful predators and pollinators.

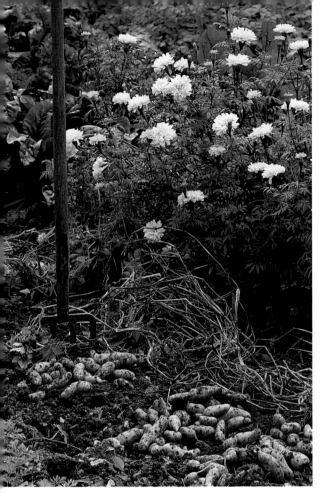

After dark Firm believers in lunar gardening have been known to dig up young potatoes at dusk when the flavour is said to be at its best.

When to harvest

Most gardeners pick their produce early in the day or at dusk, as the plants are more succulent. This is in line with gardening lore, which suggests that sap rises in response to daylight and that the leaves lose less moisture after the sun has set.

Some traditional methods of planting and harvesting have been dismissed as old wives' tales. But it is surprising how many are, in fact, forgotten pearls of wisdom.

For instance, certain plants attract beneficial insects which clear infestations of destructive pests. Try planting marigolds among your vegetables to attract hoverflies, which feed on the pollen. The female flies lay their eggs and the emerging larvae feed on whitefly that would otherwise demolish your crops.

Early morning planting

Time of day has traditionally played an important part in growing and harvesting vegetables and flowers. Experienced gardeners are always keen to get into their gardens to plant and harvest early in the day. After a dew, the soil is always more moist and, therefore, easier to work. Seeds and young plants take root more successfully if planted under these conditions.

If you sow or plant at midday, when the sun is at its hottest, watering is necessary and it is likely that a young plant's foliage will get scorched. If you leave the watering until later, the plants will be stressed and unable to establish their roots successfully.

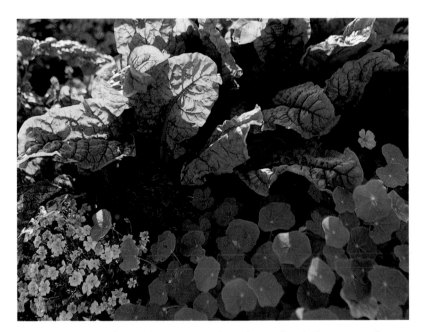

Natural deterrent Lunar planting is a traditional way of gardening to nature's rhythms. You can also use natural means of pest control, such as planting marigolds in your vegetable plot to attract hoverflies whose larvae feed on whitefly.

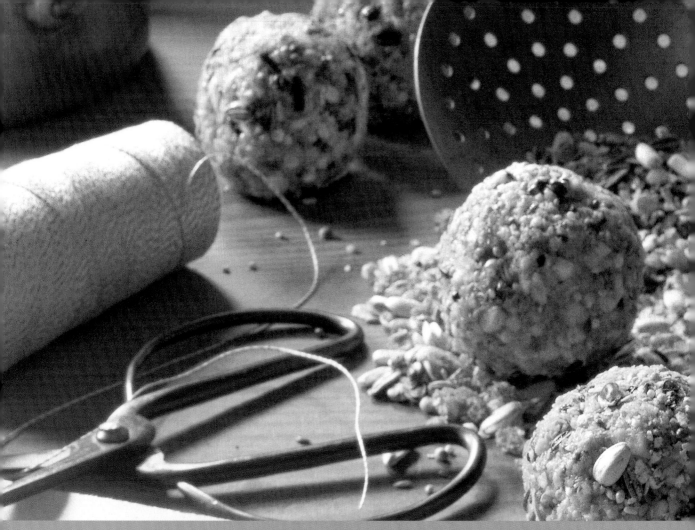

Winter bird food

Not all birds head south in the autumn. You can
make life easier for those that stay behind with
nutritious feeding balls that will help them to
survive the winter.

As winter approaches, many people
put out food for birds and derive great
pleasure from watching them feed.

While the loose seed sold in pet shops is
nourishing, it can spread disease if it mixes
with droppings on the bird table. These
feeding balls, which can be hung on strings
from your bird table or from branches, help
avoid the problem. The ingredients, including
the fat that binds the seeds together, are
highly nutritious and will help ensure that
mature birds breed successfully in spring.

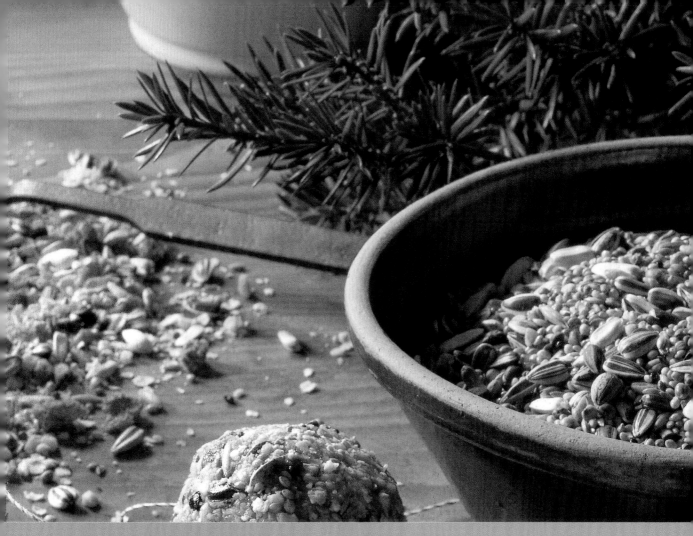

How to make bird feeding balls
Makes 12 balls, each about 100g (3½oz)

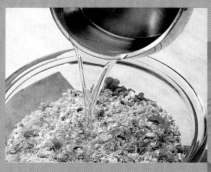

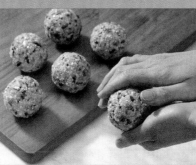

▼ Spread the remaining mixture of dry ingredients on a piece of paper and roll the balls in it. Hang the balls up by their strings.

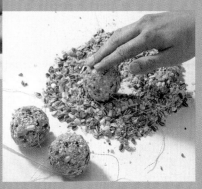

▲ Melt **250g (9oz) of vegetable lard** in a pan. Mix **200g (7oz) each of oats, chopped nuts, coarse wheatmeal, seeds** and **chopped sultanas**. Put about 5 tablespoonfuls of this mixture aside. Pour the fat over the remaining mix and leave to cool.

▲ When the fat begins to solidify, squash palmfuls of the mixture into balls. For each ball, cut a length of **string** and make a knot at one end. Thread the string through the balls using a **blunt needle** or a bodkin.

Traditional crops

Rediscover some of the vegetables that were once
a common sight in the kitchen garden and savour
the taste of times past as you add interest and
flavour to your meals.

Garden orach, May beet
and purslane are plant names
unfamiliar to most people. And yet
these vegetables were grown in
many gardens, until they made way
for the varieties more commonly
found in gardens, shops and
supermarkets today.

Some of these forgotten
vegetables were picked crisp and
fresh from the garden and eaten

raw in salads, others were cooked
and used in soups, stews and
gratins or as a side vegetable. In
addition to their culinary uses,
some plants were also used for
medicinal purposes.

Nowadays, the only way of
trying these rare delicacies is to
grow them yourself, as so few of
them are commercially available.
Luckily, most of the vegetables are
easy to cultivate, as they require no
special attention and are not

susceptible to disease. Many of
them will also make an attractive
display in your vegetable plot.

In the following pages, you'll
find out when to plant and harvest
these traditional vegetables, and
discover well-used methods of
blanching and storing them. There
are also suggestions for how to
prepare and serve them.

Seeds for the plants mentioned
can be bought from mail-order
seed suppliers who specialise in
traditional varieties (see the list of
addresses on page 339).

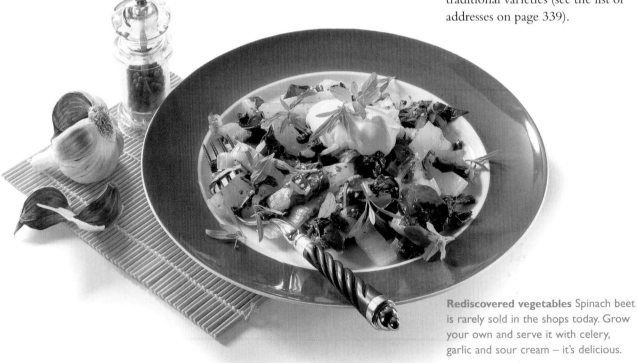

Rediscovered vegetables Spinach beet
is rarely sold in the shops today. Grow
your own and serve it with celery,
garlic and sour cream – it's delicious.

Vitamins and flavour

Old-fashioned vegetables are full of flavour and when picked fresh from your garden, they are also highly nutritious and full of vitamins. Parsnip and purslane are good sources of vitamin C, while spinach beet is rich in minerals.

These plants have therapeutic properties as well. Dandelions, for example, contain a bitter white substance that stimulates digestion.

Asparagus pea

With its velvety red flowers, the asparagus pea is a pretty sight in any vegetable patch. Sow the seeds in pots from mid March and plant out the seedlings from mid May. Harvest the pods when they are young and sweet, otherwise they will lose their flavour.

This vegetable is also known as the 'winged pea', because of its unique winged pods. Lightly cook the fleshy pods and serve them as a side vegetable or in salads.

Climbing beans

Traditional varieties of runner and French beans with colourful names such as 'Painted Lady' or 'Kelvedon Marvel' have a better flavour than the varieties usually sold in supermarkets. Climbing beans are best trained up traditional bamboo wigwams with smaller vegetables grown beneath. They like plenty of water and extra manure to thrive. Seeds are best sown in the spring after the frosts, but young plants can be overwintered in a frost-free greenhouse or frame.

Beans are a versatile ingredient. Stir fry them, part-cook for salads or serve as a side vegetable.

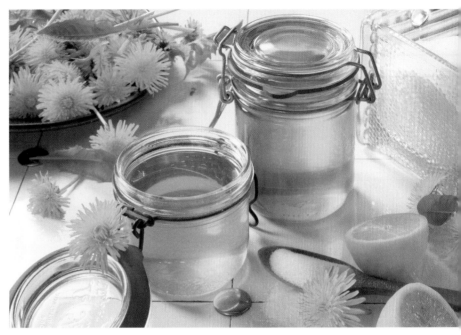

Golden syrup Bright yellow dandelion flowers can be made into a syrup to sweeten drinks and desserts.

Dandelion

The leaves of young dandelions are among the most nutritious ingredients to include in spring salads. You can also blanch them (see Tried and Trusted, page 291) as a vegetable, which was a popular way of preparing dandelions in years gone by.

The flowers can be used to make wine, while the flower buds marinated in vinegar are a spicy substitute for capers.

Dandelions are perennial plants that happily grow in all types of soil and many people consider them a weed. If you don't have a natural crop in your garden, sow dandelion seeds in spring. Pick the leaves in September. To avoid the risk of dandelions spreading all over the garden, plant them in window boxes deep enough to accommodate their long tap roots.

DANDELION FLOWER SYRUP

This piquant syrup is made using yellow dandelion flowers. Stored in jars in a cool dry place, the syrup will keep for more than a year.

I lemon
750ml (I pint 7fl oz) water
250g (9oz) fresh dandelion flowers
I kg (2lb 4oz) sugar

Cut the lemon into slices. Pour the water into a pan, then add the lemon and dandelion flowers. Simmer on a low heat for 20 minutes. Strain the liquid through a fine sieve into a clean saucepan. Stir the sugar into the hot liquid and simmer gently for another 15 minutes until the sugar has dissolved. Pour the syrup into clean glass jars and seal.

289

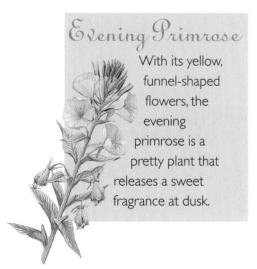

Evening Primrose

With its yellow, funnel-shaped flowers, the evening primrose is a pretty plant that releases a sweet fragrance at dusk.

Evening primrose

Sow evening primrose seeds in your vegetable patch between April and the end of May. The plant does not need fertile soil and will even thrive in sandy conditions. A gardening book published in 1887 does warn, however, against sowing in freshly manured soil.

The roots may be harvested from autumn, through the winter and into the following spring.

Fleshy red evening primrose roots are a speciality of old. They grow to a length of 18cm (7in) and have a delicate flavour. Cook them in salted water and serve them as a vegetable with white sauce or cold in a salad. Freshly cut shoot tips are used to season raw vegetable salads and potato salad.

Take care

If you want to eat the leaves and flowers of wild plants, don't pick them from roadside verges, where they will be polluted, or from waste ground where they may be contaminated by animals.

Garden orach

Known in the past as 'mountain spinach', this plant was commonly grown as a substitute for spinach. It has a more intense, spicy flavour and contains less oxalic acid – a natural substance that is harmful if taken in high concentrations. Very young leaves can be used in salads.

Garden orach can be sown throughout the year. If planted in autumn, it will be ready to pick in spring. Harvest the leaves as soon as the rosettes develop.

Garden orach tends to grow well whatever the weather and quality of the soil and will thrive in semi-shade. A fertile, well-watered and loose soil will encourage the growth of larger and more tender leaves.

Hamburg parsley

Belonging to the same species as ordinary parsley, this plant is hardier and so provides a winter crop of roots for cooking and leaves for flavouring. Whereas most smaller root vegetables taste best, with Hamburg parsley the larger roots are the most prized.

The roots have a delicate flavour said to be a cross between celeriac and turnip. They look a little like parsnips and are cooked in the same way: boiled or roasted.

Hop sprouts

In Victorian times and during the World Wars, hop sprouts were a delicacy. When the young shoots reach a length of 10cm (4in), cut them off at ground level and either add them to a salad or steam them as you would asparagus.

Fresh harvest There is nothing quite as tasty as home-grown, handpicked vegetables grown organically. Choose a traditional variety of climbing bean that is not available in the shops.

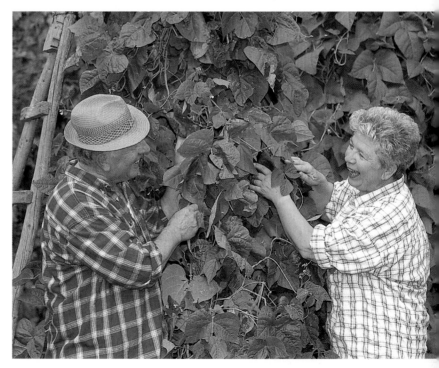

Tried & Trusted
Blanching

• **To obtain pale-coloured, or blanched, vegetables you need to exclude daylight as they grow. This process prevents the formation of chlorophyll (the green colouring matter in plant foliage). It makes the vegetables more tender. Plants that are often blanched include rhubarb, endive and celery.**

• **To blanch small plants, such as dandelions, place upturned clay flowerpots over them.**

• **To blanch larger plants, such as celery, bind the stems with raffia or garden string to conceal them from the sun. As an additional measure, you can wrap straw around them and tie it in place.**

• **Blanch curly endives by placing a large bowl on top of them for several days before harvesting.**

• **Keep cauliflowers white by shielding them from sunlight with large cabbage leaves or by bending over the leaves surrounding the central 'flower'.**

• **Earth up the lower parts of leeks with soil to keep them white.**

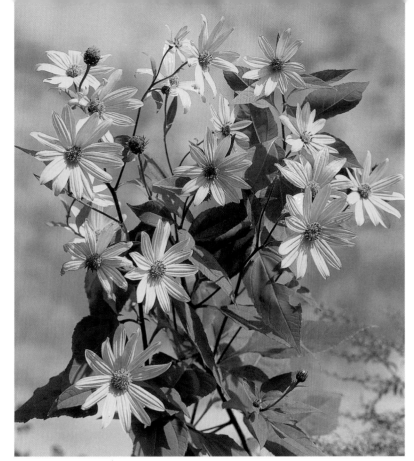

Hidden depths Jerusalem artichoke flowers make a brilliant display. The unseen tuberous roots are a versatile winter vegetable, rich in potassium.

Jerusalem artichoke

Robust and frost hardy, Jerusalem artichoke plants can reach heights of 2–3m (7-10ft). The variety 'Fuseau' has a smooth tuber which is much easier to peel for cooking than the more common knobbly tubers.

In early spring, place the tubers into the ground at a depth of about 10cm (4in). Pile up earth around the shoots as they appear. The crop takes nine months to mature and should be harvested throughout the winter.

When cooked, artichoke roots develop a nutty flavour. They can be prepared as a soup, a gratin or a purée, or blanched, coated in breadcrumbs and deep fried.

Hop

Young hop shoots are juicy, crisp and aromatic. The flower cones of this plant contain the bitter substances used to flavour beer.

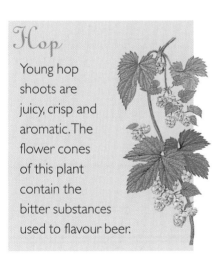

291

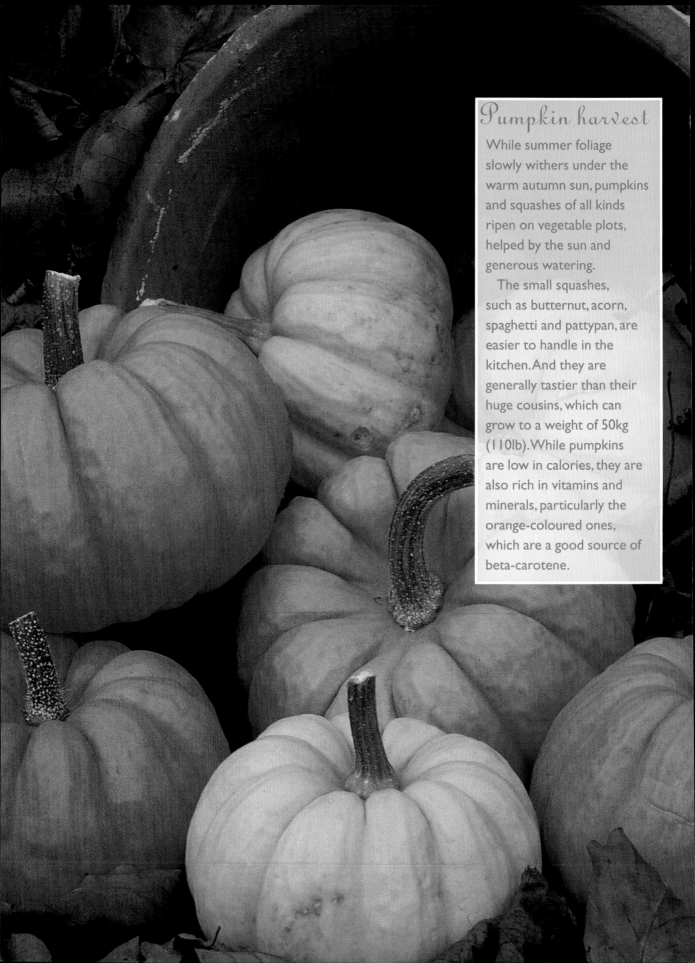

Pumpkin harvest

While summer foliage slowly withers under the warm autumn sun, pumpkins and squashes of all kinds ripen on vegetable plots, helped by the sun and generous watering.

The small squashes, such as butternut, acorn, spaghetti and pattypan, are easier to handle in the kitchen. And they are generally tastier than their huge cousins, which can grow to a weight of 50kg (110lb). While pumpkins are low in calories, they are also rich in vitamins and minerals, particularly the orange-coloured ones, which are a good source of beta-carotene.

Pumpkin and squash

Both pumpkins and squashes were among the most colourful vegetables in 19th-century gardens. These gourd-like fruits can be used in desserts, made into jams and eaten in savoury dishes.

Raise seeds of these plants in pots in April, then transfer the young plants to good-quality soil, rich in nutrients and well dug-in humus, in mid May or after the risk of frost has passed.

Pumpkins and squashes need warmth and plenty of water to grow. Depending on the variety, they can be harvested from late August to early October.

Purslane

The ancient Egyptians used purslane as a vegetable and as a healing plant.

This hardy annual requires little nurturing, but it is not a commonly-grown vegetable in Britain. The plant has red stems and is ready for harvesting during the summer months.

The lobe-shaped leaves have a sharp, vinegar-like flavour due to their high acid content. Use them in salads to complement ingredients with a stronger taste.

Rocket

Rocket has a unique, peppery flavour with a slightly bitter tang. At present this leafy salad vegetable is enjoying a revival and can be found in most supermarkets. Sow seeds in succession from March to early September. Pick the leaves after about six weeks.

ROCKET AND PARMESAN

This aromatic, spicy appetiser is quick and easy to prepare. Serves four.

115g (4oz) fresh rocket leaves
2 teaspoons balsamic vinegar
4 tablespoons olive oil
freshly ground black pepper
salt
2 tablespoons pine nuts
55g (2oz) freshly shaved parmesan

Place the rocket in a bowl. Mix the vinegar, olive oil, pepper and salt to make a dressing. Dry fry the pine nuts in a pan. Add the nuts and cheese to the bowl and pour over the dressing before serving.

Sleepy salads

Many salad plants contain a high level of vegetable milk or latex. Some, such as wild lettuce and dandelion, have long been used medicinally as a mild sedative.

It is said that a large plate of fresh leaves will calm your nerves and encourage sleep. The Greek physician Galen ate salad leaves cooked with olive oil and vinegar every evening as he got older in order to cure his insomnia.

Depending on the month in which the seeds are planted, salad leaves can be harvested either in October or the following spring.

Perfect salad partner The peppery taste of rocket goes well with shavings of parmesan cheese.

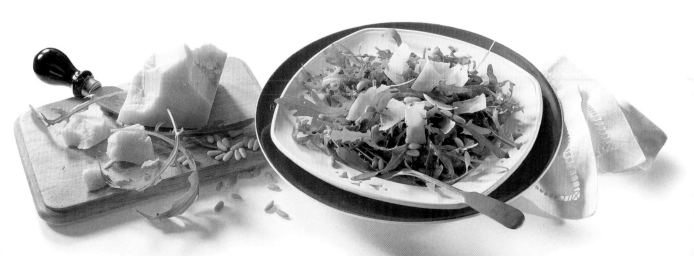

Salsify

This winter vegetable originates in central and southern Europe. Sow the seeds in April into light, well-drained soil. Water the plants generously in dry weather.

Salsify is also known as the oyster plant due to its slightly oyster-like taste. Cook it in the same way as parsnips and swedes, or blanch the roots and serve them in a salad.

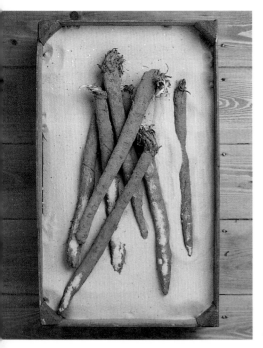

Salsify Lift the roots of salsify in late October. Cut off the leaves, then store them in boxes of sand or peat.

Spinach beet

An ornamental vegetable with large leaves and white stalks, spinach beet was once a common sight in kitchen gardens. It is sometimes called 'perpetual spinach' and is actually a form of beetroot grown for its leaves rather than its root.

Sow spinach beet at the end of April in humus-rich soil. Feed it with fertiliser and water it as the plant grows. Pick young leaves, by breaking the stems at the base, from July onwards, when they reach a length of 10-15cm (4-6in).

Both the leaves and the stems of spinach beet can be used in cooking. The leaves are slightly coarser than spinach and also more strongly flavoured.

Prepare the leaves by steaming them or boiling them in a little water for a few minutes, just as you would spinach. The stalks have a nut-like flavour and are delicious boiled, thoroughly strained and served with a béchamel sauce.

Spinach beet thrives in a semi-shaded environment and is exceptionally robust. In some regions, it is winter hardy and re-sprouts in spring.

The plant is no longer edible after the first flower appears, when the leaves become very bitter.

BRAISED SPINACH BEET

Spinach beet used to be a popular alternative to spinach in summer. Try this creamy recipe. You will need a wok or large frying pan to stir fry the vegetable.

4 tablespoons olive oil
1 small onion, chopped
750g (1lb 10oz) fresh spinach beet leaves, cut into strips
2 sprigs of fresh marjoram, chopped
150ml (5 fl oz) water
200g (7oz) double cream
salt
freshly ground pepper
grated nutmeg

Pour the oil into a pan. Add the onions and cook over a low heat until translucent. Add the spinach beet and marjoram and stir fry for 2-3 minutes. Pour in the water and cook for 10 minutes over a low heat. Stir the cream into the mixture and season with salt, pepper and nutmeg.

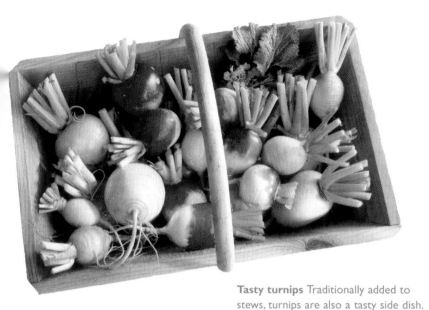

Tasty turnips Traditionally added to stews, turnips are also a tasty side dish.

Turnips, beets and swedes

Small beets known as May beets were once popular in spring and summer, because larger root vegetables, such as turnips and swedes, were not available until later in the autumn and winter.

Sow May beet seeds in early spring in a rich soil. Keep the plants well watered so they are consistently moist until harvest time. May beets were traditionally harvested in May, hence the name. However, they usually taste better if left in the ground until June. Eat them raw or braised in butter. Prepare the heart-shaped leaves in the same way as spinach.

Sow swedes and turnips from late July to early August and cultivate them like May beets. After harvesting them in October and November, store them in boxes of dry sand in a cool place.

Swedes can be puréed, added to stews or served as a side vegetable. They are delicious mashed with carrots, butter and ground black pepper. Turnips are delicious served in a gratin or glazed.

Viper's grass

Also known as scorzonera, this is a tender, delicately spicy winter vegetable with a nutty taste.

Viper's grass seeds can be sown from March to April or later in August. The plant needs a loose soil rich in humus to allow its long taproot (a long straight root, similar to a parsnip) to develop fully.

The young leaves can be used in salads, cooked as a gratin or served with béchamel sauce. The roots need to be peeled, then cut to size and boiled until tender.

Winter cress

The leaves of winter cress, also known as yellow rocket, are a good source of vitamin C. Use them in winter salads, lightly stewed, or to season your sandwiches. Winter cress can be harvested as late as early December or even beyond in a mild winter.

Taking pleasure in

Fresh or dried herbs taste best, and have the strongest, most fragrant bouquet, when they are picked from your own kitchen garden, window box or flowerpots.

It would have been unthinkable in Victorian times to keep a garden and not have a patch reserved specifically for growing herbs.

Not only are they wonderfully aromatic with delicately coloured flowers, but herbs also have so many different everyday uses.

The active substances herbs contain are ideal ingredients for teas, face creams and beauty lotions. Tied in bunches, they can be used to perfume rooms and they are invaluable for seasoning and flavouring food.

Herbs can also be used in medicinal remedies to help to alleviate pain or to promote physical and mental well-being. Whatever your ailment, there is probably a natural potion that can help. Lavender and lemon balm, for instance, may give you a good night's sleep, peppermint can help to alleviate headaches, camomile and marigold can help to reduce inflammation and sage, thyme and hyssop help to stimulate digestion.

Mixed in salad dressings, sauces or butter, fresh herbs add flavour and nutrition to all kinds of food.

When growing herbs for medicinal or beauty preparations, make sure that you grow the recommended varieties (see Garden herbs, pages 326–331).

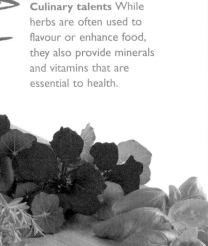

Culinary talents While herbs are often used to flavour or enhance food, they also provide minerals and vitamins that are essential to health.

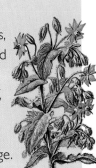

Borage

In medieval times, this plant was said to drive away sorrow and grief, to make people cheerful and to give them courage.

growing herbs

The cultivation and use of traditional herbs

Whether your herb garden has a formal layout or is a collection of pots, place your herbs close to the house, within easy reach of the kitchen. Sunny spots are ideal, since most herbs need sunshine in order to develop their full flavour. However, make sure they are watered thoroughly.

Annual herbs such as basil need to be sown every year as they are killed by frost. Biennials like parsley will flower in the second year and then die after setting seed. Perennial herbs are frost-hardy and new shoots will appear annually. If you prefer, buy the plants ready grown from a garden centre.

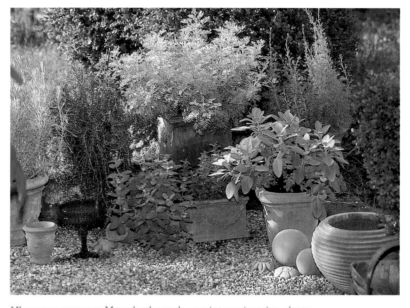

Vigorous growers Many herbs such as mint are invasive plants. Grow these herbs in pots to prevent them taking over your garden.

Basil

This culinary herb has aromatic leaves that release a warm and tangy fragrance when crushed. The flavour of basil is particularly complementary to tomato dishes, salads, cold sauces and dressings.

As a healing plant, it has a relaxing effect on the stomach and intestines and reduces cramps. The fresh leaves have a stronger aroma than when dried or cooked.

Basil is an annual herb. Sow seeds in pots in spring and place them in a greenhouse or on a windowsill to germinate. Basil grows best if taken outside when the frost has passed, in large pots with rich soil, and placed in an open porch or beside a sunny, sheltered wall of your house.

Borage

The Old Masters chose to copy the pure blue colour of borage flowers when painting the robe of the Madonna. The flowers were also used in times past to decorate food or candied as sweets. They are still used to garnish cocktails and summer drinks, especially Pimms. Young leaves can be added to salads as a garnish. They will also add spice to herb sauces and dressings.

Borage is an annual herb, sown from April to July. You can pick the first young leaves around eight weeks later.

Camomile

Probably the best-known healing plant of all, camomile can be used to cure colds and relieve sunburn. An infusion made from dried flowers can be used effectively in steam facials, inhalation treatments and eye baths. Camomile tea is one of the most popular of herbal teas. It not only aids relaxation but can also relieve stomach upsets.

Sow camomile seeds in a sunny patch in March or April. This plant prefers loamy soil rich in humus. Gather the flowerheads on dry summer days.

Dill

With its feathery leaves and delicate flavour, dill is a versatile culinary herb. It is a perfect addition to cucumber, herb butter, sauces and complements fish such as salmon. Dill is best used fresh and added to dishes only after the cooking has finished.

Dill seeds are ideal in marinades or to flavour vinegar. They can also be used in an infusion that can help to strengthen your nails.

The herb has long been used medicinally as an antispasmodic and calmative. Dill tea is an old-fashioned remedy for an upset stomach, hiccups or insomnia. The seeds are used in salt-free diets as they are rich in mineral salt.

Sow seeds each year from April until June, choosing a spot with plenty of sunlight and using soil rich in humus. Water regularly. Harvest dill leaves throughout summer and into autumn.

Fennel

The tender green leaves of fennel have a mild aniseed flavour and are used in salads and sauces and on fish. The seeds are used to season fish and meat, to flavour pickling mixtures, and are sometimes added to bread dough.

Fennel tea is an effective remedy for flatulence and can help to prevent heartburn and constipation. To ease an eye inflammation, steep a compress in the tea and place it on the eyelid.

Fennel is best sown in a warm and sunny patch in April. It will flower from July to September and seeds can be collected until October or November.

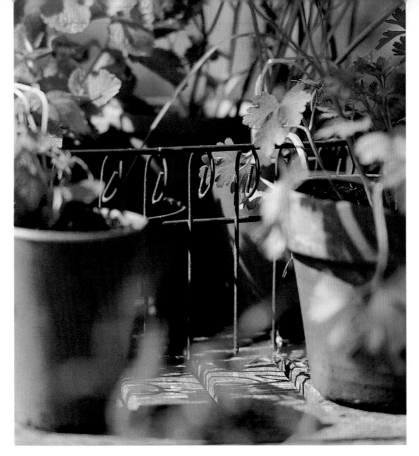

Handy for picking If you are short of space or don't have a garden, many herbs will thrive in pots on a patio or in a window box.

Garlic

Originating from India or central Asia, garlic is a member of the onion family as are chives and spring onions. It is a strong-smelling plant with numerous healing qualities. For example, it is said to kill germs, reduce blood pressure and loosen phlegm, as well as being an excellent tonic for the digestion.

In spring, use the young leaves in the same way as spring onion tops or chives – snip them over dishes for a light oniony taste.

Plant individual garlic cloves in rich, well-drained soil, about 5cm (2in) deep, in autumn or in March. Harvest the bulbs in late summer and hang in strings in a cool, airy place.

Hyssop

In the Middle Ages, hyssop was cultivated in monastery gardens. It has a harsh, slightly bitter, mint-like flavour. It grows as a small bush and usually has blue flowers but is sometimes seen with pink or white blooms.

Hyssop is used in sauces, stews and in herb-flavoured liqueur. The flowers look pretty added to a green salad and taste delicious. Hyssop stimulates digestion and can help to alleviate symptoms of colds, bronchitis and coughing.

Hyssop is a perennial. Sow seeds in pots in March and then plant out in May, choosing a sunny spot with light, well-drained soil. Trim the top shoots to encourage bushy growth.

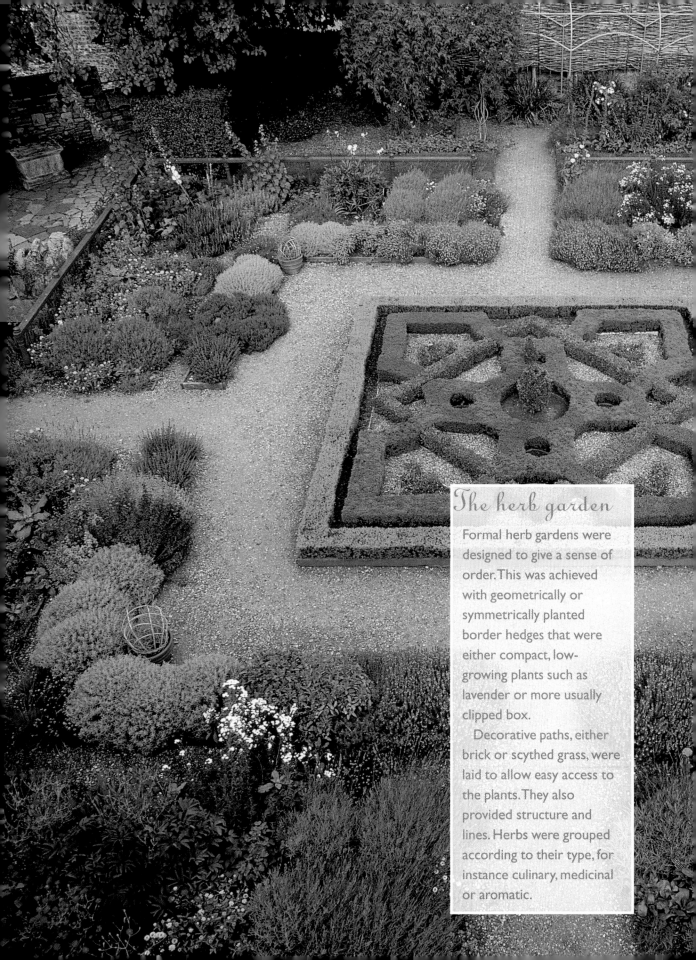

The herb garden

Formal herb gardens were designed to give a sense of order. This was achieved with geometrically or symmetrically planted border hedges that were either compact, low-growing plants such as lavender or more usually clipped box.

Decorative paths, either brick or scythed grass, were laid to allow easy access to the plants. They also provided structure and lines. Herbs were grouped according to their type, for instance culinary, medicinal or aromatic.

Lavender

The number of lavender varieties available today – French or winged, white, silver leaved – would have astounded our grandparents.

As a flavouring, lavender works well with fried or grilled meat, especially lamb. Employ its healing powers by brewing lavender tea as a relaxant, or use the essential oil to relieve headaches. A lavender bath can help to induce sleep. Bags filled with lavender flowers will also help to keep moths at bay.

Sow lavender seeds in pots in March, then plant outside in May. This plant likes plenty of sunlight, little water and a soil rich in lime. It will flower from the end of June to early August, depending on the variety and its location.

Lemon balm

Since the 13th century, when one man reputedly lived to 116 after breakfasting on lemon balm infusion for 50 years, this herb has been thought to prolong life.

Finely chopped, lemon balm adds a pleasant lemon taste to sauces, desserts and drinks. Tea made from its leaves can bring relief from chronic bronchial catarrh.

Sow lemon balm seeds in the ground in April. The herb prefers porous soil rich in humus. Harvest the leaves in summer. Self-sown seedlings can be a nuisance, but these are easy to uproot.

Herb sauce This quick, simple sauce can be on the table just hours after picking the herbs that flavour it fresh from your garden.

HERB SAUCE

This cold herb sauce is delicious on salads or served with meat or fish. It is best made using as many different herbs as possible. Ideal ingredients are basil, dill leaves, borage, nasturtium leaves, parsley, garlic tops (or garlic chives) and salad burnet.

3 tablespoons fresh herbs, chopped
2 tablespoons lemon juice
½ teaspoon finely grated lemon zest
2 drops chilli sauce (optional)
salt
freshly ground black pepper
175ml (6fl oz) olive oil

Mix the herbs, lemon juice, zest, chilli sauce and seasoning together, then slowly whisk in the oil using a hand blender set on a low speed or a fork. Leave to infuse for 3 hours. This sauce will keep for up to two days in the fridge.

Marigold

The marigold was much used in traditional medicine. Generally prepared as a tea or ointment, its orange-yellow petals can also be used to add colour to butter and cheese or to garnish green salads.

Marigold is an annual plant with modest demands in terms of soil and location. Sow the seeds in the ground in March. Once this plant has taken up residence in your garden, it will self-seed each year.

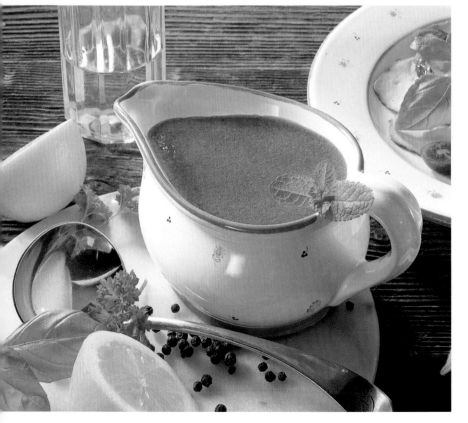

Nasturtium

This herb is also known as Indian cress. Its leaves and flowers contain vitamin C and have antibiotic properties. The slightly piquant flavour of the leaves and the colours of the flowers make it an ideal salad ingredient. Unripe seeds can be used as a substitute for capers.

The seeds can be sown in humus-rich soil in May. The herb will thrive in a semi-shaded spot, but requires regular watering.

Parsley

The leaves and stems of parsley stimulate the appetite and are rich in iron and vitamins A, B and C. They make a soothing eye bath and can be chewed to freshen the breath.

Sow the seeds in humus-rich ground in March. Parsley is a frost-hardy biennial. Cover seedlings sown in late summer with gardening fleece to protect them in winter and you will harvest fresh parsley by early spring.

Peppermint

This pungent herb can be used fresh or dried in sauces or with game, veal, fish, fruit and in drinks. It can also be used to help combat flatulence, nausea, headaches and colds.

Mint spreads prolifically, but can be propagated by offshoots planted out in April or May. It prefers moist, loamy soil in a semi-shaded location.

Harvest peppermint leaves throughout summer. Just before it flowers, cut the stems close to ground level and it will grow up again the next year.

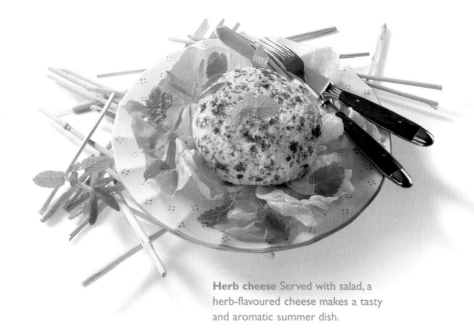

Herb cheese Served with salad, a herb-flavoured cheese makes a tasty and aromatic summer dish.

HERB CHEESE

Place this deliciously spiced cheese on a bed of salad leaves and serve with bread or jacket potatoes. Serves four.

200g (7oz) full-fat soft cheese
55g (2oz) soft butter
1 tablespoon cream
1 teaspoon each of dill,
    fennel leaves, parsley,
    salad burnet, nasturtium
    and lemon balm
marigold flowers to garnish

Mash the cheese with a fork. Finely chop the herbs. Add the butter, cream and herbs to the cheese and stir thoroughly. Shape the mixture into four rounds and serve on beds of lettuce. Garnish with the marigold flowers.

Rosemary

The powerful aroma of rosemary cooked with grilled meat, fried potatoes and tomatoes is wonderful. The stems can be scattered on a barbecue to discourage insects. The herb also contains an essential oil that helps to boost circulation and stimulate digestion.

Rosemary loves warmth and is usually only winter hardy if cultivated in a protected spot. When pot grown, keep it fully exposed to the sun. In winter, place rosemary in a cool but bright spot indoors and do not overwater it.

Rosemary

Traditionally served with lamb, rosemary can also be used in sweet dishes. It adds a distinctive flavour when infused in creams and custards.

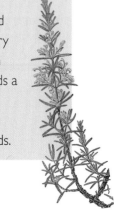

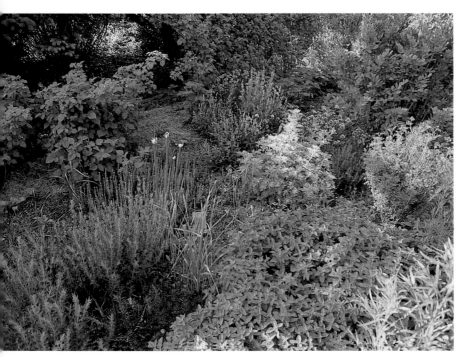

Colourful herbs A herb garden need not be a formal affair.
Grow plants for their foliage, colour and scent.

Winter savory

The leaves of perennial savory, or winter savory as it is also known, can be harvested most of the year. As it grows, it turns into a low, woody shrub. Its spicy, peppery flavour is stronger than that of the annual, or summer, variety.

Use this herb to season lamb and pork or add it to fried potatoes and stews. Savory is an ideal accompaniment to foods that may be hard to digest, such as beans.

Sow winter savory either in pots at the end of March or directly into a sunny patch of soil in May. Harvest the most flavoursome and tender leaves in July to August.

Sage

Aromatic sage is ideal for flavouring poultry, lamb, bacon or pork roasts and fish soups. It is also a versatile healing plant that is said to stimulate digestion and combat sore throats and ulcers.

Sage is an evergreen perennial that can be harvested throughout the year. Sow seeds in pots indoors in March, then plant out the seedlings in May.

Leave about 30-40cm (12-16in) between each plant, as the sage will eventually grow into small woody shrubs that dislike being pruned or cut back too hard.

St John's wort

This herb is used for healing purposes only. The leaves and flowers are harvested and added to oil or dried to make tea. Its flowers contain an essential oil that can soothe nerves, induce sleep and act as an antidepressant.

St John's wort is a perennial that thrives in the sun and on dry soil. Seeds can be sown directly in the soil in spring or it can be bought as a ready-grown plant. It flowers from mid June to the end of August.

Salad burnet

The leaves of this herb have a nutty, cucumber-like taste. Chop and add them to salads, cream cheese, herb butter, eggs, sauces and dressings. Although mainly used as a culinary herb, salad burnet leaves can be used as a tonic and a mildly diuretic tea.

The seed of this perennial plant can be sown in the ground from March and its tender leaves picked from spring to autumn.

Sage
The special medicinal properties of sage are suggested in its name, which stems from the Latin word *salvia*, meaning 'the healing plant'.

Thyme

Use thyme to season meat, poultry, pizzas and potatoes. It stimulates digestion, acts as a disinfectant and can be infused as a tea to cure hangovers.

Thyme shrubs are perennials that thrive in lime-rich soil and prefer to grow in direct sunlight. Sow the seeds in a pot in March or in the ground from May onwards or buy plants from a nursery.

HERB LIQUEUR

An assortment of herbs such as basil, camomile, lemon balm, mint, sage, rosemary, thyme and hyssop, make a delicious liqueur.

115g (4oz) fresh herb sprigs
1 litre (1¾ pints) vodka
1 unwaxed lemon
1kg (2lb 4oz) sugar
1 litre (1¾ pints) water

Place the sprigs in a glass bottle. Pour the vodka over the herbs and seal with a stopper or lid. Leave to infuse in a warm place for 12 days.

Grate the lemon zest and add to the alcohol mixture. Leave to infuse for another two days.

Place the sugar and water in a pan and bring to the boil, then simmer until the liquid makes a syrup, skimming off any froth. Remove the pan from the heat.

When the syrup is cold, pour it into the alcohol mixture. Seal the bottle and leave to infuse for two more days. Filter the liqueur through a fine sieve. Pour it into a sterilised glass bottle and seal with a stopper or lid.

Aromatic liqueur Containing an array of medicinal herbs, this liqueur is a perfect digestive drink after a rich meal.

Tried & Trusted
Herb aromas

• The aroma of most herbs becomes stronger if the plant is starved of fertiliser. A small amount of mature compost on the surface of the soil will be sufficient.

• Flat-leaved parsley is more aromatic than the curly-leaved variety. However, both make attractive garnishes.

• Herbs are a welcome addition to a low-salt diet, since their flavour penetrates most foods.

• Use fennel and dill flowers as an attractive garnish in summer salads.

• Plant herbs where you will brush by them as you walk so releasing their aroma.

Planting

• Savory seeds need light to germinate. Sow under a thin covering of soil.

• Sow borage seeds throughout the growing season to ensure a regular harvest of young leaves. The older leaves are tough and furry.

• Dill will easily self-seed after the plant has flowered, giving you plants year after year.

• Parsley seedlings do not grow well alongside mature parsley plants, which is why it is best to relocate parsley each season.

• Parsley also needs a long time to germinate. Sow seeds in pots or seed trays, then transplant the seedlings to their final destination when they are about 5cm (2in) high.

• Smaller herb varieties such as basil, thyme, chives or parsley are ideal for planting in window boxes.

Fresh-flower ring

A garland of flowers and foliage can make a colourful centrepiece or can hang decoratively on your front door. Use aromatic herb leaves and bright flowers to greet your visitors.

Decorating your front door with a welcoming garland both in summer and winter is an old tradition. This garland is easily made by simply inserting flowers in a foam base. Alternatively, you could bind twigs around a wire ring and insert the flowers and herb bundles. Buy the foam base at your local florist's or craft shop.

Use flowers with short stems or cut the stems down and then insert the flowers and sprigs of herbs into the florist's foam.

Rounded flowers such as marigolds and camomile are best. Ideal herb leaves are lemon balm, laurel, basil and rosemary. Refresh the foam with a water spray every couple of days.

How to make a fresh-flower ring

▼ Shorten the stems from the **flowers** and **foliage** using a pair of scissors or secateurs. Alternatively, buy **short-stemmed flowers**.

▼ Soak a ring of **florist's foam** in water for several minutes. The water keeps the flowers and foliage alive longer. Insert the flowers and herbs into the foam, making sure that they are attractively and evenly spaced.

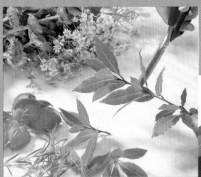

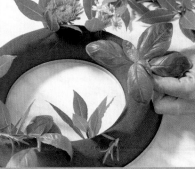

▲ Add a **decorative ribbon loop** for hanging the wreath. If you plan to use the garland as a table decoration, place it on a flat, round dish to prevent the wet foam from damaging your table or cloth.

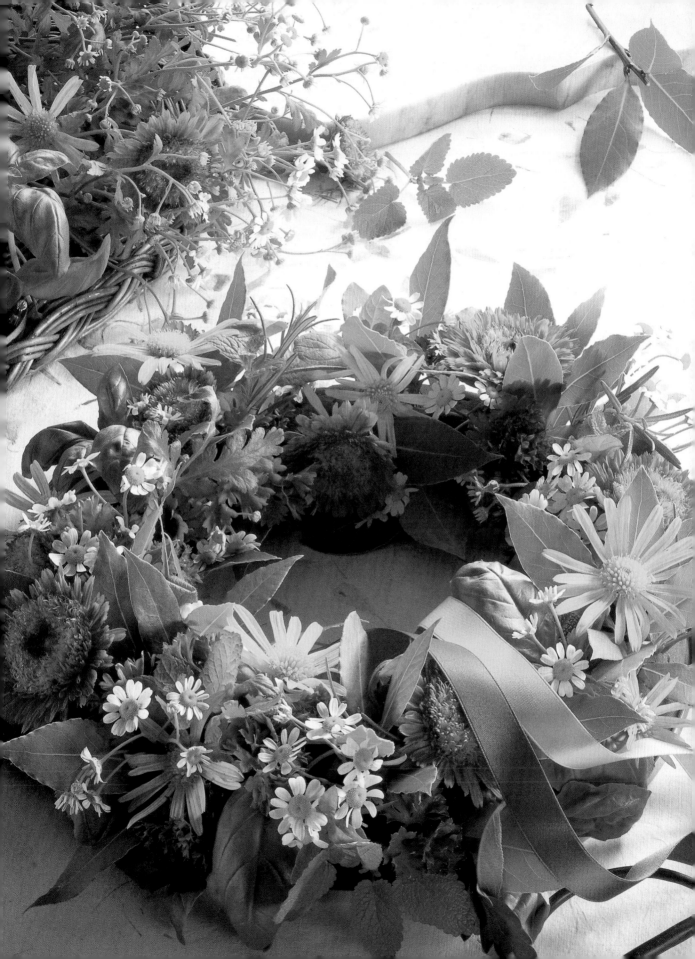

Fruit for picking

You don't have to own a vast orchard to grow your own fruit trees – many varieties can be planted in a small or modestly sized garden.

Whether you enjoy your fruit freshly picked, stewed, baked in a cake, dried or preserved to make jam, there is nothing quite as delicious as home-grown produce.

Traditionally, hardy fruit trees, such as apples and elderberries, were grown in the centre of an English garden or planted in orchards. Apricot, peach and sweet pear trees, which required more warmth, were trained along sheltered south-facing walls in mild areas. In these conditions, the tender fruit would have a better chance of ripening than if grown in unsheltered areas.

In spring, these trees were a pretty sight in the countryside, with blossoms that attracted swarms of bees. In the summer and autumn, the fruit was picked and preserved or stored to help supply the family with essential vitamins and minerals during the cold winter months. The trees in these gardens and orchards may not have borne the flawless fruits that are on sale at the supermarket today. But their taste was unrivalled.

Thanks to a multitude of specialised fruit tree nurseries, there are still a number of interesting traditional species available for planting. Many of these are easy to cultivate and require little care or attention.

Baked apples Plant a traditional tree, such as a Bramley Seedling, that produces cooking apples. Pick the fruit, core and fill, then season it with honey and nuts and bake for an old-fashioned winter dessert.

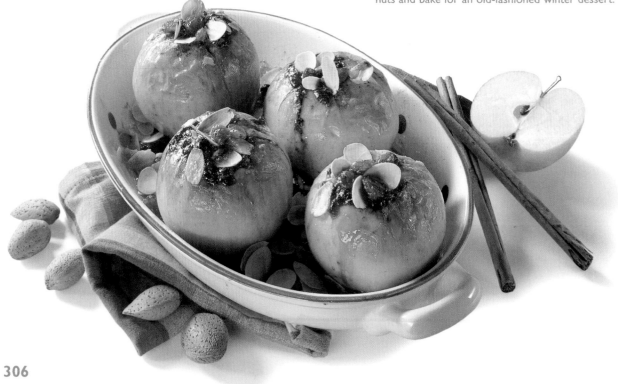

Crunchy apples to get your teeth into

Of all fruit varieties cultivated over the centuries, the apple has been most widely grown. To achieve an exceptional taste, try growing one of these traditional varieties. Plant your apple tree with another that flowers during the same period to provide cross-pollination.

Laxton's Superb

This sweet and aromatic apple has firm, juicy white flesh and a yellow-green skin, blushed with crimson. The tree grows vigorously and is a generous cropper. Harvest in September and store for eating between November and February.

Orleans Reinette

A large, high-quality apple from a strong, upright tree, the Orleans Reinette has a sweet rich flavour. The pale yellow flesh is crisp and juicy, while the skin is a golden russet. Harvest in September and store in a cool, dry place. Eat between December and February.

Tydeman's Late Orange

This apple is small to medium-sized from a tree with vigorous growth. It has aromatic crisp flesh and golden yellow skin with an orange-red blush. Harvest the fruit in September and keep in a cool, dry place for eating between January and March.

Worcester Pearmain

Worcester Pearmain is a pale yellow-green apple dappled with scarlet. The ripe flesh is strongly perfumed and sweet. The apples are small to medium, round and conical. The tree crops regularly, with moderate growth. The fruit is ready to eat between September to October.

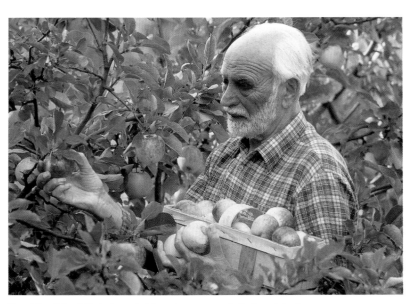

Freshly picked Fruit intended for storage needs to be picked and transported carefully to avoid bruising. Store apples in a cool, dry place such as a cellar or shed.

Fruit picker

Before the invention of extending ladders, our grandparents used long-handled fruit pickers. These devices were fitted with wire 'cages' to gently pick the fruit from the highest branches and save any prize specimens from the hungry birds.

BAKED APPLES

The ideal varieties for cooking are Bramley Seedling and Howgate Wonder, though some other sharp apples will do just as well.

8 large apples
8 teaspoons redcurrant jelly
4 tablespoons brown sugar
pinch of cinnamon
55g (2oz) flaked almonds
55g (2oz) butter

Preheat the oven to 180°C (350°F, gas mark 4). Core the apples, leaving them whole. Grease a shallow ovenproof dish and arrange the apples in it. Spoon the jelly into the apples and sprinkle a mixture of sugar and cinnamon over them. Place the almonds and small knobs of butter on top. Bake for about 20 minutes until tender but not falling apart.

Pears – fresh or preserved

Pear trees flower earlier in the year than apple trees, so they risk having their buds burnt by frost. This is why they need to be planted in a sheltered position. However, some hardier varieties have been developed to suit the weather conditions in cooler areas.

Merton Pride

This pear has an excellent flavour, with creamy white, firm and juicy flesh. The fruits are pale green, medium to large, with a conical shape. For cross-pollination, plant the tree with one early and one mid-season flowering pear tree. The fruits are ready to eat in mid to late September.

Beurré Hardy

A medium to large pear with a sweet flavour, juicy white flesh and a yellow-green skin with a brown russet blush. The tree can be planted on its own and grows vigorously, but is sometimes slow to start bearing fruit. Pick the pears when they are hard and leave them to ripen in a store – they will be ready to eat in mid October.

Conference

This juicy pear is long and thin with a dark olive green skin and sweet, creamy white flesh. Plant the tree with one early and one late-flowering pear tree. It grows quickly and is a heavy and reliable cropper. The pears are ready to eat in October to mid November.

Doyenne du Comice

The flesh of these medium to large pears is soft, white and juicy, with an excellent flavour and the skin is greeny yellow with a brown flush. Plant the tree with one early and one late-flowering pear tree on a warm and sheltered site. The pears are ready to eat in late October to late November.

Sweet and acid cherries

Cherry trees grow well in exposed areas. Plant them in pairs as most are not self-fertile. Sweet cherries will not pollinate acid cherries.

Merton Bigarreau

The sweet fruits are large and purple becoming almost black when ripe. This is a vigorous variety and a heavy cropper. The fruit ripens from mid to late July.

Morello

The best known acid cherry, with a bittersweet flavour. The skin is bright red with soft, pale flesh. This variety is self-pollinating and crops heavily and regularly. The cherries are ripe in August and September.

CHERRYADE

On hot days, this drink is refreshing served ice cold.

1 kg (2lb 4oz) sweet cherries
1 vanilla pod
2 litres (3 ½ pints) water
juice of 2 lemons
200g (7oz) granulated sugar

Stone the cherries. Take 200g (7oz) of the stones, smash them with a hammer and remove the cores. Split the vanilla pod and scrape out the seeds. Boil the water, add the cores and vanilla seeds, and simmer for 30 minutes. Add the lemon juice and sugar, stirring until the sugar has dissolved. Leave to cool.

Purée the cherries and sieve into a bowl. Sieve the stone liquid into the cherries. Mix well, pour the cherryade into a jug and serve.

Thirst quenching Fresh cherryade is a children's drink rarely seen today. Made from flavoursome varieties of cherry, such as Waterloo or Roundel Heart, it tastes very sweet.

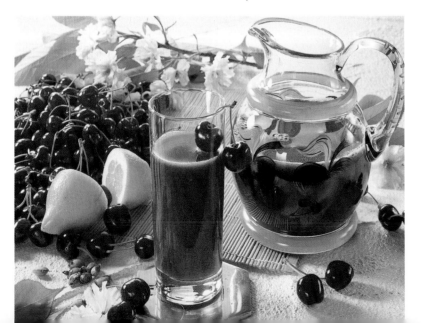

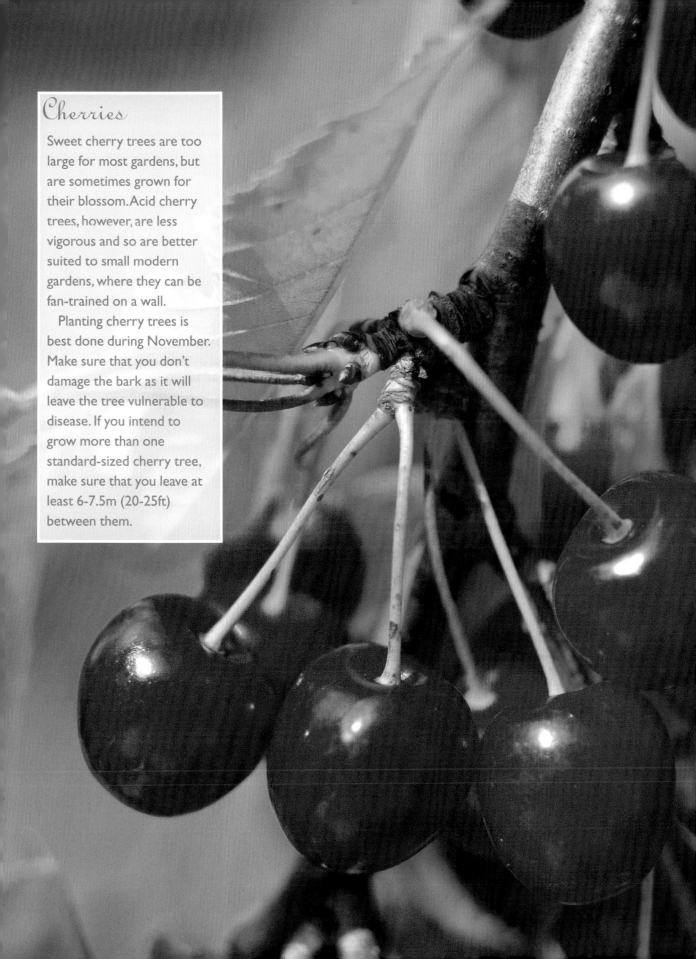

Cherries

Sweet cherry trees are too large for most gardens, but are sometimes grown for their blossom. Acid cherry trees, however, are less vigorous and so are better suited to small modern gardens, where they can be fan-trained on a wall.

Planting cherry trees is best done during November. Make sure that you don't damage the bark as it will leave the tree vulnerable to disease. If you intend to grow more than one standard-sized cherry tree, make sure that you leave at least 6-7.5m (20-25ft) between them.

Plums – abundant and versatile

Plums and damsons are every gardener's delight, for they grow easily and produce plenty of rich fruit over a long period. Cross-pollination is generally required for plum trees. However, if you want to plant only one tree, a Victoria plum is suitable.

While these trees flower early in the year, their blossom lasts for just ten days, unless killed by a late frost. Plum trees are less susceptible to attack from pests and diseases than pear and apple trees, but the fruit does get eaten by birds and wasps.

The ripe fruits cannot be stored for any length of time, but the fruit keeps its flavour when bottled or when used to make jam, juice or fruit brandy.

Kirke's Blue

This variety of plum will grow in most soils and conditions. The tree is compact and so it is perfect for small gardens.

The sweet, spicy flavour of these large, violet-coloured plums is said to be superior to all others. It also makes an ideal prune when dried. The fruit ripens from late August to early September.

Merryweather

This is a large variety of damson that is often mistaken for a plum. The fruit has a good flavour and its thick black skin has a delicate coating.

The tree is self-fertile and hardier than plum trees. The fruit is ready for eating in September and can be frozen successfully if you have a glut.

Victoria

These plums are large and red, with greeny yellow flesh. The fruit ripens from late August to early September. Both Victorias and Kirke's Blue crop heavily when fan-trained against a wall.

Greengage

This small variety of plum has a green skin and, when ripe, a yellow tinge shows through. The fruit can be poached in fruit juice, used to make jam or eaten raw.

Greengages grow best in rich, moist soil. They should be positioned on the sheltered, sunny side of larger plum trees.

GREENGAGE JAM

Greengage jam was a favourite on many tea tables after the Second World War. This quantity will make six 250g (9oz) jars.

900 g (2lb) granulated sugar
200ml (7fl oz) water
900 g (2lb) greengages

Wash the fruit and stone. Crack some of the stones to remove the kernels. Simmer the fruit, water and kernels for 30 minutes until soft and pulpy.

Add the sugar and boil until it has dissolved. Cook the mixture, skimming off any froth, until you reach the setting stage at a temperature of 105°C (221°F). Pour the jam into sterilised glass jam jars and seal.

Fruit fertility

Finding ways of maintaining and increasing the fertility of their trees has long been the aim of fruit growers.

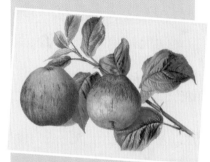

Old gardening books suggest that too much fruit in one year will result in a poor yield the next. To avoid this problem, gardeners would partially disbud their trees to prevent them from bearing too much fruit. This is still practised today.

Cherry plum

Suitable for cooking rather than eating straight from the tree, these are small, scarlet, heart-shaped plums with juicy yellow flesh. The cherry plum tree has vigorous growth and produces a good display of showy blossom.

The trees fruit best when planted in heavy clay soil enriched with nitrogen. If trained against a wall, the tree will need frequent watering in the summer.

Traditional fruit trees for the garden

Quinces and elderberries are among the oldest varieties of fruit harvested from household orchards. Today, however, the quince and the elder have become rare sights in private gardens, even though their fruits are used in a variety of interesting recipes.

Fragrant quinces

Use these aromatic, bright yellow fruits, harvested from late September to late October, to make jellies, fruit stews or baked quince slices.

Add one or two quinces to juices or fruit wines to give them a distinctive aroma. In the early years of the 20th century, people placed quinces in their linen cupboard to perfume the linen and keep pests at bay. Take care not to store quinces near other fruit, since they will affect their taste.

Tea-time delicacy Quinces contain a lot of pectin that encourages liquids to set. These quince slices were originally known as quince 'breads' because of their dough-like texture.

QUINCE SLICES

This recipe takes a little time, but it is well worth waiting for.

2kg (4lb 8oz) quinces
1 unwaxed lemon
2 litres (3½ pints) water
500g (1lb 2oz) sugar

Wash and cut the quinces into quarters. Grate the rind and squeeze the lemon. Place the quinces, water, lemon juice and zest in a pan. Bring to the boil and simmer for about 30 minutes, until the fruit is tender.

Press the mixture through a fine sieve. Return to the pan, then add the sugar and simmer for up to an hour, stirring regularly until the mixture begins to thicken and turn red. Take off the heat and cool.

Grease a baking tray, then spread a 3cm (1¼in) layer of the quince mixture over it. Place the baking tray in the oven on the lowest setting until the mixture is dry and no longer sticky.

Peel the mixture off the tray and cut into diamonds. Sprinkle with sugar to serve.

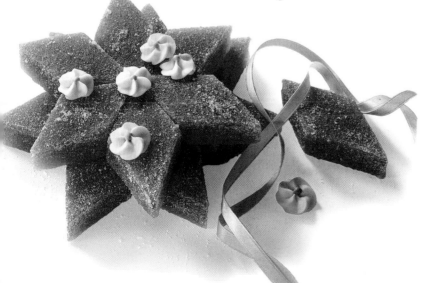

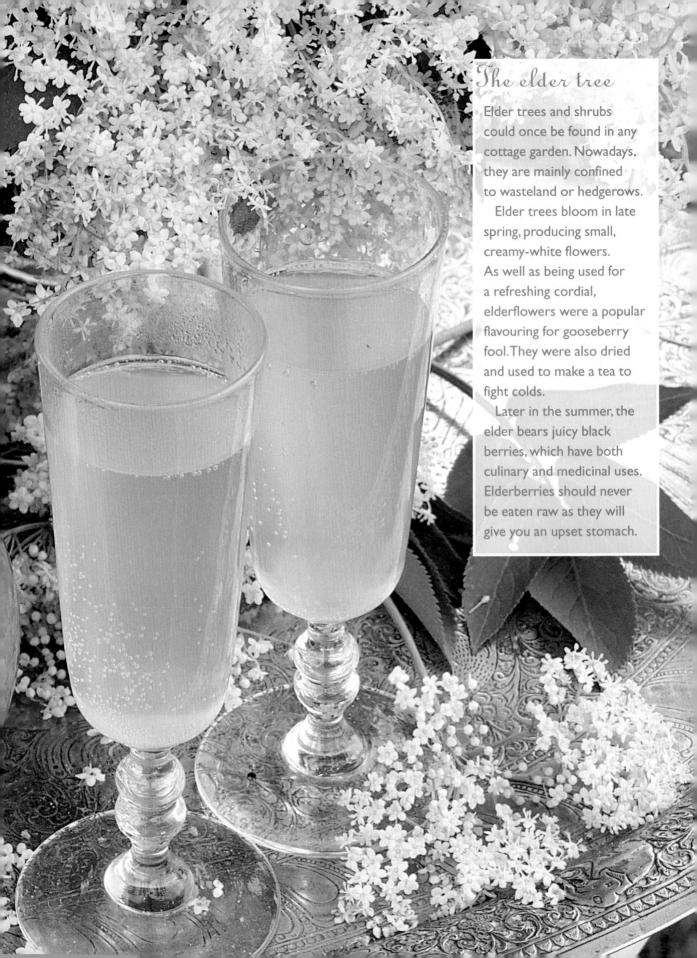

The elder tree

Elder trees and shrubs could once be found in any cottage garden. Nowadays, they are mainly confined to wasteland or hedgerows.

Elder trees bloom in late spring, producing small, creamy-white flowers. As well as being used for a refreshing cordial, elderflowers were a popular flavouring for gooseberry fool. They were also dried and used to make a tea to fight colds.

Later in the summer, the elder bears juicy black berries, which have both culinary and medicinal uses. Elderberries should never be eaten raw as they will give you an upset stomach.

Elder

Use the flowers to make an aromatic syrup, a sparkling wine or a tangy cordial. The berries make excellent juice, wine or jelly.

The flowers, berries and leaves can also be used in remedies to alleviate a number of everyday ailments such as influenza or constipation. Elder trees grow in most places, though they will bear more fruit if planted in rich soil and in a semi-shaded location in the garden.

ELDERFLOWER CORDIAL

This elderflower 'champagne' was once a popular summer drink. The recipe makes about eight 600ml (1 pint) bottles.

1 large unwaxed lemon
2 large heads of elderflowers
675g (1lb 8oz) sugar
2 tablespoons white wine
    vinegar
4.8 litres (8 pints) water

Finely pare the lemon rind and squeeze the juice. Place the elderflowers in a bowl with the juice, rind, sugar and vinegar. Pour over the water, stirring to help the sugar dissolve. Cover the bowl and leave to infuse for 24 hours.

Strain the liquid into strong bottles, such as for beer, champagne or sparkling mineral water. Cork firmly and leave for two weeks, by which time the cordial should be fizzy and ready to drink.

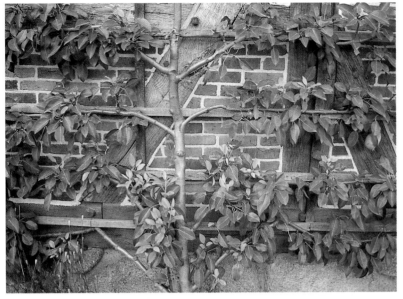

Space savers House walls and trellises lend support to fruit espaliers. The bricks store warmth from the sun and can shelter the fruit from cold winds.

Growing fruit in a small garden

Many old varieties of apples, pears and cherries are too large to grow in a small garden. But a number of these are now available grafted onto dwarfing root stocks which limit their final size. Similarly, smaller half-standard and dwarf fruit trees, with a height of 1-1.4m (3ft 4in-3ft 10in) or less than 1m (3ft 4in) respectively, take up less room.

Espalier trees are also space savers. Most stone fruit, such as peaches and cherries, as well as apples and pears, can be grown in the form of an espalier – either in a fan-shape or horizontally.

Plant apricots or peaches along warm south-facing walls, plums and greengages along walls facing south-west or south-east, and pears and sweet cherries along those facing east or west.

Apples require a more airy spot, so it's best to plant a 'step-over' – a low trained type of espalier – in the middle of the garden. If well cared for, espalier trees will yield handsome fruit.

Pruning trees

An essential tool for all gardeners and especially those planning to cultivate espaliers is a pruning knife. It will allow you to make clean cuts that will heal quickly and avoid disease.

Beautiful, fragrant

Cottage garden flowers are romantic, easy to grow and self-seed, providing endless years of colour. No wonder the old varieties of flowers are sought after today by both town and country gardeners.

In our grandparents' time, rural cottage gardens epitomised the charms of Britain's countryside. Abundant sweet-smelling wild flowers, country garden flowers and herbs created an idyllic scene.

Popular cottage garden flowers included hollyhocks, wallflowers, irises and different varieties of rose with their seductive scents and magnificent colours. These plants are now making a fashionable come-back to many gardens and are easy to obtain from nurseries as plants or seeds.

Cottage or country garden flowers are generally robust growers and, if perennial, can survive the winter

months better than more recent introductions and newly bred varieties. Old plant varieties are often more fragrant than modern species, too. Cottage garden plants often look good as cut flowers or can be dried for bowls of potpourri.

Our grandparents also enjoyed growing house plants such as sweet-scented gardenias, porcelain-like wax plants, satin Cape primroses or the exotic amaryllis with its large, trumpet-shaped flowers.

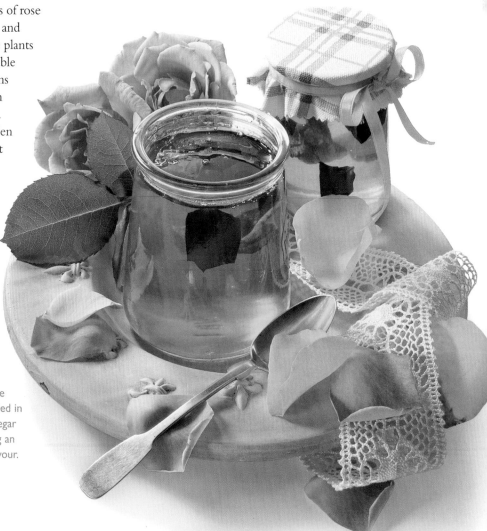

Fragrant food Rose petals can be included in recipes for jelly, vinegar and desserts, adding an unusual, delicate flavour.

garden flowers

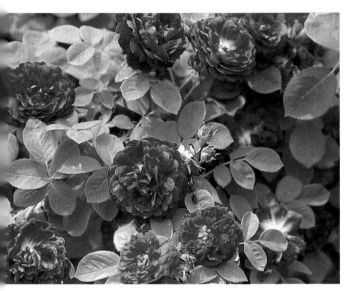

Bourbon roses
These roses form a link between old roses and modern hybrid tea varieties. They have flowers of the old rose shape and fragrance but with the ability to repeat flower.

The 'La ville de Bruxelles', with its satiny blooms, emits a fruity fragrance. The flowers are a rich pink and the plant can grow to a height of 1.5m (5ft). This rose is one of the largest old roses and has luxuriant foliage.

ROSE CREAM WITH SUGARED PETALS

This dessert is the perfect end to a special summer meal – it looks beautiful and tastes delicious. Use thin, scented petals, such as those from a Bourbon or a cabbage rose.

1 egg white
castor sugar
large, dry rose petals
1 pint double cream
4 tablespoons vanilla sugar
squeeze of lemon juice
6 teaspoons rose water
2 drops red food colouring

Whisk the egg white lightly and fill a shallow bowl with the sugar. Line several baking sheets with separating tissue. Pick up each rose petal individually and dip first in the egg white, then in the sugar. Place on the baking sheet. Leave in a warm, dry place overnight. Store between layers of greaseproof paper in an airtight tin.

Put the cream in a large bowl. Add the other ingredients and whisk until thick. Transfer to a glass bowl and strew with the sugared rose petals.

A long tradition of roses through the years

For thousands of years, the rose has seduced us with its extravaganza of blooms and fragrances. By 1870, there were already around 6000 rose species and varieties registered throughout the world. It is the old species roses, such as *Rosa primula* – the incense rose – that have a special kind of charm. They are robust and more resistant to frost than their modern counterparts.

Roses like to grow in well-drained loam soil. Add a generous mulch of compost twice a year and you will be richly rewarded with beautiful flowers. The best time to plant roses is from November to March.

Roses for potpourri should be picked when the petals first open. Hips should be harvested for syrup or wine after the first frosts.

The Bourbon rose

A chance incident of natural crossbreeding between a China and a damask rose created this hybrid plant. It flowers from June to September with large, double blooms that range from white through pink to purple.

Bourbon roses prefer to be planted in sunny positions with supports for their rather lax growth. A superb example of a Bourbon rose is 'Souvenir de la Malmaison', with pastel-pink flowers and a fruity scent.

Damask rose

It was the 13th-century Crusaders who probably discovered the damask rose. Bushes growing near the city of Damascus were brought back to Europe.

Nostalgic memories of fragrant gardens

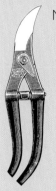
Over the years, gardeners have propagated plants and passed on their expertise. You can still buy old fashioned and well-loved varieties to create your own cottage garden.

The flowers listed here, with their swathes of colour, will all attract wildlife to your garden.

Sweet pea

A fragrant climbing plant, the sweet pea will grow up walls, fences and trellises. Originally from Sicily, it has been cultivated since the 17th century.

Its white, yellow, pink, red and violet flowers appear from June to September. Sow this annual directly into the soil from April until late May.

Stock

A summer annual, stock should be sown in pots in February and planted out when all risk of frost is passed. It produces double flowers from May to August in myriad pastel tones. Its sweet fragrance makes stock a perfect addition to summer bouquets. The plant favours a sunny or semi-shaded spot and rich soil.

Carnation

The beauty and fragrance of carnations have been popular since ancient times. Most varieties are easy to cultivate. The most strongly scented variety is the common garden pink (*Dianthus plumarius*), whose blooms can be frosted for cake decorations. Carnations like sunny flowerbeds or rock gardens. Sow seeds in spring or propagate from cuttings.

Mignonette

A fragrant annual, mignonette is not often seen in gardens nowadays. Its yellow and green flowers may look plain, but they have a very strong perfume from June to September. Sow seeds in April, spacing each one 25cm (10in) apart.

Alba rose

The alba or white cottage rose is one of the most robust types of rose. This old garden rose is probably the result of a natural cross between the wild European dog rose and the damask rose. It grows into a dense bush that can thrive in high altitudes. The sweet-smelling flowers produce sizeable rosehips in the autumn.

'Felicité Parmentier' has strong-scented, thick white-and-pink flowers that weigh heavily on their stems. The foliage is greyish-green.

Cabbage or centifolia rose

The cabbage rose gets its name from the numerous, interfolded petals that make up each bloom. Some flowers contain as many as a hundred petals.

The subtle colouring on each petal and the heavy ball shape of the overall flower make these roses look like pink porcelain.

The romance of the rose

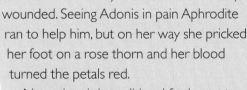

According to Greek legend, roses were always white until Aphrodite's lover Adonis was attacked by a wild boar and fatally wounded. Seeing Adonis in pain Aphrodite ran to help him, but on her way she pricked her foot on a rose thorn and her blood turned the petals red.

Nowadays, it is traditional for lovers to send red roses to their sweethearts as a romantic gesture and token of their love.

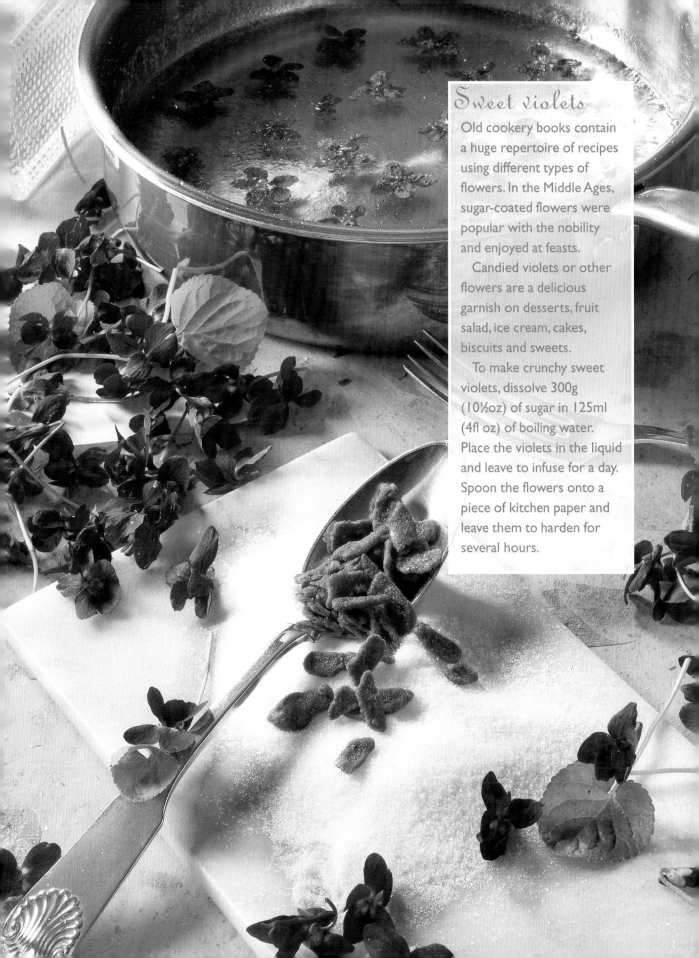

Sweet violets

Old cookery books contain a huge repertoire of recipes using different types of flowers. In the Middle Ages, sugar-coated flowers were popular with the nobility and enjoyed at feasts.

Candied violets or other flowers are a delicious garnish on desserts, fruit salad, ice cream, cakes, biscuits and sweets.

To make crunchy sweet violets, dissolve 300g (10½oz) of sugar in 125ml (4fl oz) of boiling water. Place the violets in the liquid and leave to infuse for a day. Spoon the flowers onto a piece of kitchen paper and leave them to harden for several hours.

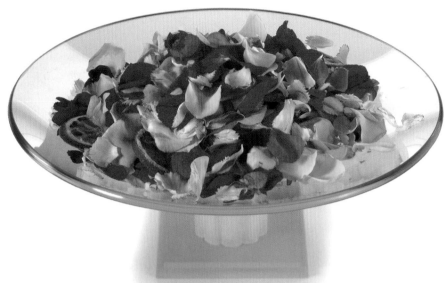

Heady potpourris Old fashioned flowers and scented herb leaves make the best potpourris. For example, use stock, lavender, carnation, rose, honeysuckle, violet and jasmine flowers with the leaves of laurel, rosemary, lemon verbena or geranium.

Violet

One of the first plants to flower in spring is the sweet-scented violet, with its dark purple flowers. It thrives beneath trees, in moist humus-rich soil. Either plant it in spring, or propagate it in autumn using seeds and offshoots.

Polyanthus and primrose

Bright polyanthus flowers in a range of colours have long been a common sight in gardens and are just as popular today. The primrose, another flower of the Primula genus, is a more subtle creamy yellow in colour. Its petals can be crystallised in the same way as those of violets.

Position these plants at the front of a border, as they are quite low growing. Sow seeds from May through to September.

SCENTED POTPOURRI

Pick the flowers early in the morning. Lay them on a piece of kitchen paper and leave to dry in a shady, warm and well-aired place. Make sure the petals and flower heads are totally dry before use.

1 litre (1¾ pints) dried flowers
25g (1oz) orris root powder
1 tablespoon mixed spices
   such as cloves, cinnamon,
   pimento, star anise or
   cardamom

Place the flowers in a decorative glass bowl. Sprinkle on the orris root powder to fix the fragrance. Gently stir in the spices, then place the bowl on a table in the centre of your room.

Tried & Trusted
Past experience
● **Do not plant a rose and a mignonette together, as the plants react badly to each other and will grow poorly or die.**

● **To improve the flower quality and shape of the bush, prune roses in the dormant season or in spring, before young shoots develop.**

● **A mixture of fish blood and bone meal is ideal as a fertiliser for roses.**

Cottage garden
● **Peonies will flower more prolifically if left to grow in their original position. They do not like to be replanted or moved.**

● **Hollyhocks are easily afflicted by rust. Prevent this by spraying them with a horsetail brew (see page 276).**

● **Irises need plenty of air circulating around their leaf bases. Do not place ground-covering plants near them as the foliage will conceal the rhizomes.**

A profusion of flowers for your cottage garden

In many villages, the cottage gardens are the showpiece of the community. They bear witness to the hours of work put in by busy gardeners.

A typical country garden will contain a vegetable patch and herb plot as well as a veritable sea of flowers to give colour all spring and summer and into the autumn.

Crown imperial

A member of the lily family, the crown imperial is a majestic spring flower. It can grow up to 1m (3ft 4in), with its crown displaying red or yellow bells. Plant bulbs in autumn in a sunny spot, with loose and porous soil.

Hollyhock

This biennial can grow to a height of 2m (6ft 8in) and bears a candle-like display of shiny, rose-like flowers. The colours range from white, pale yellow and pink right through to dark red.

Raise plants in small pots in June and July, then transfer them in autumn to a warm position protected from the wind. Hollyhocks require a rich soil.

Iris

The iris has spectacular brightly coloured, sometimes bearded, flowers with sword-shaped leaves. It originally came from the Mediterranean area and was commonly grown in medieval monastery gardens for its healing powers. The root of *Iris* 'Florentina' is known as orris root. Plant bulbs in July or rhizomes in late summer.

Madonna lily

Throughout the ages, the snow-white, sweet-scented Madonna lily has symbolised purity. Plant lily bulbs in August in well-drained soil, making sure they are embedded no deeper than 3cm (1¼in). They can also be grown in pots and tubs.

Peony

The peony has dense foliage and can grow to a height of 80cm (2ft 6in). Apart from the classic dark-red variety, pink and white flowers have also been cultivated.

Peonies like a rich humus soil and a sunny to semi-shaded position. Do not cover the roots with more than 3cm (1¼in) of soil or they won't flower.

Wallflower

The wallflower has yellow or red-gold blooms in spring. Its strong fragrance will perfume any cottage garden.

Sow seeds in June in a sunny spot protected from the wind for flowers the following year. Wallflowers grow well with bulbs and other early plants.

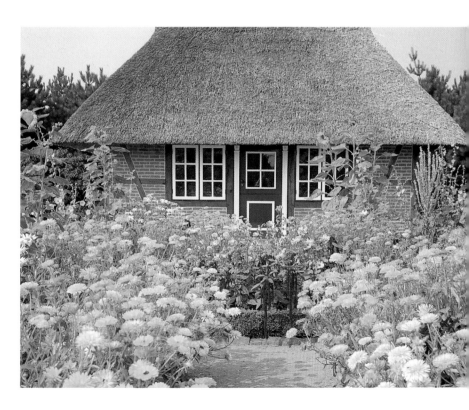

An idyllic garden Long-stemmed sunflowers and a mass of marigolds create a perfect planting arrangement for a traditional cottage garden. Long grasses and herbs also add to the freedom of the planting plan.

A flower basket

A dried arrangement of cottage garden flowers will add a charm to your home all year round. Combine bright-coloured flowers with sprigs of herbs, seed pods and different types of grass.

When you next pick summer flowers for drying, cut a supply of herbs to accompany them. Many herbs perfectly complement a floral arrangement and act as a foil to brighter colours. Yellowy green dill, grey-green southernwood, silvery white wormwood, white mayweed or the white-and-red flower heads of valerian are all traditionally used in bouquets. By using herbs as well as flowers, you can make new arrangements the whole year round.

Seed pods and different types of long-stemmed grass can also look decorative in an arrangement. Dry the plants yourself (see Drying fresh herbs, pages 278–279) or buy ready-dried material.

When you create your flower basket, spray a little water on the dried plants to prevent them from snapping. Replace soft or brittle stems with wire. A basket is an ideal way to display a dried arrangement and will make an excellent gift.

How to make a dried-flower basket
Makes one arrangement

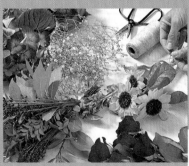

▲ Pick fresh flowers such as **roses** and **sunflowers**, **long-stemmed grasses** and **herbs**. Tie them together with raffia and hang up to dry in a warm place for two weeks.

▼ Cut a piece of **florist's foam** to fit your **basket**. Cover the foam with a layer of **moss**, using **florist's wire** to secure it in place. Insert the foam in the basket.

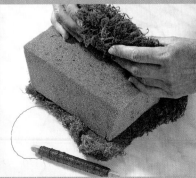

▼ Shorten the flowers, grasses, leaves and herbs to a length of 15-20cm (6-8in) and insert them in the foam. If any stems are difficult to push in, make an initial hole with a knitting needle.

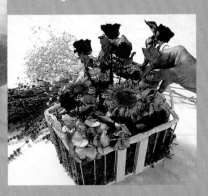

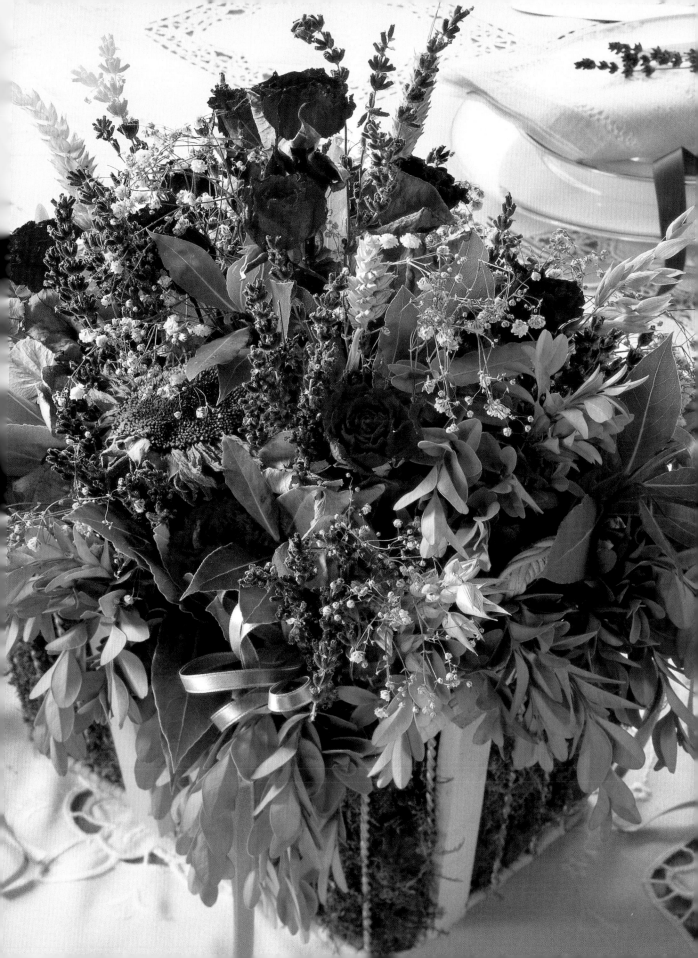

Caring for flowering and foliage houseplants

The Victorians took pride in their houseplants, displaying them on grand tiered stands in their hallways or conservatories.

These plants were not as widely available and as cheap as they are today, so they received lavish care and attention.

Houseplants that have remained popular since our grandparents' times include flowering and foliage plants, such as the aspidistra, palms and ferns, cacti and seasonal bulbs.

Gardenia

The white waxy flowers of the gardenia, or Cape jasmine, can fill a room with their powerful fragrance.

It is quite a challenging plant to grow as it needs to be placed in a bright position, but away from direct sunlight. The plant also needs to be sprayed daily with water to encourage flowering.

Jasmine

Climbing jasmine was grown by our grandparents in their greenhouses or conservatories and brought into the house to flower through the winter.

The plant produces hundreds of tiny white flowers with an attractive scent. Its leaves and stems look attractive trained around a loop, wire or decorative frame.

Wax plant

This plant is also known as hoya and is grown as much for its dark green, fleshy leaves as its waxy, star-like flowers.

The plant needs to be placed in a well-lit position and watered regularly. It should be sprayed with water to increase the humidity and placed as far away as possible from any radiators.

SPRING ON THE WINDOWSILL

Even our great-grandmothers were fond of growing early flowering bulbs to enjoy during the wintry weather.

2-3 pieces charcoal
  or
1 handful oyster shell
23cm (9in) diameter pot
bulb fibre or soil-less compost
6 hyacinth bulbs
sand
cardboard or wooden box

In early September to mid October, place the pieces of charcoal or oyster shell in the bottom of the pot. Fill it halfway with compost and position the bulbs. Add more compost to cover the bulbs and water generously.

Place the pot in the box, fill it with sand or compost and store it in a dark place for eight weeks.

Once all the bulbs have begun to sprout, take the pot out of the box and place it on a windowsill. Cover the compost with moss once the flower buds have formed.

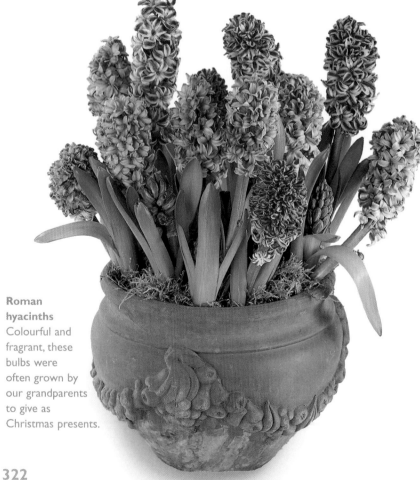

Roman hyacinths Colourful and fragrant, these bulbs were often grown by our grandparents to give as Christmas presents.

322

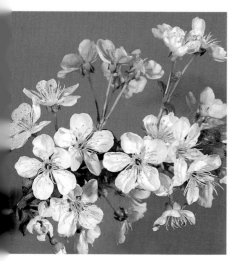

Flowering twigs Trees, such as willow and cherry produce buds in winter that will open when brought indoors.

Amaryllis

The amaryllis has long been one of the most popular winter and spring flowering plants grown indoors. Its bulb produces three huge trumpet-like flowers in white, pink or red shades. These contrast with its rounded sword-shaped leaves.

At the end of December, embed the bulb in a pot of well-drained soil, making sure that the top half is exposed. Amaryllis prefer a bright to full sunny environment, with moderate amounts of water and fortnightly feeding.

Cape primrose

The leaf rosette of the Cape primrose, or Streptocarpus, produces velvety, trumpet-shaped flowers. Their colours range from white through pink to brilliant red, or from light blue through pale lilac to a deep violet.

The plant requires plenty of light to maintain flowering but no direct sunlight. Water moderately and feed once a fortnight.

Tried & Trusted

Propagation

- Many houseplants, such as begonias, spider plants and African violets, can be propagated by taking cuttings. Cut the tips of the shoots off the parent plant and place them in multi-purpose compost.

- To prevent cuttings from drying out and dying, secure a polythene bag over the pot.

Houseplants

- Gardenia, hibiscus and camellia buds tend to fall off easily, so try not to move the plants once the first buds have appeared.

- Do not remove the old flower heads from wax plants. Even the old shoots produce new flowers.

- Regularly remove dead stems, flowers and leaves from other plants before they rot.

- When watering calcium-sensitive houseplants, such as azaleas and forest cacti, use rainwater or soften tap water by boiling it, then allowing it to cool before use.

- Position your houseplants with care. Many indoor plants do not take kindly to draughts and will die if placed near an open window in winter.

- When moving houseplants or winter-stored patio plants outdoors for the summer, gradually expose the plants to the sun. Initially place them outside in a shady spot in the morning or evening before placing them outdoors permanently.

- Kill leaf mites on houseplants with a stinging nettle brew. Infuse 100g (3½oz) of fresh nettles in 1 litre (1¾ pints) of water for 24 hours. Strain the liquid, then spray it on the leaves.

Cut flowers

- Ripe fruit emits a gas that makes cut flowers wither. So do not place fruit bowls alongside vases of flowers.

- When daffodils are cut, they secrete a slimy substance that can poison other flowers. To avoid this, place them in a separate vase of water for several hours. Once this secretion has stopped, you can put them in a vase with the other blooms.

- When you arrange flowers in a vase, pull off any small leaves and buds growing low down on the stems. If they are immersed in the water, they will quickly rot.

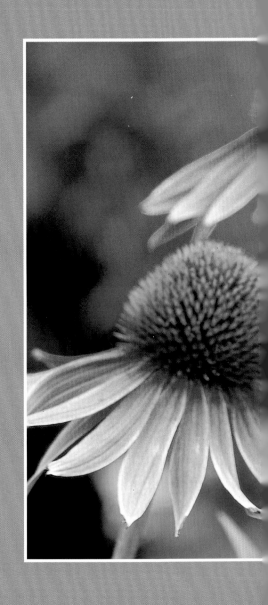

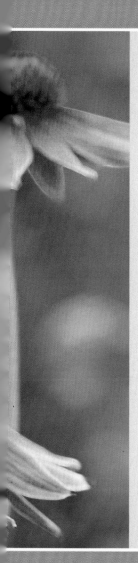

Fact file

When using our grandparents' recipes, remedies and methods, we will need to adapt them to the modern age. And a number of ingredients that were widely available just 50 years ago may now have to be tracked down.

On pages 326–331 a catalogue of herbs will help you to identify the right variety to grow when making your own treatments. Pages 332–339 list unusual products and where to buy them.

CHAPTER 6

Garden herbs

Herbs, both dried and fresh, are used for many of the recipes in this book – as cleaning agents, beauty products, for medicinal remedies or in the garden.

Most of the herbs listed here are available dried from herbalists, but others are more difficult to obtain or need to be used fresh.

Make sure that you grow the correct species and variety. This is particularly important when using herbs for medicinal remedies.

When ingesting dried herbs or dried herb mixtures, the maximum daily dosage rarely exceeds 25g (1oz) per 600ml (1 pint) of liquid a day.

If you prefer to grow your own herbs and use them fresh, a general conversion is that 15g (½oz) dried herbs is the equivalent measure to 55g (2oz) fresh herbs. You can also grow your own herbs and dry them if the dried herbs are not available commercially (see Drying fresh herbs, pages 278-9).

The types of herbs and their quantities are listed in the ingredients for each recipe. Keep strictly to these weights for the best results.

Agrimony/Liverwort
(Agrimonia eupatoria)
PART USED Leaf
TIPS AND USES The leaves have anti-inflammatory and astringent properties; may be used in footbaths.

Angelica *(Angelica archangelica)*
PART USED Whole plant
TIPS AND USES When crystallising, cut the stem in June. Harvest the leaves before the flowers appear.

Aniseed/Anise
(Pimpinella anisum)
PART USED Seed and flower
TIPS AND USES Harvest the seeds by cutting the plant to ground level when the fruit turns grey-green at the tips. Dried flowers are used in spicy potpourris.

Arnica *(Arnica montana)*
PART USED Flower
TIPS AND USES Fresh flowers are used to make tinctures and ointments. This plant is toxic if taken internally. Dried arnica flowers are not readily available.

Ash *(Fraxinus)*
PART USED Leaf
TIPS AND USES The dried leaves when taken as a herbal infusion may reduce the effect of cellulite.

Bear's garlic/Ramsons
(Allium ursinum)
PART USED Leaf and bulb
TIPS AND USES Infused leaves may improve circulation and help to combat impotence. Bear's garlic should be bought and planted as bulbs.

Bearberry/Uva-ursi
(Arctostaphylos uva-ursi)
PART USED Leaf
TIPS AND USES The leaves have antiseptic and diuretic properties.

Bilberry *(Vaccinium myrtillus)*
PART USED Fruit
TIPS AND USES Dried fruit may stop diarrhoea in teething children.

Birch *(Betula alba)*
PART USED Leaf
TIPS AND USES Dried leaves may increase the metabolic rate. Birch-leaf manure prevents mildew on roses.

Blackberry *(Rubus idaeus)*
PART USED Leaf and fruit
TIPS AND USES Dried leaves can be used to make an invigorating bath essence.

Blackcurrant *(Ribes nigrum)*
PART USED Leaf and fruit
TIPS AND USES Fresh leaves in a mouthwash may soothe a sore throat.

Bogbean *(Menyanthes trifoliata)*
PART USED Leaf
TIPS AND USES An ancient medicinal plant best grown in boggy conditions.

Borage *(Borago officinalis)*
PART USED Leaf and flower
TIPS AND USES The plant will freely self-seed in light, dry soil. The purple and blue flowers are also edible.

Burdock/Great burr
(Arctium lappa)
PART USED Leaf and flower
TIPS AND USES May help to purify the blood and to cure skin diseases.

Calendula/Marigold
(Calendula officinalis)
PART USED Leaf and flower
TIPS AND USES The flowers and leaves are used for culinary purposes. Flowers are also used in potpourris and in medicinal remedies.

Camomile, perennial
(Chamaemelum nobile)
PART USED Leaf and flower
TIPS AND USES The leaves and flowers are infused both for medicinal teas and steam facials. The leaves and flowers are also dried for use in potpourris.

Caraway *(Carum carvi)*
PART USED Whole plant
TIPS AND USES A biennial plant, the seeds are used in cooking and have medicinal properties. The aromatic leaves are eaten in salads.

Catmint/Catnip
(Nepeta cataria)
PART USED Shoot tip
TIPS AND USES The top young leaves are used in teas and potpourris. The plant prefers chalky soil.

Centaury
(Centaurium erythraea)
PART USED Leaf
TIPS AND USES A traditional medicinal herb that may help to aid digestion.

Coltsfoot *(Tussilago farfara)*
PART USED Leaf
TIPS AND USES An invasive perennial. Fresh leaves are eaten in salads. They can also be used medicinally.

Comfrey (Symphytum officinale)
PART USED Leaf and root
TIPS AND USES The roots and leaves can be infused to soften the skin. They are also used for culinary and medicinal purposes. Fresh leaves make good manure.

Coneflower
(Echinacea purpurea)
PART USED Leaf and root
TIPS AND USES An American medicinal plant that may purify the blood. The plant likes well-drained soil in full sun.

Cornflower
(Centaurea cyanus)
PART USED Flower
TIPS AND USES The dried flowers can be made into a rinse to revitalise dull grey hair. Dried flowers are not readily available.

Couchgrass/Witchgrass
(Agropyron repens)
PART USED Root
TIPS AND USES The roots may be infused with other herbs to relieve migraine and combat melancholy.

Daisy (Bellis perennis)
PART USED Leaf and flower
TIPS AND USES The flowers and leaves may alleviate gout. Dried daisies are not readily available.

Dandelion
(Taraxacum officinale)
PART USED Whole plant
TIPS AND USES The leaves are high in vitamins. The yellow flowers can be used in steam facials.

Deadnettle (Lamium album)
PART USED Leaf
TIPS AND USES An infusion of dried leaves may help to ease period pains. Liquid manure made from fresh leaves prevents mildew on roses. Dried leaves are not readily available.

Dog's mercury
(Mercurialis perennis)
PART USED Leaf
TIPS AND USES As an infusion, the leaves may help to alleviate athlete's foot. Dried leaves are not readily available.

Dogwood, Jamaican
(Cornaceae)
PART USED Bark
TIPS AND USES Powdered bark may bring relief from migraine. It is best bought from a herbalist.

Elder (Sambucus nigra)
PART USED Flower and fruit
TIPS AND USES Dried and fresh flowers and berries are used for culinary and medicinal purposes.

Elecampane/Inula
(Inula helenium)
PART USED Root
TIPS AND USES The dried medicinal roots may alleviate bronchial disorders.

Eucalyptus
(Eucalyptus globulus)
PART USED Leaf
TIPS AND USES The aromatic leaves can be used dried or fresh in potpourris and air freshening remedies.

Evening primrose
(Oenothera biennis)
PART USED Leaf, seed and stem
TIPS AND USES Oil from the seeds may combat menstrual problems. Dried evening primroses are not readily available.

Eyebright (Euphrasia officinalis)
PART USED Leaf
TIPS AND USES An annual plant that is difficult to grow. Dried leaves may be used for eye complaints.

Flag iris (Iris pseudacorus)
PART USED Root
TIPS AND USES A water marginal plant. The dried root can be infused for a relaxing herbal bath.

Fennel (Foeniculum vulgare)
PART USED Whole plant
TIPS AND USES Fresh and dried seeds and leaves are used for cosmetic and culinary purposes.

Gentian/Yellow gentian
(Gentiana lutea)
PART USED Root
TIPS AND USES The roots have been commonly used since the Middle Ages in medicinal tonics.

Golden rod
(Solidago virgaurea)
PART USED Leaf
TIPS AND USES The leaves may be used for stomach and kidney ailments and may help to heal wounds.

Greater burnet
(Sanguisorba officinalis)
PART USED Leaf
TIPS AND USES Leaves have cooling properties and may stem bleeding. Dried leaves are not readily available.

Hawthorn
(Crataegus laevigata)
PART USED Flower and fruit
TIPS AND USES The dried flowers may be used in medicinal teas to help to improve circulation.

Heartsease/Pansy
(Viola tricolor)
PART USED Leaf and flower
TIPS AND USES Gather the leaves and flowers before they are fully out and dry them immediately.

Heather (Erica)
PART USED Flower
TIPS AND USES Fresh flowers may be infused for sun oil. Never pick wild heather.

Henna (Lawsonia inermis)
PART USED Leaf
TIPS AND USES Powdered leaves are best bought from a herbalist.

Holy thistle/Blessed thistle (Cnicus benedictus)
PART USED Aerial part and seed
TIPS AND USES Dried leaves may be infused as a herbal tonic.

Hops (Humulus lupulus)
PART USED Flower/strobile
TIPS AND USES An infusion at night may prevent insomnia. Dried flowers under your pillow may promote sleep.

327

Horehound, white and black

(Marrubium vulgare)

PART USED Leaf

TIPS AND USES Dried leaves may be infused to cure coughs. A fresh-leaf infusion can prevent cankerworm in trees.

Horse chestnut

(Aesculus hippocastanum)

PART USED Leaf and fruit

TIPS AND USES Dried leaves and fruit may help to strengthen blood vessels when used as a footbath.

Horseradish

(Armoracia rusticana)

PART USED Leaf and root

TIPS AND USES The fresh roots are traditionally grated for sauce. The leaves may be infused to combat blossom rot and fungal disease in stone fruits.

Horsetail *(Equisetum arvense)*

PART USED 'Needle' and stem

TIPS AND USES A wild perennial that is extremely invasive. The herb is more potent when fresh but is available dried.

Hyssop *(Hyssopus officinalis)*

PART USED Whole plant

TIPS AND USES Grow hyssop near cabbages to deter cabbage-white butterflies. Do not take this herb during pregnancy.

Iceland lichen

(Cetraria islandica)

PART USED Aerial parts

TIPS AND USES The lichen may help to soothe skin irritation when infused in water for washing.

Ivy, ground

(Glechoma hederacea)

PART USED Leaf

TIPS AND USES Dried leaves may relieve sunburn, firm up crow's feet and possibly reduce cellulite. Fresh leaves are used in a washing treatment for silk.

Jasmine *(Jasminum)*

PART USED Flower

TIPS AND USES The flowers are used in potpourris and for decoration. They are also used in cosmetics.

Lady's bedstraw

(Galium verum)

PART USED Aerial part

TIPS AND USES The foliage is used in potpourris and for colouring cheese.

Lady's mantle

(Alchemilla vulgaris)

PART USED Leaf

TIPS AND USES Dried leaves may be used in steam facials and compresses to reduce inflammation. They can also be taken as a herbal tea.

Lavender

(Lavandula angustifolia)

PART USED Flower

TIPS AND USES The flowers can be infused. They are also added to sachets to ward off moths.

Lemon *(Citrus limon)*

PART USED Leaf and fruit

TIPS AND USES Infuse the leaves in teas to aid breathing. Lemon peel is used for medicinal and culinary purposes. Trees will not fruit outdoors. Dried leaves are not readily available.

Lemon balm/Balm

(Melissa officinalis)

PART USED Leaf

TIPS AND USES The young leaves are tasty in salads. Juice from the leaves is used in furniture polish. Dried leaves may be infused as a herbal tea.

Lemon verbena

(Aloysia triphylla)

PART USED Leaf

TIPS AND USES Dried leaves are used in potpourri.

Lime *(Tilia europaea)*

PART USED Leaf and blossom

TIPS AND USES The dried blossom is best bought from a herbalist. It may be used to relieve stress.

Lovage *(Levisticum officinale)*

PART USED Whole plant

TIPS AND USES Lovage should not be taken during pregnancy or if you have kidney problems.

Mallow, common

(Malva sylvestris)

PART USED Flower

TIPS AND USES Dried flowers contain medicinal substances that may help to soothe skin problems.

Marshmallow

(Althaea officinalis)

PART USED Leaf and root

TIPS AND USES Infuse the roots as a medicinal tea or use the roots and leaves cosmetically to combat dry hair and hands.

Masterwort

(Peucedanum ostruthium)

PART USED Root

TIPS AND USES The roots are used medicinally and to make a herbal liqueur. Dried masterwort is not readily available.

Meadowsweet

(Filipendula ulmaria)

PART USED Leaf and flower

TIPS AND USES Infused dried flowers may relieve headaches. Both the leaves and flowers are used in potpourris. The flowers are also used to freshen linen.

Mint/Peppermint/ Black mint

(Mentha)

PART USED Leaf

TIPS AND USES Pick the leaves just before the plant flowers. The plant is best grown in a pot to restrain the invasive roots.

Motherwort

(Leonurus cardiaca)

PART USED Aerial parts

TIPS AND USES A herbal infusion may reduce menopausal discomfort.

Mullein *(Verbascum thapsus)*

PART USED Flower

TIPS AND USES The flowers may relieve coughs and asthma. The leaves, stem and seeds are mildly toxic.

Nasturtium

(Trapaeolum majus)

PART USED Leaf, flower and seed

TIPS AND USES The seeds and leaves may prevent hair loss. Use the flowers to decorate salads. Infused leaves may combat woolly aphids. Dried nasturtiums are not readily available.

Oak (Quercus)
PART USED Bark
TIPS AND USES Powdered bark may be used as an anti-inflammatory. It is best bought from a herbalist.

Oat straw (Avena sativa)
PART USED Flowering top
TIPS AND USES The dried flowers are best bought from a herbalist.

Olive (Olea europaea)
PART USED Leaf
TIPS AND USES Trees are available from specialist nurseries for growing in warm conservatories.

Orange, sweet
(Citrus sinensis)
PART USED Blossom and fruit
TIPS AND USES The dried blossom is best bought from a herbalist. It may help to alleviate anxiety.

Orris root (Iris florentina)
PART USED Root
TIPS AND USES The powdered roots are best bought from a herbalist.

Parsley (Petroselinum crispum)
PART USED Leaf and seed
TIPS AND USES The seeds may be infused as an antiseptic tea for colds. The leaves are used for culinary or medicinal purposes.

Passionflower
(Passiflora incarnata)
PART USED Leaf and flower
TIPS AND USES The dried flowers and leaves may soothe colic.

Plantain (Plantago major)
PART USED Leaf
TIPS AND USES The fresh antiseptic leaves may ease insect bites or minor grazes.

Pleurisy (Asclepias tuberosa)
PART USED Root
TIPS AND USES The roots may be beneficial for lung complaints and coughs.

Poplar, white
(Populus alba)
PART USED Bark
TIPS AND USES Powdered white poplar bark is best bought from a herbalist. As a shampoo, it may combat dandruff.

Primrose (Primula vulgaris)
PART USED Flower
TIPS AND USES A flower infusion may prevent insomnia. Dried flowers are not readily available.

Quince (Cydonia oblonga)
PART USED Seed and fruit
TIPS AND USES The fruits are used to make jelly. Their high pectin content helps jam to set. Dried quinces are not readily available.

Restharrow
(Ononis spinosa)
PART USED Leaf and root
TIPS AND USES Dried leaves may be infused to promote metabolic activity. Dried leaves and roots are not readily available.

Ribwort (Plantago lanceolata)
PART USED Leaf
TIPS AND USES Dried leaves as a herbal tea may restore energy and encourage menstrual bleeding.

Rose (Rosa species)
PART USED Hip and petal
TIPS AND USES Rosehips from the dog rose are rich in vitamin C.

Rosebay
(Epilobium parviflorum)
PART USED Leaf
TIPS AND USES The leaves as an infusion may act as a diuretic. Dried leaves are not readily available.

Rosemary
(Rosmarinus officinalis)
PART USED Leaf
TIPS AND USES Dried leaves may stimulate circulation and ease pain.

Rue (Ruta graveolens)
PART USED Leaf and seed
TIPS AND USES Bathe tired eyes in a dried leaf infusion.

Sage (Salvia officinalis)
PART USED Leaf
TIPS AND USES Sage should not be taken in large doses over a long period.

**Sandalwood, red/
Sanderswood**
(Pterodarpus santalinus)
PART USED Bark
TIPS AND USES An Asian or Australasian evergreen tree. The dried bark is best bought from a herbalist.

Savory, winter
(Satureja montana)
PART USED Leaf
TIPS AND USES The leaves may be infused to relieve dry skin.

Sea buckthorn
(Hippophae rhamnoides)
PART USED Fruit
TIPS AND USES Fresh juice may stimulate appetite and is high in vitamin C. The juice is sold as an elixir.

Senna (Cassia senna)
PART USED Leaf and pod
TIPS AND USES This herb acts as a natural laxative. Do not use it regularly.

Silverweed
(Potentilla anserina)
PART USED Aerial parts
TIPS AND USES Dried leaves can be infused to cure headaches. Do not take this herb if you suffer from stomach complaints. Dried silverweed is not readily available.

Sloe/Blackthorn
(Prunus spinosa)
PART USED Flower, leaf and fruit
TIPS AND USES Infuse the flowers and leaves of the blackthorn bush for a tea that can help to relieve itchy skin. The berries are used in sloe gin liqueur. Dried flowers and leaves are not readily available.

Soapwort
(Saponaria officinalis)
PART USED Whole plant
TIPS AND USES The leaves, stem and root can be used to clean delicate fabrics. Dried leaf shampoo may be used to strengthen hair. The root is poisonous.

Sorrel (Rumex acetosa)
PART USED Leaf
TIPS AND USES Infused dried leaves may stimulate the liver. Dried leaves are not readily available.

Southernwood
(Artemesia abrotanum)
PART USED Leaf
TIPS AND USES Dried leaves are used in potpourris and to deter flies.

Speedwell/Veronica
(Veronica officinalis)
PART USED Leaf
TIPS AND USES Dried leaves may help to reduce high blood pressure.

Stag-horn sumach
(Rhus typhina)
PART USED Leaf
TIPS AND USES A cold-water extract made from fresh leaves will kill aphids and potato beetle larvae. Plants are available from garden centres.

Star anise *(Illicium verum)*
PART USED Seed
TIPS AND USES Dried seeds may aid digestion and reduce flatulence. They are also used in cooking and to flavour drinks.

Stinging nettle
(Urtica dioica)
PART USED Leaf
TIPS AND USES Astringent young leaves can be used in steam facials. Fresh leaves can also be used to clean windows without leaving marks. Infused dried leaves are a diuretic.

St John's wort
(Hypericum perforatum)
PART USED Flower
TIPS AND USES A medicinal plant used to treat sprains, relieve menopausal symptoms and ease tension.

Sundew *(Drosera rotundifolia)*
PART USED Aerial parts
TIPS AND USES Dried leaves are combined in a herbal tea that may ease asthma. Dried sundew is not readily available.

Sunflower
(Helianthus annuus)
PART USED Leaf and seed
TIPS AND USES Dried leaves may be infused to relieve fever. Dried leaves are not readily available.

Sweet cicely
(Myrrhis odorata)
PART USED Whole plant
TIPS AND USES Seeds may be tossed in fruit salads or chopped and eaten with ice cream. Fresh leaves are used to sweeten jams, sauces and stewed fruit. When the plant is infused as a herbal tea, it may aid digestion.

Tansy *(Tanacetum vulgare)*
PART USED Leaf
TIPS AND USES Dried leaves may alleviate menstrual cramp. The leaves are used to combat garden mites. Do not use during pregnancy.

Thyme *(Thymus vulgaris)*
PART USED Leaf
TIPS AND USES Dried leaves can be used as a digestive tonic and may fight viruses. It also has culinary uses and is often used to flavour lamb and roast potatoes.

Tormentil/Bloodroot
(Potentilla tormentilla)
PART USED Root
TIPS AND USES The dried roots have astringent and antibiotic properties.

Trigonella/Fenugreek
(Trigonella foenum-graecum)
PART USED Seed
TIPS AND USES The seeds may be used to make a compress on boils. They are also eaten as sprouting seeds.

Valerian
(Valeriana officinalis)
PART USED Leaf and root
TIPS AND USES Fresh leaves will enrich compost. The roots can be used in facial washes or in lotions for acne or skin rashes.

Vervain *(Verbena officinalis)*
PART USED Whole plant
TIPS AND USES Dried leaves can be infused for an eye compress. The plant may be infused as a digestive tea. Use with caution.

Violet, sweet
(Viola odorata)
PART USED Flower
TIPS AND USES The flowers can be candied as sweets. Dried flowers may restore children's energy. As an infusion, the root may relieve bronchitis.

Watercress
(Nasturtium officinale)
PART USED Leaf
TIPS AND USES Fresh juice may clear spots. The leaves can help to strengthen the immune system.

Wild strawberry
(Fragaria vesca)
PART USED Leaf and fruit
TIPS AND USES Fresh leaves can be made into a paste to calm irritable skin complaints. The tiny fruit can be eaten when picked or added to fruit salads.

Willow, white
(Salix alba)
PART USED Leaf and bark
TIPS AND USES The leaves contain salicin, a natural painkiller, and may relieve headaches. Do not ingest willow bark if you suffer from stomach complaints. Dried leaves are not readily available.

Woodruff *(Galium odoratum)*
PART USED Leaf
TIPS AND USES The aromatic dried leaves are used in potpourris.

Woundwort
(Stachys palustris)
PART USED Aerial parts
TIPS AND USES The dried leaves contain active anti-inflammatory properties. Dried leaves are not readily available.

Yarrow/Milfoil
(Achillea millefolium)
PART USED Flowering top
TIPS AND USES Dried flowers can be infused for steam facials and lotions. A herbal tea made from dried yarrow leaves may help to combat digestive problems. Fresh leaves make a good compost booster.

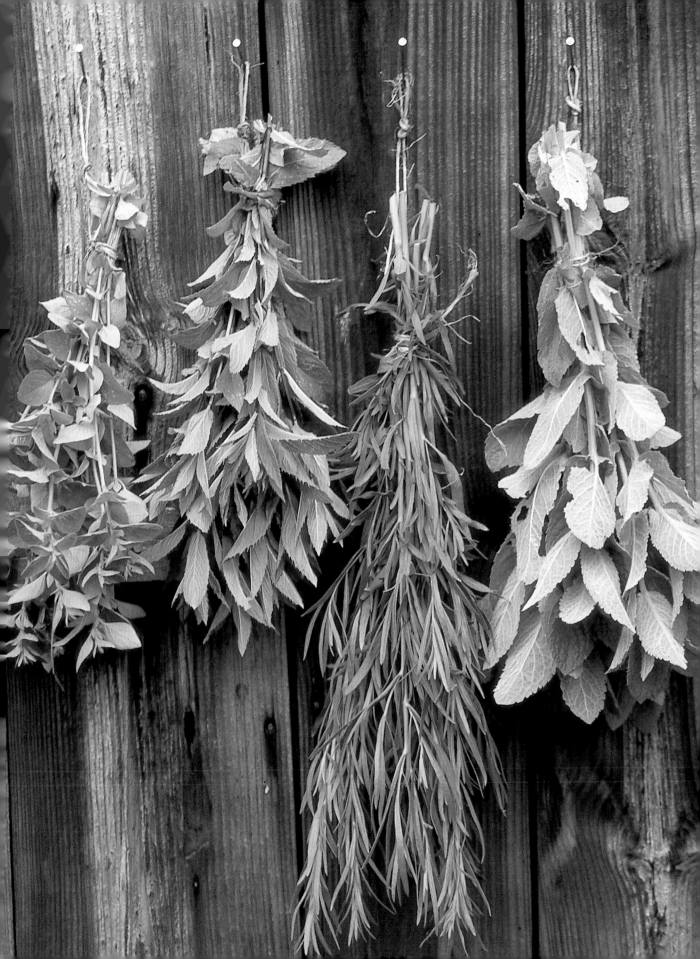

The main ingredients

On the following pages you will find an alphabetical listing of the less well-known ingredients in this book. These items were widely available in our grandparents' time and can still be found in the shops or sold by mail order suppliers if you know where to search them out. For details of mail order companies, see page 339.

Agar
A neutral-tasting product obtained from seaweed. It is available as powder or flakes.
USES It may treat excess stomach acid or act as a mild laxative. Also use as a culinary gelling agent in jellies and desserts.
AVAILABLE FROM Chemists, health shops, organic grocers and supermarkets.
LASTS Three years.

Almond oil –
SEE CARRIER OILS

Aloe vera gel
Gel extracted from the leaves of the aloe vera plant; a native to southern Africa.
USES In cosmetic creams. Medicinally it may soothe burns and minor cuts.
AVAILABLE FROM Herbalists and mail order.
LASTS Six months.

Alum
(Also known as potassium alum)
A white powder with disinfecting properties.
USES Add to bath salts and deodorants. It is also used to waterproof fabric.
AVAILABLE FROM Chemists.
LASTS See label.

Ammonia, household
Pungent-smelling solution that acts as a bleach.
USES Around the house as a cleaning agent. A caustic substance, do not splash on your skin or get in your eyes. In the event of an accident, wash the skin or rinse the eyes immediately with cold water. Never take internally.
AVAILABLE FROM Hardware stores.
LASTS Five years.

Apricot kernel oil –
SEE CARRIER OILS

Ash: wood and paper
Soft, powdery residue that remains when an item is burnt by fire.
USES In homemade cleaning and clothes washing treatments. For reviving wooden furniture. When burning wood on a bonfire, make sure that it is sited well away from other flammable items. Do not collect the ash until it is completely cold.
AVAILABLE FROM Bonfire or wood-burning stove.
LASTS Indefinitely if stored in a cool, dry place.

Attar of roses
A fragrant essential oil obtained from rose petals. You can also substitute rose otto and rose absolute.
USES To scent cosmetic creams and hair lotions.
AVAILABLE FROM Essential oil suppliers and mail order.
LASTS Nine months.

Avocado oil –
SEE CARRIER OILS

Baking soda
A fine white powder of sodium bicarbonate.
USES Take internally to calm stomach acid. Use externally to clean teeth or in bath water. It will absorb nasty smells and is the main ingredient in baking powder.
AVAILABLE FROM Chemists and supermarkets.
LASTS Two years.

Base oils –
SEE CARRIER OILS

Basil oil –
SEE ESSENTIAL OILS

Beeswax
It is obtained by melting honeycomb. Available as sheets, granules and blocks.
USES To polish furniture or for candle-making. Also used to solidify cosmetic creams.
AVAILABLE FROM Limited craft shops and mail order.
LASTS Three years.

Benzoin tincture
Alcoholic solution made from the resin of styrax trees. The tincture has anti-bacterial properties.
USES As a preservative in skin-care products and as a fixative in perfumes.
AVAILABLE FROM Chemists and mail order.
LASTS Two years.

Bergamot oil –
SEE ESSENTIAL OILS

Birchwood ash –
SEE ASH

Black pepper oil –
SEE ESSENTIAL OILS

Black radish
A black-skinned radish. Sow seeds from June to August for picking in October.
USES Eat in salads or use to make a cough remedy.
AVAILABLE FROM Seeds at garden centres and mail order.
LASTS Use the same day as picked.

Boiled linseed oil –
SEE LINSEED OIL

Bone glue
(Also called pearl glue)
A glue made from animal bones. Available as granules which become a clear jelly-like glue when mixed with water and heated.
USES To make traditional paints as used in the theatre or for furniture restoration.
AVAILABLE FROM Specialist art or restoration suppliers and mail order.
LASTS Five years if kept in a cool, dry place.

Borax
A salt that releases protein and fat, softens water and has disinfectant properties.
USES Add to skin-care products to kill germs or use around the house as a cleaning agent.
AVAILABLE FROM Chemists.
LASTS Five years.

Bran
The husks and outer layers of cereal grains that contain protein and vitamins.
USES Take internally as a roughage supplement (since bran is not digestible). It also makes an ideal exfoliant.
AVAILABLE FROM Health shops, supermarkets and chemists.
LASTS One year.

Brewer's yeast –
SEE YEAST, BREWER'S AND EASY BLEND DRIED

Buttermilk
The sour liquid that remains after the butterfat has been removed from whole milk.
USES In baking and home-made cleaning remedies.
AVAILABLE FROM Health shops and large supermarkets.
LASTS Two to three days if stored in the fridge.

Camomile oil –
SEE ESSENTIAL OILS

Camomile tincture –
SEE TINCTURES

Camphor oil –
SEE ESSENTIAL OILS

Caraway seeds
Sickle-shaped seeds from the *Carum carvi* plant. The seeds have a slight aniseed taste.
USES An infusion of the seeds may stimulate the appetite if drunk 30 minutes before a meal. The seeds are also used in cooking.
AVAILABLE FROM Health shops, supermarkets and herbalists.
LASTS One year.

Carrier oils –
(Also called base oils)
High-quality oils that are easily absorbed by the skin.
USES To dilute essential oils without harming their therapeutic effect. The oil also nourishes the skin.
AVAILABLE FROM Essential oil suppliers, chemists and mail order.
LASTS Six months if stored in the fridge.

Carrot oil –
SEE ESSENTIAL OILS

Castor oil –
SEE CARRIER OILS

Caustic soda
When using caustic soda, always wear eye shields and protective gloves. Wash it off your skin immediately.
USES As an ingredient for soap-making. Also used to unblock drains.
AVAILABLE FROM Hardware stores and chemists.
LASTS Five years.

Cedarwood oil –
SEE ESSENTIAL OILS

Celeriac
A type of celery, *Apium graveolens rapaceum*.
USES The leaves are used for freshening musty-smelling glass storage jars. The turnip-like root is eaten.
AVAILABLE FROM Organic grocers. Grow fresh in your garden.
LASTS One week if stored in the fridge.

Celery-seed powder
The spicy seeds do not come from the same variety of celery as the ones in salads. The powder is obtained by pounding the seeds.
USES To flavour soups and stews. It can also be used to treat heart palpitations.
AVAILABLE FROM Organic grocers, supermarkets and health shops.
LASTS One year.

Chalk powder
Fine grains of compacted limestone (calcium carbonate).
USES To remove verdigris and polish silver and marble.
AVAILABLE FROM Sports shops or from your garden if you live in a chalky area.
LASTS Indefinitely.

Cider vinegar
Contains vitamins and beneficial minerals.
USES Externally as an antiseptic and as a cosmetic cleanser. Take internally for arthritis, to regulate blood pressure and to aid digestion.
AVAILABLE FROM Health shops, organic grocers and supermarkets. See the recipe on pages 22-23.
LASTS Two years.

Cinnamon oil –
SEE ESSENTIAL OILS

Citric acid
Naturally found in lemon juice, but can be produced by fermenting fungus.
USES To make drinks, jams and jellies. Apply around the house to remove limescale and stains. Always dilute citric acid before use.
AVAILABLE FROM Chemists and supermarkets.
LASTS Three years.

Clove oil –
SEE ESSENTIAL OILS

Cocoa butter
Nourishing oil pressed from roasted cocoa beans during processing.
USES Add to skin-care products for a rich oily base.
AVAILABLE FROM Chemists, herbalists, health shops and mail order.
LASTS Eighteen months.

Coconut oil –
SEE ESSENTIAL OILS

Coltsfoot tincture –
SEE TINCTURES

Cream base
Pure white cream that can be removed with water.
USES As an emulsifying agent and carrier for medicinal properties in face creams.
AVAILABLE FROM Chemists, herbalists and mail order.
LASTS Fifteen months.

Cream of tartar
(Also called tartaric acid)
Substance found in grape juice after fermentation. It is refined into white powder.
USES As a raising agent when baking bread and to encourage juice to flow from ripe fruit.
AVAILABLE FROM Supermarkets.
LASTS Two years.

Cypress oil –
SEE ESSENTIAL OILS

Dried yeast –
SEE YEAST, BREWER'S AND EASY BLEND DRIED

Echinacea tincture –
SEE TINCTURES

Essential oils
Volatile oils with distinctive odours of the plants from which they were extracted.
USES Essential oils have been used for thousands of years as incense, perfumes, cosmetics and for their medicinal and culinary properties. These oils are highly concentrated and should be used with care. Most of them need to be diluted with a carrier oil before use. Many oils cannot be used during pregnancy or should be used in half the indicated amount.
AVAILABLE FROM Chemists, health shops and mail order.
LASTS Varies, see label.

Eucalyptus oil –
SEE ESSENTIAL OILS

Fennel seeds
Aromatic seeds from the *Foeniculum vulgare* plant.
USES Chew to freshen breath. Also used in steam facials for deep cleansing.
AVAILABLE FROM Herbalists and mail order.
LASTS One year.

Flower pollen
Fine powder-like material taken from the anthers of flowering plants.
USES Adds protein to herbal skin creams and masks.
AVAILABLE FROM Herbalists and mail order.
LASTS Six months.

Frankincense oil –
SEE ESSENTIAL OILS

Fuller's earth
Fine-grained clay that absorbs toxins from the body.
USES When taken internally, it may relieve heartburn, stomach complaints, diarrhoea, flatulence, constipation and mouth and throat inflammations. Apply externally to cuts and sores, swellings and eczema, but no more than twice a week as it depletes the skin's oil.
AVAILABLE FROM Health shops, herbalists and mail order.
LASTS Three years.

Galangal powder
The ground root of a Chinese medicinal plant *Alpinia officinarum*.
USES To add flavour to curries and liqueurs. May calm heart palpitations when drunk as a thick soup.
AVAILABLE FROM Asian supermarkets.
LASTS One year.

Garden lime –
SEE LIME, GARDEN

Geranium oil –
SEE ESSENTIAL OILS

Ginger oil –
SEE ESSENTIAL OILS

Glucose, liquid
A natural sugar that occurs in grapes and honey.
USES As a sweetener in confectionery and cakes. Used by athletes as a quick source of energy. Also used in the garden for speeding up decomposition.
AVAILABLE FROM Supermarkets.
LASTS Two years.

Glycerine
Colourless alcohol that absorbs moisture. Contained in all natural fats.
USES Acts as a solidifying agent and as a carrier for medicinal substances in creams and lotions. Prevents skin from becoming rough and chapped. Also used in cleaning agents and soap.
AVAILABLE FROM Independent chemists, health shops and supermarkets.
LASTS Three years.

Glycerine soap
Tub-soap made from a colourless or yellow syrupy liquid obtained from fats.
USES For cleaning leather and in cosmetics.
AVAILABLE FROM Chemists and saddlers.
LASTS Three years.

Grapeseed oil –
SEE CARRIER OILS

Ground rice
Coarse, medium or finely ground grains of rice.
USES For cleaning leather, as a sweetening agent for food and in cosmetics. Also used in milk puddings and as a thickener for sauces.
AVAILABLE FROM Health shops and supermarkets.
LASTS Six months.

Henna leaf powder
Crushed dried leaves from the henna plant.
USES To condition hair. Spring-picked leaves will not dye your hair. Check the origin of the leaves before use to avoid unwanted colouring.
AVAILABLE FROM Dried leaves from herbalists and mail order. You may need to crush them using a pestle and mortar.
LASTS Six months.

Honeycomb
Natural form of honey with wax and combs still attached.
USES May relieve hay fever.
AVAILABLE FROM Beekeepers, specialist shops and organic grocers.
LASTS Three months.

Hop flower/hop cones
The feminine pollen contains bitter substances and essential oils that have a relaxing effect and stimulate the appetite.
USES May treat menstrual complaints, sleeping problems and restlessness.
AVAILABLE FROM Herbalists and mail order.
LASTS Six months.

Household ammonia –
SEE AMMONIA

Iceland lichen
A brittle, edible moss.
USES Take internally to treat dry coughs and gastrointestinal complaints. Used externally as a gargle or rinse, it may soothe mouth ulcers. It can also be applied to cuts and sores but not to boils and abscesses.
AVAILABLE FROM Herbalists, health shops and mail order.
LASTS Two years.

Iodine tincture –
SEE TINCTURES

Isopropyl alcohol
A colourless liquid.
USES In lotions and cosmetics. It must not be consumed. Vodka can be substituted instead of isopropyl alcohol.
AVAILABLE FROM Independent chemists who have a licence to sell it.
LASTS Two years.

Jasmine absolute
The oil from jasmine flowers produced by a process of solvent extraction.
USES To scent moisturising bath oil.
AVAILABLE FROM Essential oil suppliers and mail order.
LASTS Nine months.

Jojoba oil –
SEE CARRIER OILS

Juniper oil –
SEE ESSENTIAL OILS

Kaolin
(Also called China clay)
A white or yellowish clay.
USES As an adsorbent in medicines and cosmetics. Also used for coating paper.
AVAILABLE FROM Health shops, herbalists and mail order.
LASTS Eighteen months.

Lanolin
Hydrous fat extracted from sheep's wool during the washing process.
USES The main ingredient in skin-care creams.
AVAILABLE FROM Chemists, herbalists and mail order.
LASTS Eighteen months.

Lard
Melted and clarified (with impurities removed) pork fat.
USES As a fat when baking and frying. It is also used in the traditional method of soapmaking.
AVAILABLE FROM Supermarkets.
LASTS Eighteen months.

Lavender oil –
SEE ESSENTIAL OILS

Lavender water
A fragrant liquid made by distilling lavender flowers in water. Often a by-product from the extraction of the essential oil.
USES In cosmetic creams, lotions, skin tonics and perfumes.
AVAILABLE FROM Chemists, health shops and mail order.
LASTS Nine months.

Lemon oil –
SEE ESSENTIAL OILS

Lemon balm tincture –
SEE TINCTURES

Lemongrass oil –
SEE ESSENTIAL OILS

Lemon oil, pure
Cold-pressed oil with an intense smell and flavour.
USES In cooking, as a room freshener and in cleaning remedies.
AVAILABLE FROM Mail order.
LASTS Indefinitely if stored in the fridge.

Lime, garden
A white, caustic powder.
USES In homemade cleaning remedies. Always wear protective gloves when handling garden lime. Also used for pest control and to neutralise garden soil.
AVAILABLE FROM Garden centres and hardware stores.
LASTS Three years if stored in a dry place.

Linseed
Seeds from the flax plant.
USES In firming eye gel that may reduce crow's feet.
AVAILABLE FROM Herbalists, health shops and mail order.
LASTS One year.

Linseed oil
A traditional oil used on hard or close-grained wood. Boiled linseed oil is similar to the raw oil but has an improved drying time.
USES To preserve timber furnishings. In poultices it may reduce inflammation.
AVAILABLE FROM Hardware stores, mail order and specialist art shops.
LASTS One year.

Liquid glucose –
SEE GLUCOSE, LIQUID

Liquorice root
The dried root of a herbaceous plant, *Glycyrrhiza glabra*, that has been used medicinally for centuries.
USES May loosen phlegm during bronchitis and alleviate stomach ulcers when infused as a herbal tea. It is also used to flavour beer and confectionery. Do not use for more than three to four weeks because it acts as a mild diuretic.
AVAILABLE FROM Herbalists and mail order.
LASTS Eighteen months.

Marigold tincture –
SEE TINCTURES

Marjoram oil –
SEE ESSENTIAL OILS

Mastic oil –
SEE ESSENTIAL OILS

Melissa oil –
SEE ESSENTIAL OILS

Menthol
White, organic crystals obtained from the peppermint plant.
USES In deodorants for its scent. In steam facials and inhalations it may alleviate congestion and be a mild anaesthetic. Also used for culinary purposes.
AVAILABLE FROM Chemists.
LASTS See label.

Methylated spirits
(Informally known as meths)
Highly concentrated denatured alcohol (unfit for human consumption). It usually contains methanol, pyridine and a violet dye.
USES As an additive to cleaning agents and in traditional polishes.
AVAILABLE FROM Hardware stores.
LASTS Two years.

Myrrh gum
An aromatic gum obtained from *Commiphora* trees in India and Africa.
USES As a flavouring ingredient for potpourris, incense and perfumes.
AVAILABLE FROM Herbalists and mail order.
LASTS Six months.

Neroli oil –
SEE ESSENTIAL OILS

Oak bark powder
The bark is rich in tannin, with an astringent effect.
USES Taken as an infusion, it may relieve intestinal complaints. It can also be used as a gargle, on oozing eczema, piles and minor burns. Use in the garden to speed up decomposition.
AVAILABLE FROM Herbalists and mail order.
LASTS Eighteen months.

Olive oil soap
(Also known as Savon de Marseille)
A refined, unscented soap made with olive oil.
USES In herbal shampoos.
AVAILABLE FROM Health shops and organic grocers.
LASTS Three years.

Orris root powder
A powder obtained from grinding the fragrant roots of *Iris florentina*.
USES As a fixative in potpourris and cosmetics.
AVAILABLE FROM Herbalists.
LASTS One year.

Oyster shell
Crushed, irregularly shaped shells of the *Ostrea* molluscs.
USES To prevent compost containing bulbs from turning sour or stale.
AVAILABLE FROM Garden centres and hardware stores.
LASTS Ten years.

Paper ash –
SEE ASH: WOOD AND PAPER

Paraffin

(Also called kerosene)

A mixture of hydrocarbons obtained from petrol. It boils at a very high temperature.

USES As a heating fuel and as a cleaning agent.

AVAILABLE FROM Hardware stores.

LASTS Two years.

Paraffin wax

Wax made with paraffin. It melts at 57-60°C (135-140°F). Available as pellets or granules and is usually white.

USES Mix with stearin powder to make candles.

AVAILABLE FROM Candlemaking suppliers, craft shops and mail order.

LASTS See label.

Pectin

A carbohydrate found in unripe fruit. It has gelling properties and is available in liquid and powder form.

USES To set jams and jellies.

AVAILABLE FROM Organic grocers and supermarkets.

LASTS Three years.

Peppermint oil –
SEE ESSENTIAL OILS

Petroleum jelly

(Also called Petrolatum)

A colourless gelatinous semisolid substance.

USES As a lubricant and as a basic ingredient for many medicinal ointments and cosmetic creams.

AVAILABLE FROM Chemists.

LASTS Three years.

Pine oil –
SEE ESSENTIAL OILS

Potash

Potassium carbonate is found in plant ash.

USES Add to homemade cleaning remedies. Also used in fertilisers to enrich soil.

AVAILABLE FROM Garden centres and hardware stores.

LASTS Three years.

Potato flour

A fine white flour made from cooked potatoes.

USES A thickening agent used in soups, sauces and cosmetic face masks. Also used in washing remedies.

AVAILABLE FROM Health shops.

LASTS Six months.

Potato starch

A tasteless starch powder extracted from potatoes.

USES In carpet cleaning preparations and to stiffen fabrics after washing.

AVAILABLE FROM Health shops.

LASTS Six months.

Preserving sugar

A coarser variety of granulated sugar.

USES For pickling and making preserves.

AVAILABLE FROM Supermarkets.

LASTS One year.

Propolis tincture –
SEE TINCTURES

Pumice powder

Fine abrasive powder made from porous, volcanic rock.

USES For French polishing and as an abrasive agent in cleaning remedies.

AVAILABLE FROM Furniture restorers and French polishing suppliers, mail order and hardware stores.

LASTS Ten years.

Purified water

(Also called distilled water)

Water that has been refined through a process of condensing vapour to remove impurities.

USES In homemade shampoos and rinses. Also to make cleaning remedies.

AVAILABLE FROM Chemists.

LASTS Eighteen months.

Quark

A low-fat soft cheese made from skimmed milk. Often served with fruit as a dessert.

USES For homemade face and eye packs which may alleviate swelling.

AVAILABLE FROM Health shops and supermarkets.

LASTS One week if stored in the fridge.

Raw linseed oil –
SEE LINSEED OIL

Resin

(Also called rosin)

Plant excretion of a clear or yellow gum. Different types of resin from a variety of plants are available.

USES In lacquers and varnishes. Also used to lubricate music bows.

AVAILABLE FROM Music shops, herbalists and mail order.

LASTS Ten years.

Rosemary oil –
SEE ESSENTIAL OILS

Rosemary tincture –
SEE TINCTURES

Rosewater

A fragrant liquid made by distilling rose petals in water.

USES In cosmetic creams, lotions, skin tonics and perfumes. Also used to flavour foods and potpourris.

AVAILABLE FROM Chemists, health shops and mail order.

LASTS Nine months.

Rottenstone

Very fine abrasive powder.

USES For cleaning marble as a modern equivalent to scouring sand. It is also used to 'antique' or age contemporary furniture.

AVAILABLE FROM Furniture restorers, hardware stores and mail order.

LASTS Ten years.

Rye flour

Flour made from grinding grains of rye, which are similar to wheat grains. It has a distinctive nutty taste.

USES For breadmaking and in the manufacture of alcohol, such as whisky.

AVAILABLE FROM Health shops and supermarkets.

LASTS Six months.

Sage oil –
SEE ESSENTIAL OILS

Sage tincture –
SEE TINCTURES

Salicylic acid

Scent-free crystals found in willow bark that kill germs and loosen hard skin.

USES In cosmetic ointments, powders and lotions it may treat hand and foot perspiration and loosen callous skin.

AVAILABLE FROM Chemists.

LASTS Two years.

Sandalwood oil –
SEE ESSENTIAL OILS

Sea buckthorn juice
This orange-coloured juice is high in vitamin C.
USES To make elixirs and sweets or drunk as a juice. It can also be used in jam to stimulate appetite.
AVAILABLE FROM Mail order or fresh from berries.
LASTS Three months if an elixir; two days if fresh juice.

Seaweed
Dried leaves of marine algae, usually kelp, rich in minerals.
USES As a compress it may combat oily skin. Also eaten as a vegetable.
AVAILABLE FROM Health shops, oriental supermarkets and mail order.
LASTS Varies; see label.

Sea salt
Saline crystals. Dead sea salt is high in medicinal minerals.
USES For homemade bath salts and tooth powder.
AVAILABLE FROM Chemists, herbalists, health shops and mail order.
LASTS Two years.

Sesame oil –
SEE ESSENTIAL OILS

Shellac
Reddish secretion produced by tropical lac insects.
USES As a household varnish and furniture polish.
AVAILABLE FROM Specialist art shops, hardware stores and mail order.
LASTS Two years.

Silver sand
Very fine particles of sand.
USES In sandpits as it won't stain children's clothes. Also used as a fine abrasive cleaner.
AVAILABLE FROM Builders merchants, garden centres and children's toy suppliers.
LASTS Indefinitely.

Soap flakes
Flaked curd soap; olive oil soap flakes also available.
USES To cleanse the skin and hair, or as a cleaning product around the house.
AVAILABLE FROM Supermarkets and chemists.
LASTS Three years.

Soft soap
Jelly-like substance. See recipe on pages 142-143.
USES Around the house as a cleaning agent and to wash clothes and fabrics. When using manufactured soft soap, avoid prolonged contact with the skin, protect the eyes and wash off any splashes on your skin with water. Do not swallow and keep away from children.
AVAILABLE FROM Mail order.
LASTS Three years.

Soya bean oil –
SEE ESSENTIAL OILS

Stearin powder
Stearin makes candles more opaque and raises the melting point of the wax so that candles do not bend. It also improves burning quality.
USES To make candles.
AVAILABLE FROM Candlemaking suppliers and mail order.
LASTS Five years.

Stinging nettle tincture –
SEE TINCTURES

Stock essence
A scented liquid obtained from the stock flower. Similar but not as volatile as an essential oil.
USES To scent washing soaps and perfumes.
AVAILABLE FROM Essential oil suppliers and mail order.
LASTS Nine months.

Sulphur granules
Scent-free and tasteless yellow granules.
USES Around the house as a disinfectant. Do not breathe in any of the powder.
AVAILABLE FROM Garden centres and hardware stores.
LASTS Three years.

Sunflower oil –
SEE CARRIER OILS

Swedish bitters
A bitter-tasting medicinal drink made from distilled spirits flavoured with herbs.
USES It may combat a variety of digestive problems.
AVAILABLE FROM Herbalists and mail order.
LASTS Two years.

Tea tree oil –
SEE ESSENTIAL OILS

Thyme oil –
SEE ESSENTIAL OILS

Tinctures
A traditional way of extracting the therapeutic constituents of plants using alcohol and water.
USES For cosmetic and medicinal remedies.
AVAILABLE FROM Chemists, herbalists and mail order.
LASTS Varies, see label.

Turpentine
Essential oil extracted from the balsam of a variety of pine trees. It is very volatile and should not be placed near a naked flame.
USES Around the house as a floor polish, shoe cream or as a solvent for paint.
AVAILABLE FROM Hardware stores and mail order.
LASTS Two years.

Vegetable carrier oils
SEE CARRIER OILS

Vetiver oil –
SEE ESSENTIAL OILS

Violet leaf absolute
The oil from violet leaves produced by solvent extraction from the plant.
USES In herbal remedies, which may relieve cramp.
AVAILABLE FROM Essential oil suppliers and mail order.
LASTS Nine months.

Walnut oil –
SEE CARRIER OILS

Washing soda
A mixture of soda, liquid glass, phosphorus salts and active foaming agents that soften water.
USES To pre-soak laundry, clean ovens and unblock drains. Washing soda can be an irritant for sensitive skin.
AVAILABLE FROM Hardware stores and supermarkets.
LASTS Four years.

Wax dye
Concentrated dyes, usually found in disc form. Shave a small amount onto a saucer, then add it to hot wax. These dyes are strong, but note that the colour will fade as the wax solidifies.
USES To dye clear or bleached wax when making your own candles.
AVAILABLE FROM Candlemaking suppliers, craft shops and mail order.
LASTS Two years.

Wick sustainer

The sustainers are usually sold together with the wicks and are available in different widths to suit all sizes of candle.

USES The metal base supports the wick upright in the container as the hot wax is poured in.

AVAILABLE FROM Craft shops, candlemaking suppliers and mail order.

LASTS Indefinitely.

Wheat flour

Unrefined flour ground from a variety of cereal crops.

USES The rough, grainy texture of the flour acts as a good exfoliating agent. Also used in cakes, breads and pasta.

AVAILABLE FROM Health shops and supermarkets.

LASTS Six months.

Wheatgerm

A vitamin-rich embryo of the wheat kernel, separated before milling.

USES As a cereal or food supplement. It is also added to wood-shine recipes and used as an exfoliant or to refresh the skin.

AVAILABLE FROM Health shops and supermarkets.

LASTS Six months.

Wheatgerm oil –
SEE CARRIER OILS

White spirit

A clear liquid made by distilling petroleum.

USES As a cleaning agent and paint remover. It can also be mixed into a furniture restorer for wood and used as a solvent dispersant.

AVAILABLE FROM Hardware stores, furniture restorers and art shops.

LASTS Two years.

Whiting

A plaster that is made from a pure grade of chalk. Mixed with rabbit-skin glue it forms the basis of gesso.

USES In gilding, plaster moulding and homemade cleaning treatments.

AVAILABLE FROM Art shops, furniture restorers and mail order.

LASTS Five years.

Witch hazel

A colourless medicinal alcohol containing an extract from the bark and leaves of the witch hazel shrub.

USES Not to be taken internally. Use witch hazel in face tonics and creams. Use as a compress to alleviate bruising.

AVAILABLE FROM Chemists.

LASTS Two years.

Wood ash –
SEE ASH: WOOD AND PAPER

Yeast, brewer's and easy blend dried

One-celled yeast plants are rich in protein and vitamin B. Brewer's yeast is available dried, powdered or in tablets. Easy blend dried yeast is available in powder form.

USES Yeast may help to treat skin diseases, protein deficiencies and exhaustion. Brewer's yeast may treat vitamin B deficiencies. It is also used when making cider vinegar. Use easy blend dried yeast as a raising agent for bread or in a trap for mice.

AVAILABLE FROM Brewer's yeast from specialist wine and brewing shops; easy blend dried yeast from health shops and supermarkets.

LASTS Varies, see label.

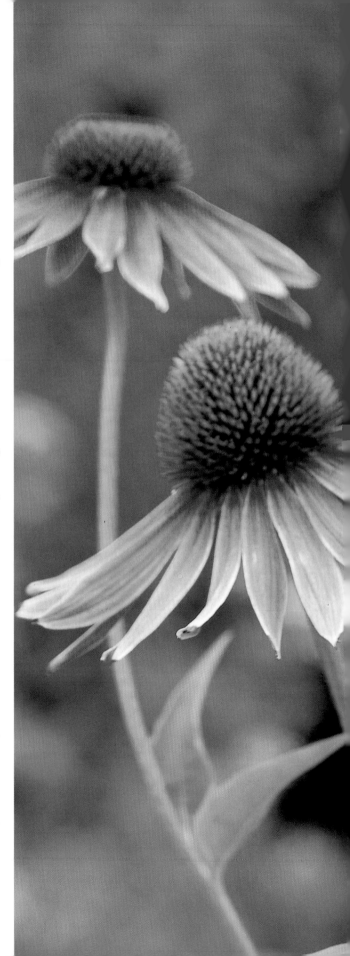

Conversion charts

These conversion charts will be useful if you find metric measurements difficult to work in. Remember that it is never wise to mix metric and imperial measurements in the same recipe as amounts given are not necessarily exact equivalents. So if you start in metric, continue in metric throughout the project.

VOLUME	
Metric	Approx imperial
30ml	1fl oz
50ml	2fl oz
85ml	3fl oz
100ml	3½fl oz
125ml	4fl oz
150ml	5fl oz ¼ pint
175ml	6fl oz
200ml	7fl oz
225ml	8fl oz
250ml	9fl oz
300ml	10fl oz ½ pint
350ml	12fl oz
400ml	14fl oz
450ml	16fl oz
500ml	18fl oz
600ml	1 pint 20 fl oz
700ml	1¼ pint 1pint 5fl oz
900ml	1 pint 12fl oz
1 litre	1¾ pints
2 litres	3½ pints
2·5 litres	4½ pints
3 litres	5¼ pints

WEIGHT			
Metric	Approx imperial	Metric	Approx imperial
15g	½oz	425g	15oz
25g	1oz	450g	1lb
40g	1½oz	500g	1lb 2oz
55g	2oz	550g	1lb 4oz
70g	2½oz	600g	1lb 5oz
85g	3oz	650g	1lb 7oz
100g	3½oz	675g	1lb 8oz
115g	4oz	700g	1lb 9oz
125g	4½oz	750g	1lb 10oz
140g	5oz	800g	1lb 12oz
150g	5½oz	850g	1lb 14oz
175g	6oz	900g	2lb
200g	7oz	950g	2lb 2oz
215g	7½oz	1kg	2lb 4oz
225g	8oz	1·2kg	2lb 10oz
250g	9oz	1·25kg	2lb 12oz
280g	10oz	1·3kg	3lb
300g	10½oz	1·5kg	3lb 5oz
325g	11½oz	1·75kg	3lb 13oz
350g	12oz	1·8kg	4lb
375g	13oz	2kg	4lb 8oz
400g	14oz	2·5kg	5lb 8oz

Mail order suppliers

MEDICAL & COSMETIC

• **NEAL'S YARD REMEDIES** Dried herbs, tinctures, oils and cosmetic supplies **0161 831 7875**

• **NAPIERS DIRECT** Dried herbs, tinctures, oils and cosmetic supplies **0131 553 3500; www.napiers.net**

• **G. BALDWINS & CO** Dried herbs, tinctures, oils and cosmetic supplies **020 7703 5550; www.baldwins.co.uk**

• **ESSENTIALLY OILS** Essential oils, tinctures, attars, floral waters and cosmetic supplies **01608 659544; www.essentiallyoils.com**

• **SUFFOLK HERBS** Herbs, cottage garden, wild flowers and vegetables **01376 572456**

• **BARWINNOCK HERBS** Culinary, medicinal and aromatic plants **01465 821338; www.barwinnock.com**

• **POYNTZFIELD HERB** Nursery Herbal plants and seeds **01381 610352; www.poyntzfieldherbs. co.uk**

• **WELEDA (UK) LTD** Sea buckthorn juice, natural medicines and toiletries **0115 9448222**

CLEANING & GARDENING

• **L. CORNELISSEN & SON LTD** Art and furniture restoration supplies **020 7636 1045**

• **HOMECRAFTS DIRECT LTD** Specialist art and craft supplies **0845 458 4531; www.homecrafts.co.uk**

• **LAKELAND LIMITED** Kitchen supplies, pure lemon oil **015394 88100; www.lakelandlimited.com**

• **LIBERON WAXES LTD** Furniture restoration supplies, Sales **01797 367555**, Technical **01797 361136**

• **ALEC TIRANTI LTD** Art and craft supplies, soft soap **020 7636 8565; www.tiranti.co.uk**

• **HDRA, THE ORGANIC ORGANISATION** **024 7630 3517; www.HDRA.org.uk**

Index

Page numbers in **bold** indicate main entries;
those in *italic* refer to illustrations only.

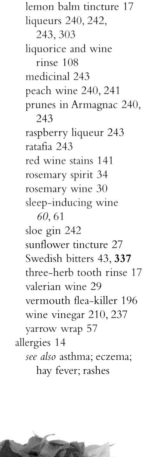

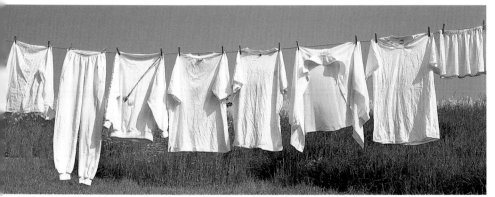

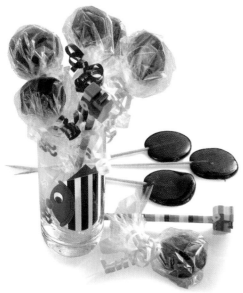

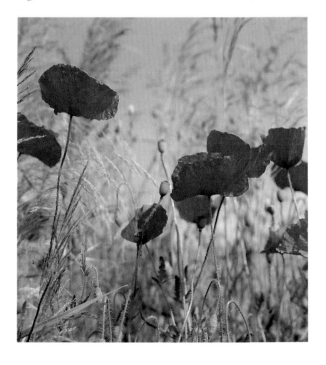

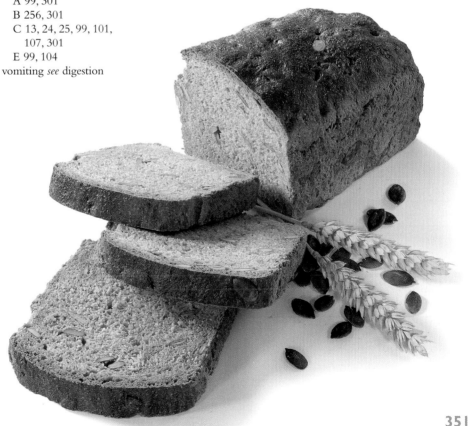

Acknowledgments

Key to acknowledgments:
t = top b = bottom l = left r = right

AGE/Mauritius 168; Monika Albrecht/Mauritius 194 l; Jacques Alexandre/IFA-Bilderteam 71; Paul Almasy/Archiv für Kunst u. Geschichte 282; Apel/Photo Press 319; Archiv Gerstenberg 184; Archiv/Interfoto 76 t; Archiv für Kunst und Geschichte 48, 168, 316 b; G. Baden/Zefa 205; Bettmann/Corbis 120; Bildarchiv Preußischer Kulturbesitz 134, 153; Bildagentur Geduldig 113; The Anthony Blake Photo Library 234, 295; Ursel Borstell 268 t; Daniel Bosler/Tony Stone 100; Dr. Helga Buchter-Weisbrodt 273, 315; Campiglio/Bavaria 94; Cephas/Tim Hill 212; Cephas/Diana Mewes 227; Cephas/Alain Proust 231; Cephas/stockfood 213, 232 l, 236-237, 256; Cortex, Fürth-Bislohe 158 (4); Craft Plus Publishing 259; Cupak/Mauritius 179; James Darell/Tony Stone 89, 127 t; Diaf/IFA-Bilderteam 115, 215; DIZ Bilderdienst Süddeutscher Verlag 228 t; Josef Ege/H. Lade 197 l; EWA/Tommy Candeler 137; EWA/Karl Dietrich-buhler 285 b; EWA/Di Lewis 167; EWA/David Markson 232 r; EWA/Spike Powell 185; First/Zefa 165 t, 343; Food Features 216, 235, 239, 252; Forbo Werke GmbH, Paderborn 158 (2); Frauke/Mauritius 33; Grafica/Mauritius 160; Siegfried Gragnato/Jahreszeiten Verlag/Zefa 146; Claus Hansmann 140; Holzförster/H. Lade 195; H. Hopp/freundin/report 26; Michael Howes/GPL 284; L. Karl/Fotex 187; Kiene/Bildagentur Schuster 157; Kohlhaupt-Sendtner/Mauritius 190 b; Ulrich Kopp 15, 21, 22-23, 31, 38-39, 44-45, 58-59, 78-79, 85, 116-117, 135, 145, 172-173, 180-181, 192-193, 200, 201, 203, 204, 208-209, 210 l, 218-219, 220, 223, 226 b, 228 b, 229, 240, 241 t, 247, 248, 250-251, 257 b, 286-287, 288, 289, 293, 300, 301 t, 303, 304-305, 306, 308, 311, 314, 317, 320-321, 351; Lambert/Zefa 155 t; Martin Ley/Mauritius 183 t; Löhr/Mauritius 197 r; Lamontagne/GPL 214; London Metropolitan Archive 263; Fotostudio Udo Loster 1, 4, 5, 10, 18, 20, 21, 24, 27, 28, 29, 32 b, 33, 34, 36 t, 40, 43, 46, 52, 53, 60, 62, 63 t, 66, 70, 72, 74, 76 b, 82, 83, 86, 88 b, 91, 95, 99 t, 101, 103, 106, 108 t, 109, 110, 114, 118, 122 t, 124, 125, 126, 129, 136, 138, 141, 144, 147 b, 148, 149, 150, 154, 156, 159, 166, 170 b, 174, 176, 177, 178, 182, 186, 188, 191, 206 t, 207, 222, 266, 270, 272, 276 b, 280, 296, 318, 340, 348; Mary Evans Picture Library 90 b, 99 b; R. Maier/IFA-Bilderteam 221 b; Mayer/Le Scanff/GPL 285 t; Meyer/Photo-Center 323; W. H. Müller/Photo-Center 189; NDS/H. Lade 14; Ginger Neumann Einband 8-9, 25, 68-69, 80 t, 130-131, 132, 133, 198-199, 264-265; Ulrich Niehoff 35 t, 67; André Perlstein/Tony Stone 121; Clay Perry/GPL 299; Peter Pfander/Carina/report 101; Pfander/Zefa 111; Phototeque SDP/Mauritius 49; Reader's Digest 11, 12 t, 13, 42 t, 47 b, 63 b, 72 t, 80 b, 87 b, 89 t, 122 b, 124 t, 127 b, 155 b, 158 (2), 190 t, 226 t, 245, 246, 249, 258, 267 t, 268 b 281, 290 t, 291, 294 t, 296 r, 301 b, 302 b, 345; Reader's Digest/Martin Brigdale 242, 262; Reader's Digest/Tony Robins 2, 142-143, 152, 162-163, 211, 230, 238, 243, 244, 255, 260, 261, 278-279, 294 b; Reader's Digest/Richard Surman 292; Reader's Digest/Pia Tryde 312; Reader's Digest/Francesca Yorke 298; Wolfgang Redeleit 55, 202, 277, 283, 331, 302 t, 313 t; Hans Reinhard 19 t, 30, 42 b, 50, 65, 73, 87 t, 90 t, 96, 108 b, 291 t, 324-5, 338; L. Reupert/H. Lade 84; Howard Rice/GPL 36 b; D. Rose/Fotex 139; Rosenfeld Images Ltd./Mauritius 307 b; Rosen-Union 119 t; H. G. Rossi/Zefa 54, 128; Ernie S./IFA-Bilderteam 64, 290 b; Dieter Schinner/allOver 164; Hannah Schwarz-Böhm 47 t; H. Schwarz/Mauritius 57; J. Silverberg/Mauritius 112; S.K./H. Lade 175; Jörg Steffens/freundin/report 12 b; Friedrich Strauß 269, 275, 297, 309, 322; Susan/Mauritius 41; Telegraph Colour Library 75 t, 171, 233, 271; VCL/Bavaria 77, 81; Kristiane Vey/Jump 56, 107; Voigt/Bildagentur Schuster 150; Weststock/Mauritius 161.

HINTS AND TIPS FROM TIMES PAST was published by The Reader's Digest Association Limited, London

First edition Copyright © 2001 The Reader's Digest Association Limited, 11 Westferry Circus, Canary Wharf, London E14 4HE
www.readersdigest.co.uk

We are committed to both the quality of our products and the service we provide to our customers. We value your comments, so please feel free to contact us on **08705 113366** or by email at:
cust_service@readersdigest.co.uk

If you have any comments or suggestions about the content of our books, email us at gbeditorial@readersdigest.co.uk

Copyright © 2001 Reader's Digest Association Far East Limited.
Philippines Copyright © 2001 Reader's Digest Association Far East Limited

Reader's Digest production credits:
Book production manager
Fiona McIntosh
Pre-press manager
Howard Reynolds
Pre-press technical analyst
Martin Hendrick
Origination
Colour Systems Ltd
Printing and binding
MOHN Media, Germany

For **Grossmutters Hausmittel Neu Entdeckt** (Germany)

Editorial
**Annegret Diener-Steinherr,
Dr Angela Meder,
Hildegard Mergelsberg,
Erwin Tivig,
Joachim Wahnschaffe,
Joachim Zeller**

Design
**Gabriele Stammer-Nowack,
Peter Waitschies**

Picture research
**Christina Horut,
Ute Noll**

ISBN 0 276 42559 6
BOOK CODE 400-051-01
CONCEPT CODE GR 0927/IC